PLANTING
THE FUTURE

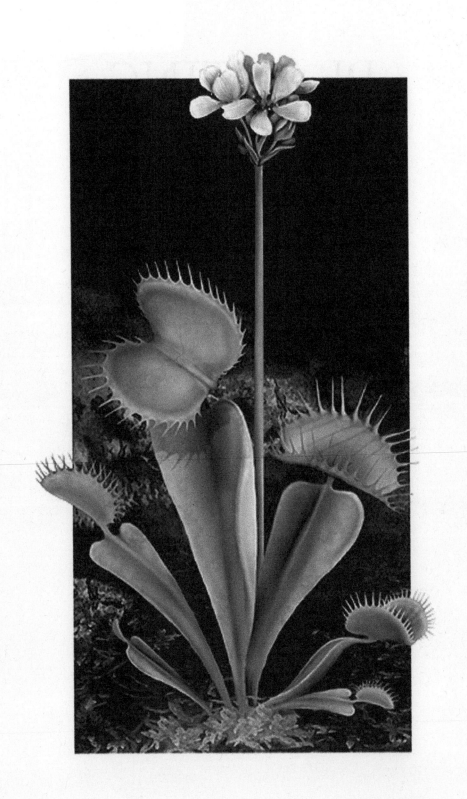

PLANTING THE FUTURE

Saving Our Medicinal Herbs

Edited by

ROSEMARY GLADSTAR
and PAMELA HIRSCH

Healing Arts Press
Rochester, Vermont

Healing Arts Press
One Park Street
Rochester, Vermont 05767
www.InnerTraditions.com

Healing Arts Press is a division of Inner Traditions International

Frontispiece: Venus's-Flytrap © 2000 by Ajana Green
Insert Photographs: Arnica, Black Cohosh, Bloodroot, Blue Cohosh, Calamus Root, Echinacea, Eyebright, American Ginseng, Threeleaf Goldthread, Goldenseal, Helonias, Kava, Pink Lady's Slipper, Lobelia, Oregon Grape, Partridgeberry, Pleurisy Root, Slippery Elm, Spikenard, Trillium, Stoneroot, Roundleaf Sundew, Venus's-Flytrap, Virginia Snakeroot, Wild Indigo, American Wild Yam, and Yerba Mansa © 2000 Martin Wall; Cascara Sagrada, Lomatium, Cultivated Lomatium Seedling, Cultivated Osha Seedling, and White Sage © 2000 by Richo Cech; Osha © 2000 by David Bunting; Pipsissewa © 2000 by Ed Smith; Yerba Santa © 2000 by Deb Soule.

Note to the reader: This book is intended as an informational guide. The remedies, approaches, and techniques described herein are meant to supplement, and not to be a substitute for, professional medical care or treatment. They should not be used to treat a serious ailment without prior consultation with a qualified health care professional.

This book, though compiled by United Plant Savers, represents each author's personal view of the plant he or she chose to write about. UpS edited for technical accuracy, but not for the authors' styles or opinions. We feel that the chapters offer a cohesive collection on medicinal plant conservation, but the authors' opinions are their own and do not always represent the views of UpS.

Library of Congress Cataloging-in-Publication Data

Planting the future : saving our medicinal herbs / edited by Rosemary Gladstar and Pamela Hirsch.
     p. cm.
  Includes bibliographical references and index.
  ISBN 978-0-89281-894-5 (alk. paper)
   1. Medicinal plants. 2. Materia medica, Vegetables. 3. Herbs. I. Gladstar, Rosemary.

SB293 .P53 2000
633.8'8—dc21

00-039573

Printed and bound in the United States

10 9 8

Text design and layout by Priscilla H. Baker
This book was typeset in Janson, with Avenir as a display face.

CONTENTS

❧

Acknowledgments		viii
Foreword	RICHARD LIEBMANN, N.D.	ix
Introduction	ROSEMARY GLADSTAR	1
What You Can Do to Make a Difference	ROSEMARY GLADSTAR	13
Creating Botanical Sanctuaries	CHRISTOPHER HOBBS, L.Ac.	17
Wise Old Plants	ROBYN KLEIN	24
The American Extra Pharmacopoeia	DAVID WINSTON	39
Flower Essences	KATE GILDAY and SHATOIYA DE LA TOUR	55
Arnica	BRIGITTE MARS	60
Black Cohosh	MATTHEW WOOD	64
Bloodroot	PAM MONTGOMERY	72
Blue Cohosh	RICHO CECH	78
Calamus Root	DON BABINEAU	84
Cascara Sagrada	RICHO CECH	88
Echinacea	STEVEN FOSTER	93
Eyebright	SARA KATZ	100
American Ginseng	KATHI KEVILLE	105
Goldenseal	MARK BLUMENTHAL	111
Goldthread	NANCY and MICHAEL PHILLIPS	123
Helonias Root	DEB SOULE	127
Kava	TANE DATTA	130

Lady's Slipper Orchid	ROSEMARY GLADSTAR	139
Lobelia	CASCADE ANDERSON GELLER	150
Lomatium	KRISTA THIE	159
Oregon Grape	RYAN W. DRUM, PH.D.	167
Osha	GREGORY L. TILFORD	176
Partridgeberry	SUSUN S. WEED	182
Pipsissewa	STEPHEN HARROD BUHNER	191
Pleurisy Root	JOANNE MARIE SNOW	197
Slippery Elm	PAUL STRAUSS	203
Spikenard	KATE GILDAY	210
Stoneroot	MARTIN WALL	215
Sundew	JANICE J. SCHOFIELD	221
Trillium	PAMELA HIRSCH	226
Venus's-Flytrap	JAMES GREEN	231
Virginia Snakeroot	DOUG ELLIOTT	241
White Sage	JANE BOTHWELL	247
Wild Indigo	DAVID BUNTING	252
American Wild Yam	RICHO CECH	259
Yerba Mansa	TIM BLAKLEY	266
Yerba Santa	SHATOIYA and RICK DE LA TOUR	272
Appendix 1: Sea Vegetables	RYAN W. DRUM, PH.D.	277
Appendix 2: Concern for European Medicinal Plants	CASCADE ANDERSON GELLER	285
Appendix 3: Planting Guides and Resources		287
About the Authors		294
Join United Plant Savers		301
Index		302

ACKNOWLEDGMENTS

Though every book is a collective effort of sorts, the fruition of *Planting the Future* was completely dependent upon a group of fellow beings who have committed their lives fully to the green medicine of plants. All these people contributed their time and expertise with no recompense other than the satisfaction of knowing they were contributing to a worthwhile cause. The list is long. First and foremost our thanks go to Pamela Hirsch. Her tireless and talented editing skills and ever bright personality were the magic that wove more than forty chapters into an inspiring cohesive whole. The beautiful photographs of at-risk plants were generously donated by Martin Wall, botanical photographer and avid supporter of UpS. Richo Cech and David Winston, aside from writing excellent chapters of their own, contributed much expertise and experience in helping others write their chapters with necessary technical data. Christopher Hobbs graciously offered to review the manuscript for technical accuracy. Special thanks are needed for the marathon efforts of Sara Katz, Cascade Anderson Geller, Richo Cech, and Tammi Hartung, who worked together to compile the conservation guidelines; for Kathi Keville for her undaunting support on due day; and for Nancy Scarzello and Richard Liebmann for their continuous efforts toward this project. We'd also like to acknowledge all of the contributors, who in the midst of their busy lives took the time to write informative chapters on their favorite herbs. And, finally, special thanks to Rosemary Gladstar and Deb Soule; it was their initial vision that inspired this book project for United Plant Savers.

United Plant Savers

FOREWORD

RICHARD LIEBMANN, N.D.,
Executive Director, United Plant Savers

As we enter the new millennium, a twenty-year, sixteen-organization study reports that thirty-four thousand plant species—12 percent of plants worldwide and 29 percent of plants in the United States—have become so rare that they could easily disappear. This potential catastrophic loss of plant life is directly attributable to loss of habitat caused by urban sprawl and deforestation. Native medicinal plants in the U.S. are additionally being stressed to fuel the skyrocketing growth of the herbal industry both at home and abroad. Worldwide, more than 80 percent of the population uses herbal medicine as their primary form of health care. In the U.S. herbs are a $4-billion-plus industry; worldwide, at least $20 billion. Many of the most important native medicinal plants—those used for human healing for thousands of years—are threatened with extinction. United Plant Savers is a non-profit grassroots membership organization whose mission is to conserve and restore native medicinal plants and their habitats while ensuring an abundant renewable supply of medicinal plants for generations to come. United Plant Savers was formed in the spirit of hope, by people committed to protecting and replanting native medicinal plants and to raising public awareness about the plight of native medicinal plants. United Plant Savers' activities include:

- Identifying which native medicinal plants are at risk

- Raising public awareness of the current plight of at-risk native medicinal plants

- Creating and managing botanical sanctuaries

- Providing seeds and rootstock and information for replanting at-risk species

- Replanting and restoring at-risk medicinal plants

- Consulting with those who grow and harvest medicinal herbs regarding sustainable land-use practices

- Sponsoring programs for school systems and communities to replant at-risk medicinal species back into their natural habitats

- Carrying out focused research to help accomplish the above goals

We have many exciting projects. One is working with government, industry, and the public to establish and implement a strategy for the long-term sustainability of goldenseal *(Hydrastis canadensis).* Another is working at a grassroots level throughout the country sponsoring native plant giveaways; providing small grants for community planting projects; hosting workshops and conferences; establishing the UpS Botanical Sanctuary Network in people's backyards, farms, and woodlands; and creating a living greenway of native medicinal plants throughout North America.

United Plant Savers recently established its first center on 378 acres of fertile and beautiful land in the Appalachian foothills of southeastern Ohio. This botanical sanctuary serves as a research and education center where many come to interact with and learn about native medicinal plants in their natural habitat. We offer diverse learning opportunities for children, university students, farmers, scientists, and the general public. Research focuses on native medicinal plant population studies, cultivation studies, and wild-harvesting and sustainability studies. The sanctuary also serves as a repository of native medicinal plant germ plasm, as a propagation facility for native medicinal plant seeds and live planting material, and as model of sustainable land use.

With the publication of *Planting the Future,* United Plant Savers has taken a major step forward in disseminating up-to-date and comprehensive information on conservation, cultivation, and usage of at-risk native medicinal plants. What's special about this book is that it is a collaborative effort by some of the most respected names in American herbalism. All the contributors are deeply impassioned about native medicinal plants and committed to the health and well-being of these species and their natural habitats.

Our plant brothers and sisters have been essential healers for humans since the beginning. Today the very survival of native medicinal plants is symbolic of the challenge we face as humans. United Plant Savers is taking both the short and long view of protecting native medicinal plants. We understand that the issues are complex, and that much research will be needed if we are to understand the full implications of our present actions. As a grassroots organization, we plan to stay intimately involved with planting and protection efforts across the United States. The words of Margaret Mead ring true: "Never doubt that a small group of thoughtful, committed citizens can change the world; it is the only thing that ever has." We all must work together to protect at-risk native medicinal plants. At the same time we must champion sustainable organic cultivation and sustainable wild-harvesting to ensure an abundant, renewable supply of native medicinal plants for future generations.

INTRODUCTION

ROSEMARY GLADSTAR

It was early winter when I moved to the Northeast. I'd missed the renowned autumn splendor of the Vermont woodlands by only a few weeks. Instead, I was greeted by the first cold blasts of winter and the promise of several more months of the most penetrating cold I'd ever known. As it turned out, it was the perfect opportunity for me, wrapped in warm woolens by the woodstove, to study. The entire landscape was new to me, and I was ready to delve into my botanical references and learn as much as I could about the neighborhood before the spring thaw awoke the plants in the forest.

These eastern deciduous forests were a different world from the ancient redwood groves of northern California where I'd grown up. The first thing I noticed in the earliest days after my arrival in New England was that there were few truly old trees in the forest. The surrounding forest, though beautiful, was young, lacking the craggy bark and towering pitch of the old ones. Those elders that had managed to survive past one or two hundred years were all marked by the blessings of imperfections that saved them from the frenetic logging activities of the past

three hundred years. At the time, I was too new to the language of these particular woods to realize fully what the lack of forest elders was stating so surely about the missing understory plants, or to read the message clearly written in the landscape about the history of these forests.

For the first couple of years, I wandered through our woodlands in a state of happy anticipation. There was an endless variety of new greenery to discover as the northern woods slowly revealed their secrets to me. And, of course, I was ever on the lookout for those mysterious and oh so famous eastern woodland medicinals: ginseng, goldenseal, bloodroot, black cohosh. These illustrious eastern woodland plants had been present in my materia medica since I first began reading Jethro Kloss in the early 1970s. But I had never encountered them in the wild. A couple I had seen only as glossy prints in plant identification books. But, after several seasons passing with nary a sighting, I began to doubt that any of these native medicinals remained, though tales of recent harvests were still told by my elderly neighbors.

During my third spring in Vermont, I came

1

The plants are calling you. They have a rich and diverse vocabulary and speak in many tongues. For the scientist the plant may speak in the complex language of chemicals and isolates; to the medicine person they speak in the multiversed language of healing; to the poet, they speak of beauty. No matter what language you speak or comprehend, the plants will converse in a manner that you can understand, though it may take a listening ear and an open heart to hear them. Through their color, scent, medicine power, and beauty they seduce and entice us into the realm of our senses where we hear best their subtle language. Many people, when they first begin working with plants, don't recognize the language that plants use. They are listening for familiar words. But words are only one method of communication and, as most people discover, they are not always the best way to convey feelings or thoughts. Ask anyone who has dug their hands deep in the dirt, planted seeds, harvested medicine, and taken time simply to get to know plants on their own turf, and they will tell you that plants communicate clearly if we but choose to listen. And the plants are calling us now, asking us for help. The wild gardens are in trouble, and the precious medicines of the earth are being lost.

to realize that many of the oldest plants of the eastern deciduous forests, including many important medicinal plants, had either completely disappeared or were in short supply. I was mind wandering, stepping over the wake robins and adders tongues of early spring, feeling a certain despair, an abiding loss at the disappearance of these sweet earth medicines, when I heard a voice rising from the forest around me. It was plain and directive and said rather simply, "Plant us. Bring us back to our communities." Having listened to plants all my life, I had no doubt what to do. That fall I ordered several pounds of ginseng, goldenseal, black cohosh, and bloodroot and reintroduced them into my woodlands. I planted them back among the native landscape where once—before logging, before sheep farming, before haying and mowing, before the stone walls that marked the activities of the early New England farmers—these plants had thrived in abundant communities. I really had no idea how to go about this project and, admittedly, many of the earliest plantings faired poorly. Soil conditions, pH factors, the changing overstory as well as the rootstock I ordered were all factors I hardly thought to consider. I was acting from pure enthusiasm and ignorance, an impractical combination, but it lit a fire in my heart and fueled me on.

Those early efforts were the beginning of a project that reshaped my life work and became a driving passion. Having spent the greater part of my life studying medicinal plants, working within my community as a practicing herbalist, wildcrafting, making herbal products, and educating others about this marvelous ancient system of herbal medicine, I suddenly found myself thrust into new territory: the intricate village system of the wild plant communities. How were they thriving, these healing plants, in their native landscape? How did other plant communities fare when important members of the medicinal clan disappeared from their ecosystem? After all, these were the powerful medicine plants, medicines as valued for the earth's well-being and the vitality of the wild plant communities as for the health of the two leggeds, the humans, who have been dependent on them for thousands of years. What happens when the balance is lost? When the medicine is removed from the community? Is the ever diminishing population of these powerful medicine plants perhaps one of the reasons why there are so many more diseases attacking native plant communities as well as the human population?

Scientists are just beginning to understand the delicate relationship plants have to one another and to their environment. Many plants—perhaps all of them—have a symbiotic relationship with the soil microorganisms that they grow in and a specialized method of communicating with one another through soil microbes, or mycorrhizae. Botanists and foresters are beginning to recognize that forest plants communicate through a complex underground grafting network, and that this highly sophisticated communication system may warn plants of approaching disease, spread nutrients, and serve to connect the forest biomass. Indigenous people have long recognized that all things in life are connected through a great web and that disturbing one small plant in the ecosystem, in the great web of life, can cause the whole to become unbalanced. This concept is familiar to most herbalists as well, who through their close relationship with plants have experienced the interconnectedness of life.

As I planted, I began to talk to other people: students, fellow herbalists, naturalists, farmers, locals, the woodland people who were long-time residents, those "seers" of the forested landscape. It was as I expected; others, too, were concerned about diminishing native medicinal plant populations. My coworkers, many of whom have been friends since our earliest herbal forays, had noticed similar disturbances in their own areas. Many of our old-time favorite wild plants were no longer found in the lush abundance we remembered from our youth. We had to travel farther to find them and often found fewer population stands than we might have several years earlier. Most notably, the shy woodland plants were becoming harder to find.

In the past fifteen years little attention has been paid to the loss of plant species except in the tropical rain forest. As well-known author and plant photographer Steven Foster commented, "Plants, unlike animals, are not warm, cute, or fuzzy and, therefore, don't catch the public's attention so readily." Yet, the World Wildlife Fund estimates that more than thirty thousand varieties of plant life worldwide are in imminent danger of extinction. In 1992 the First World Congress on Medicinal and Aromatic Plants for Human Welfare met in the Netherlands to address this situation. At this important gathering it was noted that while 80 percent of the world's population depends on traditional herbal medicine, the accelerating need for phytomedicines, pharmaceutical drugs, and other industrial applications has caused over-exploitation of medicinal plants, resulting in genetic erosion and increasing the threat of extinction.

> Frances Thompson, the English poet, once wrote that one could not pluck a flower without troubling a star. If we cannot pluck a flower without troubling a star, what then if we lose a species?
>
> Loren Israelson

Diminishing habitat is certainly one of the more obvious reasons for plant loss. Recent statistics suggest that more than 2,500 acres of native land is disturbed each day by human activity. We all can—and do—lament about those wild places we wandered as children that have relentlessly been transformed into shopping centers, housing developments, or factories (so inappropriately called "plants"). Most of us have experienced feelings of helplessness as we've witnessed the teaming biomass of the earth's surface being buried beneath those abysmal layers of cement and asphalt. Habitat loss is without doubt the greatest threat to plants as well as to other forms of life. But what effect does the sudden resurgence of interest in herbal medicine have on our dwindling plant resources?

A gypsy at heart and by blood, I've traveled a fair amount in my life to places of botanical beauty and interest. In many countries one can find the rich traditions of herbalism alive and well, especially in the hearts of the country people. However, on my travels I have observed, especially in the most heavily populated areas, that though the herbal traditions were generally alive and well in the hearts of the people, the native plant populations upon which these traditions were based were often in dire straits.

For instance, China, long regarded for its enduring herbal tradition, is devoid almost entirely of its most important wild medicinal plants. In the 1950s China embarked on an ambitious program to integrate traditional Chinese medicine into the public health policy. Within a few short years traditional Chinese medicine had become the primary mode of health care for more than 40 percent of the population. But in the ensuing years shortages in supplies of the most popular medicinal plants began to result from overharvesting of wild populations. In response, China began a massive effort to cultivate medicinal plants and now has more than one million acres of medicinal plants under cultivation. But the wild plant resources were almost completely annihilated and have been slow to recover.

India also boasts one of the world's oldest systems of traditional herbal medicine, Ayurveda. India is also considered the largest producer of medicinal plants in the world. With more than two million acres of herbs under cultivation, India not only provides herbs for its own herbal tradition but also for the rest of the world. Even so, one seldom finds large stands of wild herbs growing on this vast continent. India, too, has experienced severe shortages of wild medicinal plants from the overharvesting of wild medicinals.

Many of our favorite plants originated in the Mediterranean. Greece, particularly, had a major influence on Western medicine as well as on our modern herbal tradition. However, traveling through modern Greece one is hard pressed to find the fields of wild herbs or the great majestic forests described so poetically in the *Iliad*. Though the rocky cliffs and barren hillsides of the Grecian terrain are ruggedly beautiful, they are sorely lacking in great forests or carpets of wild herbs. One must go to the highest mountains to encounter the last vestiges of the great forests that were so famous in the days of Homer and Hippocrates. Where are the fields of wild herbs that these ancient men so fondly wrote of—herbs that form the basis of much of the modern herbal tradition?

In England, always a rich repository of herbal tradition and history, medical herbalist and author David Hoffmann reported recently that it is illegal to pick wild medicinal plants from the English countryside because they are threatened in their native landscape. Furthermore, English herbalists have created an organization to conserve North American medicinal plants because these plants are so important in their herbal practices.

After my travels when I return home to my own wild woodlands, I marvel anew at the great expanse of wilderness that stretches out before me. I've come to fully appreciate the wealth of biodiversity that still remains in this young, eager land and the degree to which it is changing before our very eyes. As elsewhere in the world, habitat loss, overpopulation, and poor logging practices are contributing to diminishing plant populations in the United States. Likewise, overappreciation of medicinal plants can be detrimental to their health. Perhaps the fact that herbal medi-

cine became widely unpopular—actually illegal to practice—in the U.S. from 1940 through the late 1980s may have been the saving grace not only for the wild heart-centered tradition of American herbalism, but also for the wild plants themselves. Forced underground, herbs and herbalism set deep roots and flourished quietly.

The last ten years of the twentieth century saw an American herbal renaissance, the ramifications of which are still being explored. This sudden burgeoning interest in herbal medicine in America may account for a much greater loss of plant species than we've yet recognized. The American herbal industry is expected to reach the $5 billion mark by the end of this year. Large drug companies have entered the herbal marketplace with a gung ho attitude and goals sharply aimed at profit. Small herbal companies, most of which boast ethical business practices and wildcrafted products, can be found all across the landscape of America. Today, finding an herb store in most towns is as simple as opening a phone book.

While positive on one hand, this situation has engendered a unique set of challenges for wild medicinal plants and for the people who love and use them. Where do all the plants needed for this vast amount of product originate? Until very recently, almost all of the resources used in botanical medicine came either from Third World countries that have far from ideal growing conditions or from our native wild gardens. Large-scale cultivation of medicinal herbs is slowly becoming more common in the United States, but we have a long way to go before there are enough herb farms to meet the demands of manufacturers.

I can't help but reflect on the hundreds of students my fellow herbalists and I have trained over the years to identify and harvest wild medicinals. Generations of herbalists have emphasized the quality of wild versus cultivated plants. This bias was not based on plant constituency, which is often higher in cultivated species, but rather on the energetics of wild plants. There is a spirit, an energy inherent in wild things, both fauna and flora, that is apparent to anybody who has visited the last remaining wilderness areas of this country. That essence is hard, if not impossible, to capture. However, concurrent with the growing awareness of diminishing plant populations is the increasing awareness of the need for organic cultivation of medicinal herbs. Gardeners and farmers are discovering means to energize and potentize their cultivated varieties of medicinal plants by incorporating not only good soil management, but also the forces of nature to grow crops of medicinal plants that equal or exceed the life force and power of their wild counterparts.

I've yet to meet the unethical wildcrafter. Each person feels he or she is using sustainable harvesting practices. We have each developed our own special methods and techniques of sustainable harvesting. Many of us were trained by our elders in "conscious collecting." Prayer and a sacred connection with the spirit of the plant are an important part of our gathering ritual. However, no matter how ethical or sustainable our wildcrafting techniques, and how heartfelt our prayers, if evermore people and greater numbers of companies continue to depend on our wild resources, the supplies will diminish as surely as did the great herds of buffalo that once graced the plains and passenger pigeons that once darkened the sky.

> The beauty and genius of a work of art
> May be reconceived,
> Though its first material expression be destroyed;
> A vanished harmony may yet again
> Inspire the composer;
> But, when the last individual of a race of living beings
> Breathes no more,
> Another heaven and another earth must pass
> Before such a one can be again.
> **Belize City Zoo for Endangered Species**

Many of the plants—in fact, most—that are wild harvested are wholly renewable. These common "weeds" of the North American landscape, many of which are nonnatives, settled the continent readily and became as tenacious as the white settlers in whose footsteps they followed. Equipped with amazing survival skills, they grow prolifically and abundantly throughout the countryside and, though they may require future monitoring, it would be absurd not to harvest them at this juncture. Of great concern, however, are our native medicinals that are habitat specific, have a limited range, and reproduce more selectively. Some of these natives, such as ginseng, bloodroot, blue and black cohosh, and goldenseal, are found growing nowhere else in the world and are in great demand not only by the herbal industry but also by pharmaceutical companies. It is these plants we need to safeguard and protect, seeking sustainable herbal practices such as organic cultivation of important medicinal crops, limiting or restricting the use of those plants that are severely at-risk, and incorporating better health practices into our lives so that reliance on herbal medicine—and medicine of any kind, for that matter—is reduced.

One of the greatest challenges facing us in the twenty-first century is the notion that we live in the age of abundance. Life is measured in excess. Many people using herbal medicine have a difficult time comprehending that demand is outpacing supply. We measure abundance by bioregional plentitude—what we see out our own back door. How can we talk of a plant being endangered, at-risk, when the numbers seem so wonderfully plentiful in our own hunting grounds. Wake robin (*Trillium* spp.), or bethroot, is an excellent example of bioregional abundance. If you live in the Pacific west, midwestern states, or the Northeast you may have witnessed hundreds of wake robins rising their chocolate-red blossoms in the early spring. So why is it included on the UpS At-Risk List? Trillium, an important medicinal plant with a long history of use, is a slow-growing perennial with a limited habitat and restricted range. It takes more than seven years for a single trillium to mature, set seed, and reproduce. Each trillium produces only a limited number of seeds and the insects required to pollinate it are becoming scarce. Thus far, large-scale cultivation of trillium for medicinal purposes has not been undertaken. However, if trillium was targeted for the herbal "best seller" list, like several other of its woodland neighbors have been, conceiv-

ably thousands of pounds of trillium could be removed from the forested landscape. *How long would it be able to withstand the demand? How long before trillium became a rare jewel of the forest?*

LOCAL ABUNDANCE

So you know a place where ginseng is common. Sustainable harvest in such an area (that is, harvesting no more than the additive growth increase of all the ginseng plants in this niche) might seem ecological, but given the paucity of ginseng in other areas, it may not be a good idea. Better to create a wild garden and harvest plants you have grown yourself, and allow increase to occur in areas of local abundance.

Though *our* marshlands may be teeming with thousands of sundews, or the mountains where *we* live be carpeted with the bright yellow flowers of arnica, though the prairies surrounding *us* may be resplendent with the fiery orange of butterfly weed, or *our* woodlands be rich in cohoshes, bioregional abundance is not an insurance of a plant's long-term sustainability. Consider how many of these seemingly abundant plants are needed to fill the tonnage required by the ever growing demand of the herbal marketplace. Consider the propagation mechanisms of each particular plant. How long does it take to mature and set seed and what is its survival rate in the best of conditions? Consider the plant's range. How specific is its habitat and is it threatened by urban sprawl, logging, or other human activities? Is the plant in high demand in other countries? And how much is exported yearly? Consider the message from the plant itself. What is it saying to us?

In 1994 at the Third International Herb Symposium a group of concerned individuals came together to discuss the issues of medicinal plant preservation and conservation. We met again that following autumn at the Green Nations Gathering in the Catskills of upstate New York. United Plant Savers was born from these meetings. A nonprofit grassroots organization, UpS is dedicated to preserving native medicinal plants and the land they grow on and, ultimately, to ensuring an abundant renewable supply of organically cultivated medicinal herbs. Formed in the spirit of hope, our membership reflects the great diversity of American herbalism and includes herbalists, botanists, health professionals, organic farmers, business owners, wildcrafters, seed savers, manufacturers, and plant lovers from all walks of life.

UNITED PLANT SAVERS

Why did UpS select a name that's often confused with America's most well-known delivery service? We often joke that we should adopt as our motto "We'll plant anywhere." When herbalism first resurfaced in the early 1970s, it was embraced eagerly by the emerging hippie culture. Few of us differentiated in those early days the difference between good or bad quality herbs. The term *organic* was hardly coined at the time. In fact, sources were so limited, we were just happy to have plants of any kind.

When Ed Smith and Sara Katz, city herbalists from Boston, first moved to the lovely Applegate Valley in Oregon in 1978, they were astounded to discover the obvious difference in the freshly harvested plants. Their small herb company, Herb Pharm, soon reflected this quality in their products. Ed, in his efforts to educate the rest of us about the differences in quality used to travel around in his red van to the small herbal gatherings and lecture us about using wildcrafted organic plants, of course, selling his own all the while! His statement, "We're all like a bunch of UPS herbalists; we think the plants are grown on the UPS truck, delivered by UPS, and shipped UPS," addressed the problems we were faced with at the time: lack of quality herbs, few herbal products, and lack of herbal education. Thirty years later, *organic* is almost synonymous with the herbal industry, herbal educational opportunities are widely available, and herbal products flood the marketplace. United Plant Savers (UpS) was chosen as the name for our newly formed group to identify the current issues and problems facing herbs and herbalists today, especially the depletion of our wild plant resources. We remain as hopeful as we were then that we can and will make a difference helping to ensure that our medicinal plant populations are here for our grandchildren and their grandchildren to enjoy and even more importantly, that they remain an integral part of the great web of life.

ALTERNATIVES

If an herb is on the At-Risk List:

- Manufacturers should be reducing use, and cultivating or substituting instead.

- Consumers should be aware of how valuable it is and use it sparingly, or opt for cultivated material or substitutes.

- Herbalists and doctors should be aware of the implications of their recommendations and take plant protection into account.

- Retailers can look at this list and make decisions about what extracts to stock based on plant protection as well as saleability, and they can make plant protection a positive selling point.

To date United Plant Savers has initiated a number of replanting projects, including our "Plant Give Aways" in which more than fifty thousand goldenseal roots and several thousand other at-risk plants—black cohosh, blue cohosh, bloodroot, slippery elm, white oak saplings, and others—have been distributed to members to plant on their land. UpS does not advocate randomly planting at-risk species into wild areas unless privately owned. We do encourage the stewarding of existing wild medicinal plants by spreading their seed within the habitat and by weeding out nonnative species. We also encourage gardeners to propagate at-risk medicinal plants in their backyards, gardens, farms, and privately owned lands, and to monitor their status from season to season thus helping to protect the germ plasm of these important medicinal species. Like Margaret Mead, we believe that the most positive changes are often the result of thoughtful, committed citizens taking action. Though large planting projects, scientific research, and biological studies are an important part of plant conservation, equally important is individual participation by lay persons. Often it is those people out there living and working with the plants for decade after decade who have the most information. We support the grow-your-own-medicine mentality and encourage our members both to plant medicinal herb gardens and to help reestablish the wild gardens on their land.

Our largest and most complex task to date was defining and developing the Medicinal Plant At-Risk List and the accompanying To-Watch List, which have become the guiding source for the herbal industry, herbal community, and for the public (see pages 11–12). These lists, though nondefinitive in nature and continuously reviewed and examined, identify the native medicinal plants that are most at risk in their native habitat or those that have the potential to become at risk within the near future. Rather than assume these plants are impervious to human activity, we have developed a conservative attitude and chose to err in favor of the plants. Necessary scientific research and data, important to confirm that these plants are, in fact, endangered, can take years to accumulate. We are choosing to act before these plants disappear from the native landscape forever. Herbs included on the lists are those that are most sensitive to human activity. Inclusion is based on current market analysis, increased demand, habitat specificality, a plant's sensitivity to human activity, and lack of known propagation techniques or large-scale cultivation. Our hope is that—by acting before it's too late—each of the designated plants can be removed from the At-Risk and To-Watch Lists in our lifetime.

With the generous support of green angels Judy and Michael Funk, United Plant Savers established a 370-acre botanical sanctuary in southeast Ohio that serves as model farm for medicinal plant conservation, research, and education and as a seed repository for American medicinal plants. This beautiful farm is rich with native at-risk medicinals and has a number of research and educational projects underway. We have also established the Botanical Sanctuary Network, a program that helps members create botanical sanctuaries on their land.

Planting the Future, another United Plant Savers project, is the collective effort of many concerned herbalists and represents professional wildcrafters, practitioners, manufacturers, and community herbalists. Each contributor brings a personal knowledge and love of the plants as well as a sincere concern that these plants continue to flourish in their native landscape and remain an intricate part of the great web of life.

Through these and other projects we are seeking solutions, optimistic that our efforts are making a difference. Our mission is to ensure the perpetuation of important medicinal plants and the habitat they thrive on so that when future generations of plant lovers walk upon this planet, they, too, will know and appreciate the medicines of their ancestors and the healing power that grows from the heart of the earth. The good news is that it is not too late; none of these important North American medicinal plants is yet extinct. You have the opportunity and skills needed to make a difference.

If we choose to use plants as our medicine, we then become accountable for the wild gardens, their health, and their upkeep. We begin a co-creative partnership with the plants, giving back what we receive—health, nourishment, beauty, and protection. We have reached a time in history when to not consider our relationship with the resources we use on this small and beautiful planet will be disastrous. We invite you to join our efforts to help Plant the Future.

NORTH AMERICAN INDIGENOUS MEDICINAL PLANTS

For the benefit of the plant communities, wild animals, harvesters, farmers, consumers, manufacturers, retailers, and practitioners we offer this list of wild medicinal plants that we feel are currently most sensitive to the impact of human activities. Our intent is to assure the increasing abundance of the medicinal plants that are presently in decline due to expanding popularity and shrinking habitat and range. UpS is not asking for a moratorium on the use of these herbs. Rather, we are initiating programs designed to *preserve* these important wild medicinal plants.

We ask wildcrafters to consider the ecological impact of taking these herbs from the wild. Replanting in the wild, as well as careful stewarding of your collection areas is of tantamount importance if the trade of wildcrafting is to continue. Although the herb may be abundant in your locality, it has probably already disappeared from other areas. Wildcrafters are among those who have the best understanding of wild plants, and you can contribute greatly by providing seed and advising others on how to plant and grow these herbs.

We ask manufacturers and consumers to assist in the transition from wildcrafted sources to those that are organically grown. If there is demand for wild herbs, then we will continue to lose them. If there is demand for cultivated herbs, then we will create environmentally friendly jobs while saving the wild plants. Although it is an expensive proposition, the time is ripe to assure sustainability of the herbs we love.

AT-RISK LIST

American Ginseng (*Panax quinquefolius*)

Black Cohosh (*Actaea racemosa*, syn. *Cimicifuga racemosa*)

Bloodroot (*Sanguinaria canadensis*)

Blue Cohosh (*Caulophyllum thalictroides*)

Echinacea (*Echinacea* spp.)

Eyebright (*Euphrasia* spp.)

Goldenseal (*Hydrastis canadensis*)

Helonias Root (False Unicorn) (*Chamaelirium luteum*)

Kava, Hawaiian Wild (*Piper methysticum*)

Lady's Slipper Orchid (*Cypripedium* spp.)

Lomatium (*Lomatium dissectum*)

Osha (*Ligusticum porteri, L.* spp.)

Peyote (*Lophophora williamsii*)

Slippery Elm (*Ulmus rubra*)

Sundew (*Drosera* spp.)

Trillium (Beth Root) (*Trillium* spp.)

True Unicorn (*Aletris farinosa*)

Venus's-Flytrap (*Dionaea muscipula*)

Virginia Snakeroot (*Aristolochia serpentaria*)

Wild Yam (*Dioscorea* villosa, *D.* spp.)

TO-WATCH LIST

Arnica (*Arnica* spp.)

Calamus *Root (Acorus calamus)*

Cascara Sagrada *(Rhamnus purshiana)*

Chaparro *(Castela emoryi)*

Elephant Tree *(Bursera microphylla)*

Gentian (*Gentiana* spp.)

Goldthread (*Coptis* spp.)

Lobelia (*Lobelia* spp.)

Maidenhair Fern *(Adiantum pendatum)*

Mayapple *(Podophyllum peltatum)*

Oregon Grape (*Mahonia* spp.)

Partridgeberry *(Mitchella repens)*

Pink Root *(Spigelia marilandica)*

Pipsissewa *(Chimaphila umbellata)*

Pleurisy Root (Butterfly Weed) *(Asclepias tuberosa)*

Spikenard *(Aralia racemosa, A.californica)*

Stillingia (Queen's Delight) *(Stillingia sylvatica)*

Stoneroot *(Collinsonia canadensis)*

Stream Orchid *(Epipactis gigantea)*

Turkey Corn *(Dicentra canadensis)*

White Sage *(Salvia apiana)*

Wild Indigo *(Baptisia tinctoria)*

Yerba Mansa *(Anemopsis californica)*

Yerba Santa *(Eriodictyon californica)*

Note: Read "spp." as "all North American species in the genus." We are using this category when: (1) all North American members of the genus fit the "at risk" definition or (2) there is reason to believe that either through inability to locate the commonly used species, or through misidentification, or through intentional collection, species besides the commonly used species in the genus might also be at risk. We see this situation clearly with the harvest of *any* trillium species to be sold as "bethroot," or in the harvest of *any* echinacea species to be sold as *"E. angustifolia."*

WHAT YOU CAN DO
TO MAKE A DIFFERENCE

ROSEMARY GLADSTAR

BE A CONSCIOUS AND
RESPONSIBLE CONSUMER
Know the Herb Products You Use and the Herb
Companies You Purchase From

It seems that everyone these days is interested in learning how herbal medicine can benefit them. But equally important, if not more so, is the welfare of the plant communities themselves. When you're planning to use plants for herbal medicine, know where these products came from. Were they organically cultivated? Or wild-harvested? If wild-harvested, are they on the UpS At-Risk or To-Watch Lists? If so, can they be cultivated? (Refer to the Propagation and Cultivation section in each herb chapter.) If an herb is considered at risk and is not being cultivated, your plants are coming from an unsustainable wild-harvest. Do not purchase these products. Take a few minutes to write to the company and inform them of your concern. Consumer letters do have impact; they are the only way you really have of letting a company know your concerns about or appreciation for a product. And don't neglect to write those companies that are cultivating their own medicinal plants and/or using weedy species in place of the more sensitive species.

STAY AWAKE, BE MINDFUL
Know Your At-Risk Herbs

Keep a copy of the At-Risk List tacked on your cupboard door or on the refrigerator. Ask the local store where you purchase your herbs to post the list next to its herb section for quick customer reference.

GROW YOUR OWN MEDICINES
It's an Heirloom Art

Most of the plants you need for herbal medicine are easily grown, and many are extremely adaptable. Why do you think so many of our most popular and effective herbal medicines are the weedy species? If you have a small garden space, consider planting those herbal medicines you use most: echinacea, valerian, chamomile, goldenseal, cayenne, mints, and the like. Plant as many of the at-risk herbs in your garden as will grow in your habitat (see the Propagation and Cultivation section in each herb chapter).

Even those you may not use will benefit from being planted in your garden. And don't forget the weedy plants. They often make the best medicines. Weedy species are quite prolific and are famous for showing up uninvited in your garden. And often, these prolific growers make appropriate substitutes for the more sensitive and at-risk herbs.

RESTORE WILDNESS ON YOUR LAND

Whether you own a city lot, an acre, or 1,000 acres, help restore biodiversity by restoring at least part of the land you caretake to its wild state. Find out what species of plants, birds, animals, and insects inhabited your neighborhood before people moved in and houses were built; then set about restoring this habitat as much as possible. You may be amazed at the results this simple effort rewards you with. The act of allowing a small section of a garden or acre to return to its wild state is an invitation to a variety of species that don't normally survive in the sterile environment of lawns. Read *The Man Who Planted Trees* by Jean Giono for a glimpse into the magnitude of the changes that such a small action can effect—and be inspired to start your own story. Don't be nervous if your neighbors get antsy about the weeds and other wild things that may start moving back. Use it as an opportunity for education.

PLANT A NATIVE MEDICINAL PLANT TRAIL

This is a wonderful project and can be far less daunting than it sounds. A native plant trail doesn't need to meander through a large plot of wilderness. It is just as effective and perhaps more educational winding through a backyard garden, where it's accessible to family and friends. Do a little research (see the resources at the end of this book) into which native medicinal plants, as well as other native plants, grow (or grew) in your area. Also, research cultivation requirements. The nursery directory (located in the back of this book), a land consultant, or a local native plant group can be helpful with this aspect of planning your trail.

Allow the trail to have a natural curve; if there are streams, rocks, and other natural features nearby, include them in the design. It's helpful to make signs identifying the plants. These can be simple, inexpensive signs painted on wood or plastic, or you may decide to invest in professional-quality signs made especially for botanical identification (see the resources). Invite friends, family, or the neighborhood to help plant the trail. Once it's well established, invite your helpers back to enjoy it with you.

If you've been searching for ways to interact and share with your community, a garden is a natural place to start. Add to it the special feature of native medicinal plants and you've got a sure winner. Native plant trails featuring medicinal plants are great in local parks, schoolgrounds, and other public places. Check with your community for possibilities.

CREATE A BOTANICAL
SANCTUARY ON YOUR LAND
It Already May Be One

The dictionary defines *sanctuary* as "a holy place, a place of refuge or protection, a reservation for people, animals, and plants." Creating a botanical sanctuary is a simple act of purpose. Begin by caretaking the land you live on as sacred space, preserving or restoring the rich biodiversity that resides there. One of the goals of United Plant Savers is to establish botanical sanctuaries in people's backyards, farms, and woodlands, creating a living greenway of native medicinal plants patchworked throughout the landscape of North America. These botanical sanctuaries will serve as repositories of at-risk native medicinal plants and germ plasm and as educational centers for medicinal plant conservation and propagation. For information on becoming a member of the UpS Botanical Sanctuary Network, write:

UpS
P.O. Box 98
East Barre, VT 05649

HERBS FOR WELLNESS,
NOT JUST ILLNESS

Almost every herb on the At-Risk and To-Watch Lists is used for specific medicinal purposes; several are restricted to more serious illnesses and imbalances. Many of our most plentiful and weedy species are those herbs considered tonics, or food herbs. Herbs such as burdock root and dandelion, chickweed and cleavers, nettle and red clover grow in abundance across the landscape of America. These herbs have long been considered superior tonic medicines and are used to maintain wellness, prevent illness, and restore vitality. Most are hardy; they grow prolifically and in a wide variety of habitats and bioregions. These are the herbs we should celebrate and use daily to maintain and restore health and well-being. Grow a garden and many of these herbs will pop up—just like weeds—in it. Cultivate a field and there they are again. Unpampered, mostly unappreciated, these feisty weeds are full of vitality themselves and offer us a path to well-being.

LARGE OR SMALL
HERBAL MANUFACTURER
Does It Matter?

We don't think so. Whether an herbal company is small or large, using plants that have been identified as at-risk is not a wise choice for the health and ecology of the earth. Small companies collecting small amounts of at-risk plant material from the wild can have an impact on a plant community, even though the amounts collected may be smaller. Soil disturbance and improper collecting techniques can lower yields in ensuing years. The all-too-common practice of collecting the largest of the plants can also reduce the viability of the plant populations, because it is often these "grandmothers and grandfathers" of the plant communities whose genetic material is healthiest.

Often, small herbal companies metamorphose into large ones. It's better to start with good environmental practices from the get-go. Use organically cultivated plants and weedy species in your formulas. Support herbal sustainability by helping responsible companies to prosper and grow.

WHAT YOU DON'T TEACH MATTERS

If you're one of the many herbal educators out there these days teaching others about the wonders of green medicine, it is imperative to address the issues of plant conservation and propagation in your program. Even teachers who deal strictly with clinical therapeutics should consider including plant conservation as an important aspect of the educational program. We need future herbalists who are not only well trained in the medicinal applications of herbs but also deeply and keenly aware of conservation issues. It is these future herbalists who will carry on the tradition of herbalism and serve as plant caretakers. United Plant Savers offers an educational package and slide show of at-risk plants to help with this process of educating future herbalists to be conservation minded.

BE MINDFUL OF GROUPS ON WILDCRAFTING EXPEDITIONS

Though wildcrafting forays are valuable learning experiences and an important part of the tradition of herbalism, it may be time to de-emphasize them in favor of gardening and propagation classes. Even with the best inten-

tions and a skilled leader, a group of ten or twenty students foraging in the same area can leave the soil impacted, plant communities disturbed, and populations decreased beyond sustainable levels. In addition, twenty students wildcrafting in one area this year could mean up to eighty there next year if each student showed only two other people the spot.

Many wildcrafting educators follow a practice they learned from Native teachers: leaving an offering of tobacco, cornmeal, or some other token to honor plants for providing us with their sacred medicine. Such wisdom! But this offering turns to folly when it is not accompanied by wise sustainable practices. Tobacco and cornmeal offerings will not grow good crops of osha or bloodroot, ginseng or goldenseal. Neither will sprinkling seeds in the area of harvest—not unless you have a working knowledge of the germination and viability of the seeds you're planting. In addition to passing on the traditions of our Native elders by continuing the practices of offerings and prayers, we must teach future wild-harvesters proper cultivation and propagation techniques for the plants collected. That way, when offerings are made, seeds and crowns planted, the gesture of renewal will be more than token.

CREATING BOTANICAL SANCTUARIES

CHRISTOPHER HOBBS L.Ac.

The world is changing at an accelerating rate. The Internet, jet travel, and satellite links have helped facilitate this change with increasing fervor. Growing up in southern California in the 1950s, I became used to the kind of change that is quickly reshaping the surface of the earth. I watched chaparral-covered hillsides at the foot of the Sierra Padre Mountains plowed and planted with vast orange and lemon groves, only to be cut and plowed twenty years later for tract housing and strip malls. When I was fifteen, we moved to a 5-acre piece of land that was full of quail, deer, coyotes, aromatic shrubs, and huge two-hundred-year-old live oaks. I used to roam this land—smelling, touching everything, feeling very much a part of the wild animals and plants that called this place home. Several years later, preparations were made to put a major freeway through our backyard; the small country lane that wound peacefully along the front of our house was widened and became a four-lane freeway for frantic travelers. The native habitat with its trees and plants were paved over, buried beneath layers of concrete. But despite these immense disruptions, the wild spirit of the land and of the plants that grew a mile above us on steeper slopes could still be felt.

A few winters ago in the desert where I grew up, the hundred-year bloom happened. In all the years I had walked through this desert, imbibing the essence of flowers and the pungent aroma of the chaparral bush under the bluest of skies, I could not, even in my wildest imagination, have pictured the vast ocean of purple sand verbenas and desert evening primrose sweeping as far as the eye could see. They had been waiting quietly for just the right moment to burst forth in such splendor and were literally blooming their hearts out.

In the Coachella Valley, near Palm Desert, most of the extensive chaparral and mesquite-studded dunes had slowly been flattened, plowed, and made into golf courses, trailer parks, or strip malls. Here and there, however, a few hundred-acre squares were still untouched, more a testament to the outrageously steep price of land than lack of interest by developers. It was here in these untouched lots scattered amid the malls and golf courses that the flowers bloomed most intensely. Since many of the lots had for sale signs on them, it was only a matter of time before these too would be paved over, sealed in crypts of concrete. Did the intelligence of the flowers know what was to come? Were they reveling in the sheer joy of being with such bloom in one last majestic effort? It was then that the poignancy of it all struck me. After a half-million years of evolution, these flower species—and all the insects and animals that flourished with them—would be no more, soon to be buried beneath malls and roadways. Standing among the transitory beauty of a thousand plus blossoms in full glory, witnessing what might never be seen again in my lifetime, I felt a great surge of tears.

It's likely that you have seen similar changes in the areas where you grew up and have experienced similar feelings. Perhaps the woods or fields you ran in as a child, the places where you built forts, climbed trees, and breathed in the fresh scent of spring wildflowers are gone now. Perhaps, too, the old forests that you knew as a child have been replaced by a maze of buildings. If you ever experienced walking in an old-growth forest, it's a feeling you'll never forget. It is impossible to fully describe such an experience. The delicate and complex web of life found in an old-growth forest is vital, so perfect that one feels completely at home and at peace. Truly, one has entered the ultimate cathedral or temple containing all the beauty and inspiration that is earthly possible. Surely these rare old forests provide an intelligence pattern, a blueprint, for life to continue. But of the vast ancient forests that once carpeted the earth and provided a home for countless species, only a small por-

tion remains. In North America, it is estimated that as little as 4 to 5 percent of these original forests remains intact.

It's impossible not to imagine what will happen to the land, the plants, animals, insects, and other life-forms that are being systematically destroyed in our lifetime and replaced by our vision of a convenient world, a world re-created to optimize our shopping opportunities. But this scenario is not inevitable. The land where you live is sacred and alive, even if it lies buried under concrete or has had toxic chemicals poured into it. It is our personal responsibility to protect the earth and the creatures and plants who share our home and to nurture and protect the expansion of the intelligence of nature. The land will regenerate; the first soil microorganisms and plants will detoxify, purify, and sanctify it. But we need to be willing to help.

Following are three important ways you can help expand, protect, and reclaim the landscape and thus preserve the rich diversity of life that occupies native land. Though these steps in themselves may seem small in view of the vast amount of habitat destruction taking place daily, they are among the most important ways we can turn the tide and create a greener world because at the deepest level they empower us to make the difference.

1. **Green belts.** Consider coordinating land purchases, even small lots of land, with neighbors to create "corridors," or "green belts," which are so important to the health and continuance of the wild plants and animals. Encourage family, friends, and community members to do likewise.

2. **Become educated about land conservation.** Educate yourself about local land trusts, conservation easements, and environmental legislation in your area. Consider placing conservation easements on your land to protect its natural environment and resources in perpetuity.

3. **Create a botanical sanctuary on your land.** Though it may sound daunting, creating a sanctuary is relatively simple. Buy as much land as you can, whether it is a city lot, an acre homestead, or a 100-acre wilderness parcel, and create a sanctuary for life. Though gardens and cultivated fields are lovely, it is important to restore wilderness, even to a small parcel of land. Begin restoring the native species that once grew in your area. This may require some investigation and research on your part. Talk to local wildflower societies; they are often great resources for plant information. Replant the native trees, shrubs, flowers, and medicinal plants that once inhabited your area and witness the rich diversity that begins to return to your acreage, your sanctuary, within a few short seasons. In the process, you will find out much about health, vitality, and your own family's well-being.

United Plant Savers has created a Botanical Sanctuary Network to support others in creating their land as sanctuary. Our vision is to see a network of private and public botanical sanctuaries spread across the landscape of America and to help ensure that the rich tradition of American herbalism and the plants that comprise it

continue for our children and our grandchildren to enjoy. UpS has put together an informative Sanctuary Workbook that gives resources for creating a sanctuary on private land. For further information contact UpS at our home office or visit our Web site at www.plantsavers.org.

CREATING A BOTANICAL SANCTUARY

You can create a botanical sanctuary on any amount of land—a city lot, suburban backyard, or 700 acres of forests and fields, which is exactly what herbalist-farmer Paul Strauss did. An inspiration to those who meet him, Paul embodies the essence of the Green Man. Three decades of keen observations and commitment to the land has instilled in him a knowledge deeper and more profound than any amount of book learning. In the early 1970s, Paul settled on a small farm in southeastern Ohio. Beginning modestly with only a few acres, Paul continued acre by acre to purchase this inexpensive but lushly abundant land. Land purchase and stewardship became an overriding passion as his relationship with the land developed. Unable to sit back and watch the surrounding forests be clear-cut, displacing the plants and animals that lived there, Paul mobilized family, friends, and community members to purchase land. More than 700 acres of farmland and forest were preserved in the ensuing years. Strip mines that had devastated the land were reclaimed, the land replanted, and ponds created. The sanctuary evolved naturally as Paul replanted, restored, and reclaimed the land.

In 1998 Paul donated 70 acres of his land to United Plant Savers to help form the first UpS Botanical Sanctuary. Shortly thereafter, Michael and Judy Funk of Mountain People, a natural products distributor, made a considerable donation that enabled UpS to buy 300 adjoining acres, completing the first United Plant Savers Botanical Sanctuary. This 370-acre farm has many of the elements of a plant sanctuary already in place. The land is 50 percent mature, diverse, native hardwood forest and 50 percent fields. Extensive botanical assays have been performed to determine the resources present on the land. To date more than 500 species of plants, 120 species of trees, and 200 species of fungi have been identified. Half of the UpS at-risk native medicinal plants are thriving in abundance on this land. Large communities of goldenseal, American ginseng, black and blue cohosh, and grand old medicinal tree species such as white oak and slippery elm flourish in abundance on this reclaimed land. The UpS sanctuary is a living model for protecting diversity and ensuring that the rich traditions of the North American and Euro-American folk medicine continue to thrive.

But one doesn't need a large parcel to steward land and/or create sanctuary. UpS member Katherine Yvinskas has created a different and equally valuable model of a Botanical Sanctuary in her backyard in Morris County, New Jersey. On a small plot of land, Katherine has created an enchanted sanctuary for plants and people. Her garden landscape abounds with native plant species and in a wooded corner of her lot she has planted several of the at-risk

THE UNITED PLANT SAVERS BOTANICAL SANCTUARY: MANY FACETS, MANY FUNCTIONS

- Educational Center: Diverse learning programs are being offered to children, university students, herbal products industry members, and scientists.

- On-site Research Center: Research of native medicinal plants in the wild focuses on population studies, wild-harvesting sustainability studies, and seed germination studies. Research focusing on the cultivation of native medicinal plants (i.e., soil and shade requirements, disease challenges, etc.) is critical to ensure abundant renewable supplies.

- Repository of Native Medicinal Plant Germ Plasm: Healthy wild medicinal plant populations serve as repositories of germ plasm, or genes, which is essential for genetic diversity and ensuring the long-term survival of medicinal plant species.

- Propagation Facility: The planting material for propagation is being generated through the various research projects and would be used to supply farmers wanting to grow native medicinal plants commercially.

- Sustainable Land Use Model: The UpS Botanical Sanctuary is cultivated as a model of sustainable land use to others within the local community and beyond.

herbs. Goldenseal, American ginseng, blue and black cohosh, mayapple, and bloodroot are thriving where the former owners grew only grass. In her community, Katherine's botanical sanctuary offers a quiet respite for the weary, a reflective place to ponder, a joyous gathering spot to share with friends, and an educational center where others come to learn about the medicinal uses of native plants. Even on this small plot, Katherine is able to offer workshops and herb walks to raise her community's awareness of native plant conservation.

She's planned her sanctuary to be a welcoming spot for more than the "two legged" visitors. By simply installing a birdbath and a small pond, an increase in birds, butterflies, and bees was noted in the first season. "The sanctuary reflects my love affair with the Tao, the complementary forces of nature. There is an ebb and flow to the garden. To me, it's a living sculpture, always changing, beautiful to watch as it unfolds season by season. I feel blessed. The garden sanctuary is truly paradise . . . am I in heaven?" reflects Katherine.

Rosemary Gladstar, president and founder of United Plant Savers, created yet another model of sanctuary. Living in the midst of thousands of acres of wilderness in the Green Mountains of Vermont, Rosemary became acutely aware of the necessity of maintaining the integrity of wilderness and the importance of protecting large green belts for wildlife and plant preservation. When a 100-acre parcel of old-growth forest abutting Sage Mountain, Rosemary's 500-acre retreat center and botanical sanctuary, was slated for clear-cutting, Rosemary appealed to friends and family for help. Through a lengthy and complex transaction, the land was purchased and placed in a UpS land trust with strict conservation easements ensuring that it remains forever wild. This old-growth forest, home to black bear, moose, white tail deer, and beaver, as well as a rich variety of native plants, remains in its pristine state.

But the story didn't end there. In talking with surrounding landowners, Rosemary discovered that there was a great deal of interest in land preservation. Several other landowners in the area are now considering placing large tracts of land in forever wilderness conservation easements. A small community-supported nature center is in progress, and a mile-long self-guided medicine trail has been established. It has become a popular place for community members to hike, to learn about the native plants and wildlife, and to become more aware of habitat preservation and plant conservation.

The possibilities are infinite, but what it takes is people willing to make a difference. Whether you have a small backyard like Katherine, a working farm like Paul, or a tract of wilderness, imagine it as a sanctuary, a haven for plants, wildlife, and people. The idea of ownership of land was unheard of by the native people. How could one own land, own the heart of Mother Earth? We are stewards of the land, caretakers in the deepest sense of the word. By creating sanctuary, we begin to restore the idea that land belongs to all life, that it is life, and that our job is to restore it to its richest diversity.

GROWING AWARENESS
The Practical Side of a Botanical Sanctuary

Once you decide to establish your own botanical sanctuary, what practical steps can you take to help it grow and flourish? Focus on these four areas: identification, restoration, preservation, and education.

LEARN TO IDENTIFY PLANTS

Before this century, herbalists were also botanists. Begin by identifying as many plant species on the land as possible. Enlist the aid of a friend who knows some of the plants, and buy several identification guides. When we moved onto our 40-acre piece in the Soquel hills near Santa Cruz, California, I roamed the land observing every plant and tree. As I recognized the plants, one by one, I began a list, which eventually grew to more than 200 species. For the eastern United States, I recommend the *Peterson Field Guide to Medicinal Plants of the Eastern U.S.* by Steven Foster and James Duke. Terry Willard's identification guide to Rocky Mountain medicinal plants is very helpful, and Michael Moore's excellent books cover the western United States. Many flower identification books offer full-color photos specific to your area and are available at your local bookstore or local wildflower society. For the more technically minded, order a flora, or technical identification manual, for your bioregion or state.

LEARN WHERE PLANTS COME FROM AND WHERE THEY ARE GOING

Pay special attention to whether a plant is a native plant to your area, an ornamental from some exotic place, or a weedy species. Many weedy plants, though valuable and often lovely to look at, tend to take resources such as water and light that native plants require to live. In establishing a botanical sanctuary, you will want to limit the number of weedy species that thrive on your land, especially if they are obviously widespread. Herbalists love dandelion and milk thistle, valuable medicinal plants, but try to limit their growth to specific areas.

One of the first things I did on our land in the Santa Cruz Mountains was to establish a good weed patch. I collected weedy seeds and plants from all over the county and actually brought them to the land; first because I love their tenacity and survivability, and second, so I could observe them more closely and begin to understand how they fit into the whole botanical tangle on the land. I removed many other weedy plants around the land, especially in those areas that were most conducive to the native wild species.

Don't forget about the UpS consultant service. We can put you in touch with a consultant who can help you learn more about your ecosystem and how to go about establishing and managing a sanctuary.

PLANT NATIVES

Identify as many plants and trees that originally came from your ecosystem as possible. The more you learn about the ecosystem where you live, the better able you will be to help the land regenerate. In the process, you will be renewed and regenerated. Get to know your land intimately. Wander all over it and, with permission, the surrounding areas. Get your neighbors involved! Locate a local native plant nursery, wildflower society, or call one of the suppliers listed in the nursery directory in the back of this book.

Whenever possible use local sources. This preserves the purity, precedents, and intelligence of the original ecosystem where you live. You can order the same species from a supplier or nursery, but these may be genetic hybrids or carry the genes of some other species. We do a lot of seed collecting and propagation through cutting of local plants. I carry those little brown coin envelopes with me all the time, to store, identify, and organize weedy and native seeds. These are available from a craft store or stationery store.

Preserve and protect the land

Join the UpS Sanctuary network and be your own sanctuary manager. In today's world, the land needs a champion, a steward, and a manager to reduce interference, bring natives back to the land, and allow the intelligence of nature to work its magic. Signs are available through UpS that can be hung around the perimeter of your land to help people to honor and preserve the sanctuary.

Allow your sanctuary to become the educational center it naturally is

Teaching and learning about the land is a lifetime study. Within every community you'll find knowledgeable people who are often willing to share. Invite them to your land, and always be willing to share with others what you have learned about land management, wild plants, and the importance of biodiversity.

Create a medicine trail on your land as part of your educational effect

It can be a path through your front yard, or as on Rosemary's land, a self-guided mile-long trail. Make signs for the trail that give the Latin binomial, common name, origin, and uses of the plants.

Lead herb walks or encourage others to give classes on the land

You'll often find knowledgeable and willing people through the local forestry service, wildflower society, herb clubs, or senior center.

Create a nature center on your land

Teach others how to grow wild plants, ethical wildcrafting techniques, preservation, medicine making, and herbal therapeutics.

Help create and preserve serene places

Allow spaces among the plants and trees for communion with the green spirits and devas.

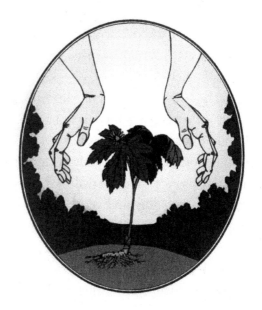

WISE OLD PLANTS

ROBYN KLEIN

We easily accept the fact that a tree might be hundreds of years old. But discovering that a wild herbaceous plant can grow for forty or even three hundred years is quite a surprise to most people. Take, for example, the case of green gentian. *Peterson's Field Guide to the Rocky Mountain Wildflowers* lists green gentian (*Frasera speciosa*) as a biennial. Biennials develop a rosette of leaves in their first year or two, and then produce a large flowering stalk with thousands of seeds the following year, after which the whole plant dies. Herbalists in the western United States consider *F. speciosa* a good digestive-bitters substitute for yellow gentian (*Gentiana lutea*), which is the European species commonly found on the herb market.[1]

What is new and disturbing information, however, is that green gentian is not a biennial at all, but a perennial that has been estimated by some biologists to remain in the rosette stage for up to sixty years.[2] That herbalists have been unwittingly harvesting these very old roots suddenly presents the possibility that other wild herbs are likewise much older than we have realized. Such discoveries could be crucial to determining sustainable harvesting methods.

OTHER GROWTH-PATTERN FACTORS

Yet it is not just the potential age of these wild herbs that is of importance. Plants are intricately attached to a web of life that can falter or shift for many reasons. Among those factors is the question of how many years a plant takes to become a reproductive individual.

Biologist Ellen O'Callaghan has studied the reproduction of the glacier lily in Colorado. *Erythronium grandiflorum* is a long-lived perennial found at various altitudes from British Columbia to California to Colorado. This species spends its first five to six years as a nonflowering juvenile with only one or two leaves. It then produces a flower (and seeds) at around year seven. Adult plants, which usually have two leaves of unequal size, have been known to revert back to the nonflowering stage for a year or more.[3] Thus, we don't know the full life span of the glacier lily, but we do know that mature individuals are at least seven to ten years old. This information is important because it suggests that other medicinal genera related to the glacier lily, such as *Trillium, Chamaelirium,*

Aletris, and *Lilium*, may have similar growth stages. So in estimating their ages, we must consider that they, too, may revert to a nonflowering stage when conditions require conservation of energy and resources.

Other characteristics of perennial plants are important in considering their ability to withstand continued harvest. Paulette Bierzychudek has studied the jack-in-the-pulpit *(Arisaema triphyllum)*, a long-lived perennial that changes sex during its life. This ability to change sex throws off all calculations when we're trying to decipher whether seeding individuals exist in a population![4]

Lady's slippers also have a complex life cycle that includes several stages of below-ground growth that are difficult to assess in the field. Anecdotal accounts from greenhouse experiments have shown that it takes fifteen years to grow an adult, reproductive plant from seeds. Though the life span of these herbs is difficult to ascertain, some biologists estimate that some grow for thirty-nine years.[5]

Not all herbaceous plants reproduce primarily from seeds. Many reproduce predominantly from underground root systems, which create new individual plants that are each exact genetic replicas of the parent. Individuals that sprout from clonal rhizomes and produce leaves are called *ramets*, while the root system itself is called the *gamet*. Rhizomes may connect all the individual plants in this clonal population, or sometimes the underground connection dies and rots, leaving an individual separate. Such underground clonal root systems can live for a very, very long time. Thus, most of the oldest plants known are clonal species.

For instance, the largest living organisms in the world are quaking aspens, which have been estimated to be more than one million years old![6] Many of the oldest species known are herbaceous plants. One chaparral organism living near the Colorado River has been carbon-dated at ninety-four hundred years old.[7]

Yet age determination for clonal plants can be very complicated. This is because this type of root system moves and intermingles so much that it is difficult to follow the genetic material. Thus, many biologists consider clonal species to be problematic in figuring age. As a result, they tend to ignore them as chosen specimens in life-span research.[8] Unfortunately, this means that there is a lack of life-history information for clonal plants, many of which have a history of medicinal use.

Cain and Damman studied the medicinal wild ginger *(Asarum canadense)*, which grows from clonal root systems. They discovered that the underground roots that connect the individual plants persist for up to ten years.[9]

HARVEST OF MATURE INDIVIDUALS

Still other population biology factors become very important once we understand their implications. Consider, for instance, that many wildcrafters collect the largest (and thus the most mature) individuals, because the heavier weight brings more income. It is usually assumed that the smaller, juvenile plants within a harvested population will continue to survive or that enough seeds will already be present in the soil to maintain a healthy population. However, myriad crucial environmental and biological factors can alter this utopian attitude.

Take, for example, the pink lady's slipper, *(Cypripedium acaule)*. Observational research indicates that individuals in the seed and seedling stages (ending at around the fourth year of growth) have a very high mortality.[10] That is, many juveniles do not survive to reproductive age at all. Harvesting older plants—which are therefore the most successful survivors, with the strongest genes—results in less of these individuals in the population. This practice may likely lead to a disproportionately large number of smaller plants. If these do manage to survive and produce seeds, they may produce more plants with less robust genes. The results of

harvesting older individuals from a population may not be evident for decades. Perhaps there is a very good reason for the herbalists' adage, Leave the grandmother plants.

THE UNITED PLANT SAVERS LISTS

Let us now consider the particular species found on the United Plant Savers At-Risk and To-Watch Lists. *At risk* is defined as "those herbs broadly used in commerce that are—due to factors such as loss of habitat and overharvest—diminishing in population and viability within their current ranges." Table 1 lists crucial facts about these species.

TABLE 1

VITAL STATISTICS OF AT-RISK SPECIES*

UPS AT-RISK SPECIES	LATIN NAME	PART USED	PERENNIAL?	CULTIVATED?	PLANT FAMILY
Black cohosh	*Cimicifuga racemosa*	Root	X	X	Buttercup (Ranunculaceae)
Bloodroot	*Sanguinaria canadensis*	Rhizome	X	X	Poppy (Papaveraceae)
Blue cohosh	*Caulophyllum thalictroides*	Root	X	X	Barberry (Berberidaceae)
Echinacea	*Echinacea* spp.	Root	X	X	Aster (Asteraceae)
Eyebright	*Euphrasia* spp.	Whole plant			Figwort (Scrophulariaceae)
American ginseng	*Panax quinquefolius*	Root	X	X	Ginseng (Araliaceae)
Goldenseal	*Hydrastis canadensis*	Rhizome	X	X	Buttercup (Ranunculaceae)
Helonias	*Chamaelirium luteum*	Root	X		Lily (Liliaceae)
Kava	*Piper methysticum*	Root	X	X	Pepper (Piperaceae)
Lady's slipper	*Cypripedium* spp.	Root	X		Orchid (Orchidaceae)
Lomatium	*Lomatium dissectum*	Root	X		Parsley (Apiaceae)
Night-blooming cereus	*Cactus grandiflorus*	Leaf/stem	X		Cactus (Cactaceae)
Osha	*Ligusticum* spp.	Root	X		Parsley (Apiaceae)
Partridgeberry	*Mitchella repens*	Leaf/stem	X		Madder (Rubiaceae)
Peyote	*Lophophora williamsii*	Whole plant	X		Cactus (Cactaceae)
Slippery elm	*Ulmus rubra*	Bark	X	X	Elm (Ulmaceae)

27

UPS AT-RISK SPECIES	LATIN NAME	PART USED	PERENNIAL?	CULTIVATED?	PLANT FAMILY
Sundew	*Drosera* spp.	Whole plant	X		Sundew (Droseraceae)
Trillium	*Trillium* spp.	Root	X		Lily (Liliaceae)
True unicorn	*Aletris farinosa*	Root	X		Lily (Liliaceae)
Venus's-flytrap	*Dionaea* spp.	Whole plant	X		Sundew (Droseraceae)
Virginia snakeroot	*Aristolochia serpentaria*	Root	X		Birthwort (Aristolochiaceae)
Wild yam	*Dioscorea* spp.	Root	X	X	Yam (Dioscoreaceae)

*This list is current as of August 2000.

From this table you can see that 82 percent of the species listed are treasured for their roots or rhizomes. Thus harvest destroys not only the individual, but also the seeds these plants would have produced for many years to come. Notably, most are perennials and not in mass cultivation—an option that would reduce the pressure on their wild populations. Species on this list are from an assortment of plant families with myriad evolutionary strategies and growth characteristics.

A second category of plant species has been compiled by United Plant Savers that may not fit into the at-risk category but are still worthy of closer scrutiny due to their popularity in some instances. Assessment of whether these species should be added to the At-Risk List would be greatly enhanced if we considered not only the part of the plant collected, but also the plants' age at reproductive maturity and their possible life span.

TABLE 2					
VITAL STATISTICS OF TO-WATCH SPECIES*					
UPS TO-WATCH SPECIES	LATIN NAME	PART USED	PERENNIAL?	CULTIVATED?	PLANT FAMILY
Arnica	*Arnica* spp.	Flower	X	X	Aster (Asteraceae)
Butterfly Weed	*Asclepias tuberosa*	Root	X	X	Milkweed (Asclepiadaceae)
Calamus	*Acorus calamus*	Root	X		Arum (Araceae)
Chaparro (Simaroubaceae)	*Castela emoryi*	Stem/leaf	X		Quassia
Elephant tree	*Bursera microphylla*	Resin	X		Bursera (Burseraceae)
Gentian	*Gentiana* spp.	Root	X		Gentian (Gentianaceae)
Goldthread	*Coptis* spp.	Root	X		Buttercup (Ranunculaceae)
Lobelia	*Lobelia* spp.	Root/leaf	some	X	Lobelia (Lobeliaceae)
Maidenhair fern	*Adiantum pedatum*	Stem/leaf	X		Fern (Polypodiaceae)
Mayapple	*Podophyllum peltatum*	Root	X		Barberry (Berberidaceae)
Oregon grape	*Mahonia* spp.	Root	X		Barberry (Berberidaceae)
Pinkroot	*Spigelia marilandica*	Root	X		Logania (Loganiaceae)
Pipsissewa	*Chimaphila umbellata*	Root/leaf	X		Wintergreen (Pyrolaceae)
Queen's delight	*Stillingia sylvatica*	Root	X		Spurge (Euphorbiaceae)
Spikenard	*Aralia* spp.	Root	X	X	Ginseng (Araliaceae)

UPS TO-WATCH SPECIES	LATIN NAME	PART USED	PERENNIAL?	CULTIVATED?	PLANT FAMILY
Stoneroot	*Collinsonia canadensis*	Root	X	X	Mint (Lamiaceae)
Stream orchid	*Epipactis gigantea*	Stem/leaf	X		Orchid (Orchidaceae)
Turkey corn	*Dicentra canadensis*	Stem/leaf	X		Fumitory (Fumariaceae)
White sage	*Salvia apiana*	Stem/leaf	X		Mint (Lamiaceae)
Wild indigo	*Baptisia* spp.	Root/leaf	X	X	Pea (Fabaceae)
Yerba mansa	*Anemopsis californica*	Root	X		Lizard's-tail (Saururaceae)
Yerba santa	*Eriodictyon californicum*	Stem/leaf	X		Waterleaf (Hydrophyllaceae)

*This list is current as of August 2000.

You can see from table 2 that roots are still the highly valued part of the herbs. Most of these species are perennial, and most are not in cultivation. Again, these species represent many diverse plant families. In fact, it is apparent from both the lists that medicinal plant species most in danger are those that are perennial, whose roots are collected, and for which cultivation is difficult or uncommon.

The important information missing from these lists is the estimated life spans of these species. But first, how do biologists estimate the life spans of plants?

GROWTH STAGES

Plants cannot be carbon-dated unless they are hundreds of years old. But aging an individual can be accomplished by simply observing its growth stages and how many years it stays in these stages. Much of this research involves complicated mathematical analysis that is impractical for laypeople. However, close estimates can be accomplished through simpler means.

For example, you might select plots that can be revisited for at least five years. Individual plants in these plots can be measured and tagged. From this a number of growth stages can be ascertained by noting the unique characteristics and sizes of the individuals. For example, a juvenile with one leaf would be in a younger growth stage than a juvenile with two leaves, and so on. Once the stages are ascertained, then it is a matter of recording how many years an individual stays in that growth stage. Finally, you can add up the number of years spent in each growth stage to estimate the minimum age of a mature individual. The difficulty, of course, is in estimating the age of mature individuals. But this is still possible with continued observation over a period of many years or decades.

Biologists Margaret E. Cochran and Stephen Ellner have calculated many plant ages using the growth-stage technique.[11] For example, they compared the growth stages of two plants—a perennial weedy species called teasel (*Dipsacus sylvestris*) and the wild and delicate pink lady's slipper (*Cypripedium acaule*), both of which reproduce by seeds. Table 3 compares their growth stages.

TABLE 3		
GROWTH STAGES OF TEASEL AND PINK LADY'S SLIPPER*		
STAGE	*DIPSACUS*	*CYPRIPEDIUM*
1	Dead or dormant seeds	Year 1, seeds
2	Dead or dormant seeds	Year 2, corms (year 1)
3	Small rosettes	Corms (year 2)
4	Medium rosettes	Corms (year 3)
5	Large rosettes	Dormant
6	Flowering plants	1 leaf
7		2 leaves, no flower
8		Flowering plants

*Excerpted from Cochran and Ellner 1992.

Dipsacus must grow for six years and *Cypripedium* for eight years before developing the first flowers and seeds. This is much longer than it takes to get a college education!

Herbalists and wildcrafters need not be mathematical geniuses to estimate the growth stages and ages of hundreds of long-lived perennial plants. It takes only the dedication of at least five years to record sizes of various individual plants in more than several plots to get some fair estimates.

Though how long a plant species stays in a growth class is not always known, we can sometimes find information on the number of growth stages known for a species. Table 4 offers growth-stage information that could be used to estimate life spans of some wild medicinal herbs.

TABLE 4

SPECIES	COMMON NAME	FAMILY	GROWTH STAGES
Cypripedium acaule	Pink lady's slipper	Orchidaceae	8*
Arisaema triphyllum	Jack-in-the-pulpit	Araceae	7*
Dipsacaceae sylvestris	Teasel	Dipsacaceae	6*
Gentiana pneumonanthe	Gentian	Gentianaceae	6†
Pedicularis furbishiae	Lousewort	Scrophulariaceae	4*

*Cochran and Ellner 1992.
†Oostermiejer et al. 1996.

COUNTING RINGS AND LEAF SCARS

Other simple ways to determine the ages of long-lived perennials include counting leaf scars. Estimating the age of a ginseng (*Panax* spp.) root is a tradition going back thousands of years. This technique should also work well for members of the Lily family, such as trillium and helonias.

Annual rings can be counted in a cross section of a root. Dietz and Ullmann published a list of wild plants for which ring counting is or is not a viable technique.[12] For example, the growth rings found in comfrey roots (*Symphytum officinale*) and horseradish are clear and easy to read. However, the growth rings in the roots of mugwort (*Artemisia vulgaris*), chicory (*Cichorium intybus*), and snakeroot (*Eryngium campestre*) are only weakly readable. Thus, this technique is applicable to some plant families but not others.

In reviewing the population biology literature, one very important plant family is absent—the Parsley family (Apiaceae or Umbelliferae). The ages of important wild medicinal plants, such as osha (*Ligusticum* spp.) and biscuit root (*Lomatium dissectum*), are not known. But while the rings of the roots in these species are all but nonexistent, the leaf scars are quite evident.

One species of osha, *Ligusticum filicinum*, common in parts of the Rocky Mountains provides a clue. The root of one small specimen, measuring 1/2 inch in diameter, 8 inches long, and weighing approximately 0.4 ounce, evidenced more than eighteen leaf scars. Even considering that one year's growth might be represented by up to three leaf scars, this example still suggests that larger specimens are at least ten years old, and probably much, much older. It is folly to assume that continued digging of wild osha and *Lomatium* root is a practice without finite limits.

LIFE SPANS OF SOME PERENNIAL PLANTS

The known estimated life spans of more than fifty species could be very useful in determining the ages of our wild medicinal herbs. Table 5 provides a compilation of the estimated life spans found in the literature.

TABLE 5

ESTIMATED LIFE SPAN OF SELECTED PLANTS

SPECIES	FAMILY	COMMON NAME	ESTIMATED LIFE SPAN (IN YEARS)	CITATION
Larrea tridentata	Zygophyllaceae	Chaparral	9,400–9,411; 700*	Mabry 1979; Vasek 1980
Ginkgo biloba	Ginkgoaceae	Ginkgo	3,000+	Del Tredici 1991
Convallaria majalis	Liliaceae	Lily-of-the-valley	670+*	Oinonen 1969
Silene acaulis	Caryophyllaceae	Silene	100–300	Benedict 1989; Morris 1998
Carnegiea gigantea	Cactaceae	Saguaro cactus	175–300	Pierson and Turner 1998
Narcissus pseudonarcissus	Amaryllidaceae	Wild daffodil	120–180	Barkham 1980
Ceanothus greggii	Rhamnaceae	Redroot, snowbrush	85–155	Zammit and Zedler 1992
Teucrium scorodonia	Lamiaceae	Germander	50–100	Hutchinson 1968
Frasera speciosa	Gentianaceae	Green gentian	60–80	Inouye 1997
Chamaelirium luteum	Liliaceae	Helonias	30–80	Meagher 1982
Trillium ovatum	Liliaceae	Trillium, bethroot	72	Jules 1995
Panax quinquefolius	Araliaceae	Ginseng	50–60	Anderson 1993; Charron 1991
Yucca filamentosa	Agavaceae	Yucca	30–50	Massey and Hamrick 1998
Clintonia borealis	Liliaceae	Bead lily	20–50	Pitelka et al. 1985
Helianthella quinquenervis	Asteraceae	Aspen sunflower	40	Inouye 1984
Balsamorhiza sagittata	Asteraceae	Balsamroot	40	Treshow and Harper 1974
Cypripedium acaule	Orchidaceae	Lady's slipper	39+	Cochran and Ellner 1992

SPECIES	FAMILY	COMMON NAME	ESTIMATED LIFE SPAN (IN YEARS)	CITATION
Polygonatum multiflorum	Liliaceae	Solomon's seal	35	Ernst 1979
Aralia nudicaulis	Araliaceae	Spikenard	30	Thomson, pers. comm., 1/98
Anemone hepatica	Ranunculaceae	Windflower	6–30	Persson 1975
Wyethia amplexicaulis	Asteraceae	Wyethia	28	Treshow and Harper 1974
Veratrum tenuipetalum	Liliaceae	False hellebore	25+	Inouye 1997
Arisaema triphyllum	Araceae	Jack-in-the-pulpit	15–25	Bierzychudek 1982a
Corydalis aquae-geldii	Fumariaceae	Corydalis	17–25+	Goldenberg 1997
Hedysarum boreale	Fabaceae	Sweet vetch	20	Treshow and Harper 1974
Liatris cylindracea	Asteraceae	Gayfeather	19	Schaal and Levin 1976
Mitchella repens	Rubiaceae	Partridgeberry	15	Bierzychudek 1982b
Centaurea maculosa	Asteraceae	Spotted knapweed	11–12+	Good, pers. comm., 2/16/98
Arnica cordifolia	Asteraceae	Arnica	12	Treshow and Harper 1974
Primula vulgaris	Primulaceae	Primrose	10–30	Valverde and Silvertown 1998
Viola sororia	Violaceae	Violet	10–14	Cook 1979; Solbrig 1980
Asarum canadense	Aristolochiaceae	Wild ginger	10*	Cain and Damman 1997
Allium ursinum	Amaryllidaceae	Onion	8–10	Ernst 1979
Dipsacus sylvestris	Dipsacaceae	Teasel	5+	Werner and Caswell 1977

*The age of the rhizomes (genets) that connect the ramets in this clonal species.

These estimated ages suddenly make us recognize that many of the medicinal plants being harvested from the wild are most likely very old. How many individuals should we harvest from a population? How soon could that population return to its current size? Thoughtful consideration of the life spans of our medicinal herbs should change our appreciation of them. It should also change the way we harvest them.

We can use this information to make valuable decisions. For instance, from this list we might deduce that many perennials in the Lily family tend to be long lived; populations of any lily species should thus be carefully managed. The presence of helonias (*Chamaelirium luteum*), trillium (*Trillium* spp.), and true unicorn (*Aletris farinosa*) on the UpS At-Risk List therefore should not be surprising. Collection of the underground parts of these species may, in fact, irreparably damage a population that cannot rebound when future seeds are removed. Remember that a plant in the Lily family does not form a flower for some seven to ten years. And we cannot assume that reseeding will occur. Research shows that the disappearance of genetic material and the lack of food (nectar) available to pollinators can both have a great impact on a plant population's ability to survive. If the flowering individuals in a population become too sparse, the pollinators may not be able to find enough plants to cross-pollinate any of them.[13]

Herbalists and wildcrafters have not traditionally considered issues of reproductive cost, stage-structured models, and life demographics. This is the territory of academia, with unfamiliar technological terms and rather daunting mathematical equations. But we must bravely delve into these issues if we are to discover facts crucial to the continuance of our wild medicinal herbs.

ESTIMATING AGES FOR HERBS

Between 1995 and 1998 some seven to ten thousand pounds *per week* of dried *Echinacea angustifolia* was shipped out of eastern Montana to feed a growing U.S. and international demand.[14] Very little is understood about how such massive harvesting affects these wild populations.

Another wild medicinal plant used in herbal medicine, though not as commonly, is *Balsamorhiza sagittata*, or arrow-leaved balsamroot. It, too, exists only in locally abundant populations. Very little is known about the growth stages and life spans of either species. There are no recorded estimated ages for *Echinacea* or *Balsamorhiza*.

But perhaps we can make use of the published estimated ages for related plants. Both species are from the Aster (Compositae or Asteraceae) family. Various species in the Aster family have been aged at eleven, nineteen, and forty years (*Centaurea maculosa, Liatris cylindracea*, and *Helianthella quinquenervis*, respectively). Therefore, could we not estimate that the oldest *Echinacea* individuals are in excess of twenty years of age? In comparison, the very stout and much larger taproot of a mature *B. sagittata* must surely be between forty and eighty years old.

Lomatium dissectum is another wild herb that has a questionable ability to meet the demands of the world's herbal market. Estimating its age is a little more problematic, since age estimations for species in the Parsley (Apiaceae) family are lacking in the literature. However, the Parsley family is very closely related to the Ginseng (Araliaceae) family.[15] Therefore, the fact that *Aralia* spp. can grow to be thirty years of age and *Panax* spp. can grow to fifty or sixty should offer us some guidance. It would be conservative to suggest that mature *L. dissectum* individuals in stable populations are most likely between twenty and forty years old—especially considering that dried sliced roots found on the market are often 3 inches in diameter.

CONCLUSION

It should now be clear that any herb whose roots are highly prized on the herbal market is potentially at risk if it is a long-lived perennial harvested primarily from the wild. Efforts to encourage sustainable harvesting practices and to protect these valuable resources must continue. If we do nothing, we can expect that many other wild medicinal herbs will fall into a decline similar to that of the rare sixty-year-old ginseng root—something only our grandparents now remember.

ACKNOWLEDGMENTS

I benefited greatly from the many biologists who helped me locate information—especially Joan Maloof and David W. Inouye, who unwittingly started this quest. And of course *Frasera speciosa*, whose patience and determination have not gone unnoticed.

NOTES

1. Moore, *Medicinal Plants of the Pacific West.*

2. Inouye, "Variation in generation time in *Frasera speciosa.*"

3. O'Callaghan, "Reproductive costs in *Erythronium grandiflorum.*"

4. Bierzychudek, "The demography of jack-in-the-pulpit."

5. Cochran and Ellner, "Age-based life history parameters for stage-structured populations."

6. Mitton and Grant, "Genetic variation and the natural history of quaking aspen."

7. Mabry, "Creosote bush"; Vasek, "Creosote bush: long-lived clones."

8. Bierzychudek, "Shade-tolerant temperate forest herbs."

9. Cain and Damman, "Clonal growth and ramet performance in the woodland herb."

10. Cochran and Ellner, "Age-based life history parameters for stage-structured populations"; Cook, "Patterns of juvenile mortality and recruitment in plants."

11. Cochran and Ellner, "Age-based life history parameters for stage-structured populations."

12. Dietz and Ullmann, "Age-determination of dicotyledonous herbaceous perennials."

13. Kearns and Inouye, "Pollinators, flowering plants, and conservation biology."

14. Kolster, "The Echinacea craze."

15. Plunkett, Soltis, and Soltis, "Relationship between Apiaceae and Araliaceae."

REFERENCES

Anderson, R. C., J. S. Fralish, J. E. Armstrong, and P. K. Benjamin. "The ecology and biology of *Panax quinquefolium* L. (Araliaceae) in Illinois." *American Midland Naturalist* 129 (1993): 357–72.

Barkham, J. P. "Population dynamics of the wild daffodil *(Narcissus pseudonarcissus)*." *Journal of Ecology* 68 (1980): 607–33.

Benedict, James B. "Use of *Silene acaulis* for dating: The relationship of cushion diameter to age." *Arctic and Alpine Research* 21 (1): 91–96 (1989).

Bierzychudek, P. "The demography of jack-in-the-pulpit, a forest perennial that changes sex." *Ecological Monographs* 52 (4): 335–51 (1982a).

———. "Life histories and demography of shade-tolerant temperate forest herbs: A review." *New Phytologist* 90 (1982b): 757–76.

Cain, Michael L., and Hans Damman. "Clonal growth and ramet performance in the woodland herb, *Asarum canadense*." *Journal of Ecology* 85 (1997): 883–97.

Charron, D., and D. Gagnon. "The demography of northern populations of *Panax quinquefolium* (American ginseng)." *Journal of Ecology* 79 (1991): 431–45.

Cochran, M. E., and S. Ellner. "Simple methods for calculating age-based life history parameters for stage-structured populations." *Ecological Monographs* 62 (3): 345–64 (1992).

Cook, R. E. "Patterns of juvenile mortality and recruitment in plants." In *Topics in Plant Population Biology*, edited by O. T. Solbrig, S. Jain, G. B. Johnson, and P. H. Raven, 207–31. New York: Columbia University Press, 1979.

Dietz, H., and I. Ullmann. "Age-determination of dicotyledonous herbaceous perennials by means of annual rings: exception or rule?" *Annals of Botany* 80 (1997): 377–79.

Del Tredici, P. "Ginkgos and people—a thousand years of interaction." *Arnoldia* (summer 1991): 2–15.

Ernst, W. H. O. "Population biology of *Allium ursinum* in northern Germany." *Journal of Ecology* 67 (1979): 347–62.

Goldenberg, D. M., and D. B. Zobel. "Allocation, growth and estimated population structure of *Corydalis aquae-gelidae*, a rare riparian plant." *Northwest Science* 71 (3): 196–204 (1997).

Good, W. Personal communication with author, Western Agricultural Research Station, Corvallis, Mont., 16 Feb. 1998.

Hutchinson, T. C. "Biological flora of the British Isles: *Teucrium scorodonia*." *Journal of Ecology* 56 (1968): 901–11.

Inouye, David W. "Variation in generation time in *Frasera speciosa* (Gentianaceae), a long-lived perennial monocarp." *Oecologia* 47 1980: 171–74.

———. "The ant and the sunflower." *Natural History*, June 1984, 49–52.

———. "An unusual flowering display." *Crested Butte, [Mont.] Chronicle and Pilot*, 11 July 1997.

Jules, Erik J. "Consequences of forest fragmentation for the understory plant, *Trillium ovatum* (Liliaceae)." In *Proceedings of the Conservation and Management of Native Plants and Fungi*, n.p.: Native Plant Society of Oregon, 1995.

Kearns, Carol Ann, and D. M. Inouye. "Pollinators, flowering plants, and conservation biology." *Bioscience* 47 (1997): 297–306.

Kolster, Monique K. "The Echinacea craze: a case study." Master's thesis, University of Montana, 1998.

Mabry, T. J., J. H. Hunziker, and D. R. DiFeo. *Creosote Bush: Biology and Chemistry of Larrea in New World Deserts*. Strousburg, Penn.: Dowden, Hutchinsen, and Ross, 1979.

Massey, Lisa K., and J. L. Hamrick. "Genetic diversity and population structure of *Yucca filamentosa* (Agavaceae)." *American Journal of Botany* 85 (3): 340–45 (1998).

Meagher, T. R. "The population biology of *Chamaelirium luteum*, a dioecious member of the Lily family: two-sex population projections and stable population structure." *Ecology* 63 (6): 1701–11 (1982).

Mitton, Jeffry B., and Michael C. Grant. "Genetic variation and the natural history of quaking aspen." *Bioscience* 46 (1996): 25–31.

Moore, Michael. *Medicinal Plants of the Pacific West.* Santa Fe: Red Crane Books, 1993.

Morris, William F., and Daniel F. Doak. "Life history of the long-lived gynodioecious cushion plant *Silene acaulis* (Caryophyllaceae), inferred from size-based population projection matrices." *American Journal of Botany* 85 (6): 784–93 (1998).

O'Callaghan, E. "Reproductive costs in *Erythronium grandiflorum* (Lileaceae)." Master's thesis, University of Maryland, 1998.

Oinonen, E. 1969. "The time table of vegetative spreading in the lily-of-the-valley (*Convallaria majalis* L.) and the wood small-reed (*Calamagrostis epigeios* [L.] Roth.) in southern Finland." *Acta For. Fenn.* 97 (1969): 1–35.

Oostermeijer, J. G., M. L. Brugman, E. R. De Boer, and H. C. N. Den Nijs. "Temporal and spatial variation in the demography of *Gentiana peneumonanthe*, a rare perennial herb." *Journal of Ecology* 84 (1996): 153–66.

Persson, H. "Deciduous woodland at Andersby, Eastern Sweden: field-layer and below-ground production." *Acta Phytogeographica Suecica* 62 (1975): 1–71.

Pierson, Elizabeth A., and Raymond M. Turner. "An 85-year study of saguaro (*Carnegiea gigantea*) demography." *Ecology* 79 (8): 2676–93 (1998).

Pitelka, L. F., S. B. Hansen, and J. W. Ashmun. "Population biology of *Clintonia borealis*." *Journal of Ecology* 73 (1985): 169–83.

Plunkett, G. M., D. E. Soltis, and P. S. Soltis. "Clarification of the relationship between Apiaceae and Araliaceae based on MATK and RBCL sequence data." *American Journal of Botany* 84 (4): 565–80 (1997).

Schaal, B. A., and D. A. Levin. "The demographic genetics of *Liatris cylindracea* Michx. (Compositae)." *The American Naturalist* 110 (1976): 191–206.

Solbrig, O. T., S. J. Newell, and D. T. Kincaid. "The population biology of the genus *Viola*. I. The demography of *Viola sororia*." *Journal of Ecology* 68 (1980): 521–46.

Thomson, James D. Personal communication with author, 22 Jan. 1998.

Treshow, M., and K. Harper. "Longevity of perennial forbs and grasses." *Oikos* 25 (1974): 93–96.

Valverde, Teresa, and Jonathan Silvertown. "Variation in the demography of a woodland understorey herb (*Primula vulgaris*) along the forest regeneration cycle: Projection matrix analysis." *Journal of Ecology* 86 (1998): 545–62.

Vasek, Frank C. "Creosote bush: Long-lived clones in the Mojave Desert." *American Journal of Botany* 67 (2): 246–55 (1980).

Werner, P. A. and H. Caswell. "Population growth rates and age *versus* stage-distribution models for teasel (*Dipsacus sylvestris* Huds.)." *Ecology* 58 (1977): 1103–11.

Zammit, C. A., and P. H. Zedler. "Size structure and seed production in even-aged populations of *Ceanothus greggii* in mixed chaparral." *Journal of Ecology* 81 (1992): 499–511.

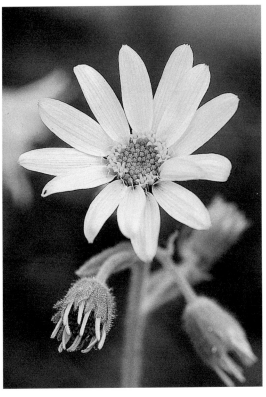

Arnica (*Arnica acaulis*)

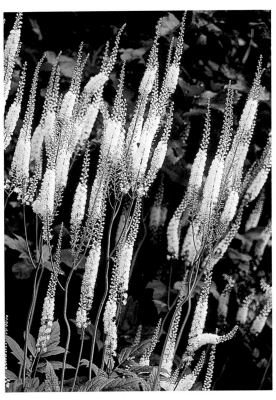

Black Cohosh (*Cimicifuga racemosa*)

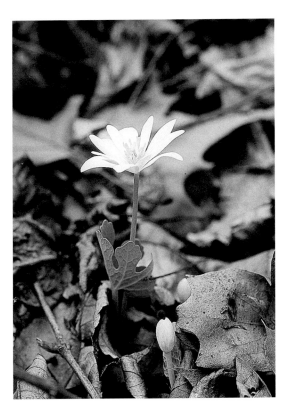

Bloodroot (*Sanguinaria canadensis*)

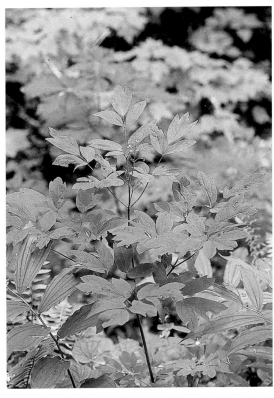

Blue Cohosh (*Caulophyllum thalictroides*)

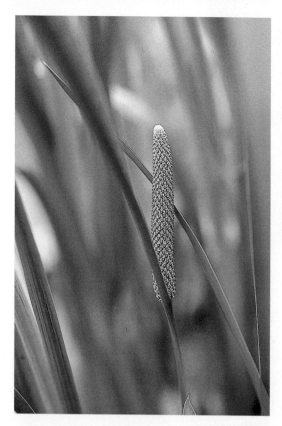

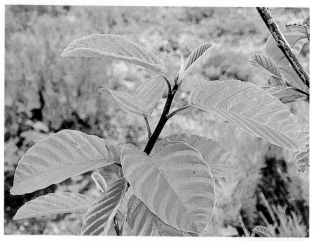

Cascara Sagrada *(Rhamnus purshiana)*

Calamus Root *(Acorus calamus)*

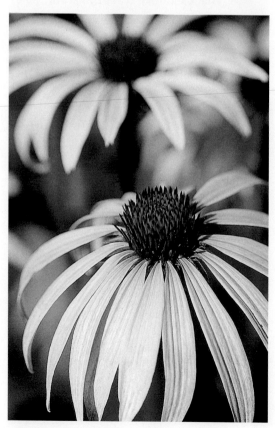

Echinacea (*Echinacea* spp.)

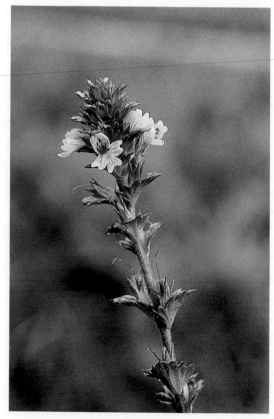

Eyebright (*Euphrasia nemorosa*)

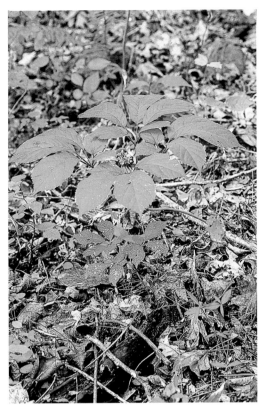

American Ginseng *(Panax quinquefolius)*

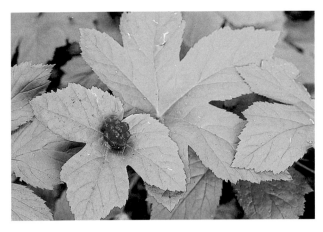

Goldenseal *(Hydrastis canadensis)*

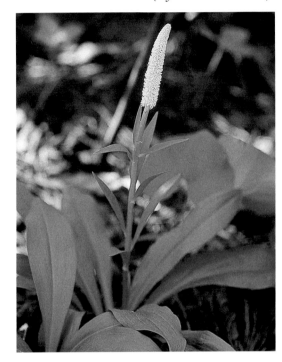

Helonias Root *(Chamaelirium luteum)*

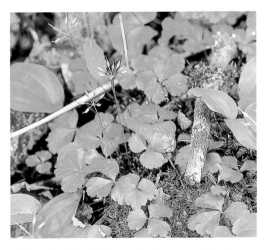

Threeleaf Goldthread *(Coptis trifolia)*

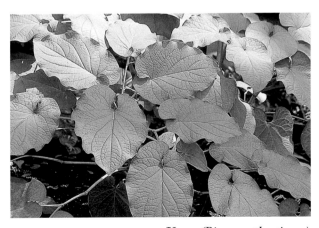

Kava *(Piper methysticum)*

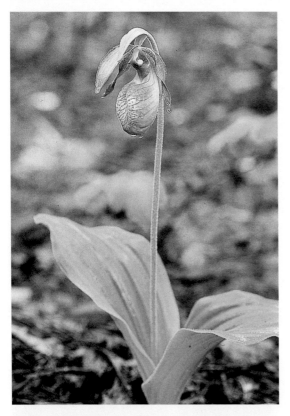

Pink Lady's Slipper *(Cypripedium acaule)*

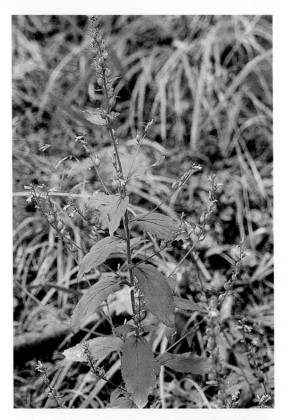

Lobelia *(Lobelia inflata)*

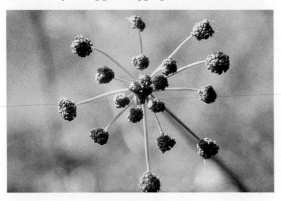

Lomatium *(Lomatium dissectum)*

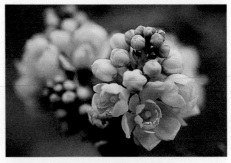

Oregon Grape *(Mahonia aquifolium)*

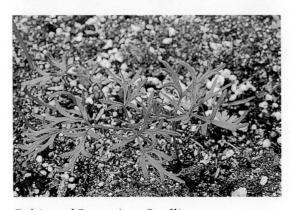

Cultivated Lomatium Seedling

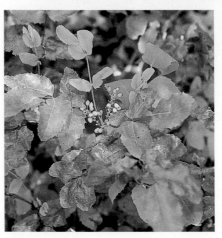

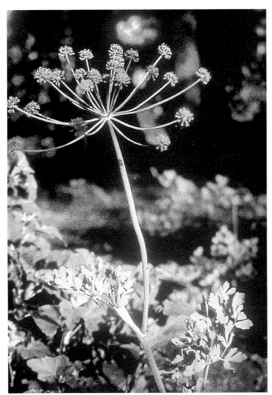

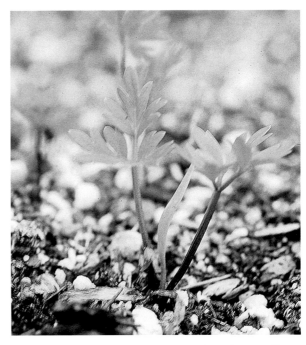

Cultivated Osha Seedling

Osha *(Ligusticum porteri)*

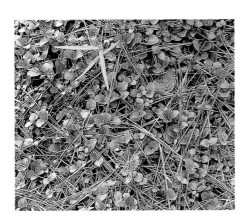

Partridgeberry *(Mitchella repens)*

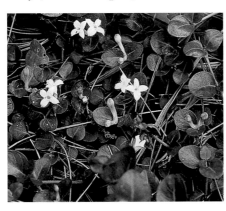

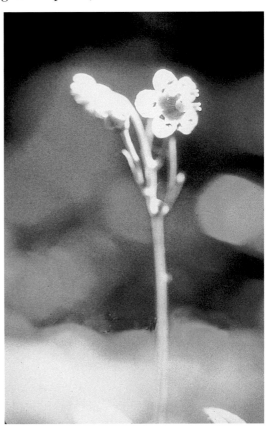

Pipsissewa (*Chimaphila* spp.)

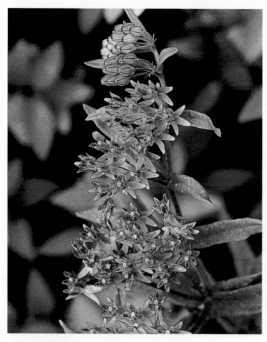

Pleurisy Root *(Asclepias tuberosa)*

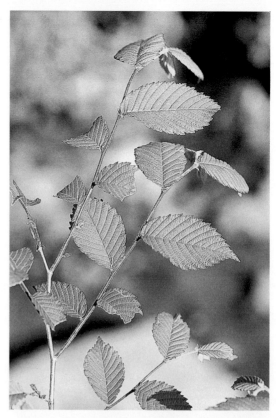

Slippery Elm *(Ulmus rubra)*

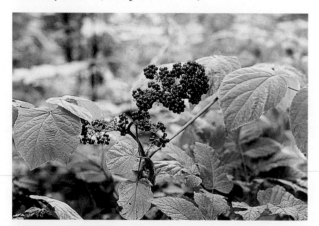

Spikenard *(Aralia racemosa)*

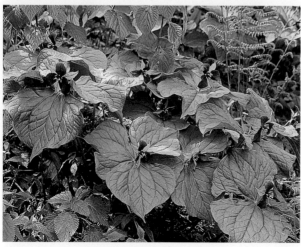

Trillium *(Trillium erectum)*

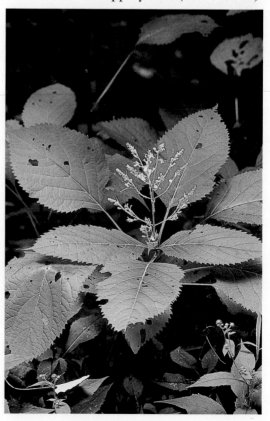

Stoneroot *(Collinsonia canadensis)*

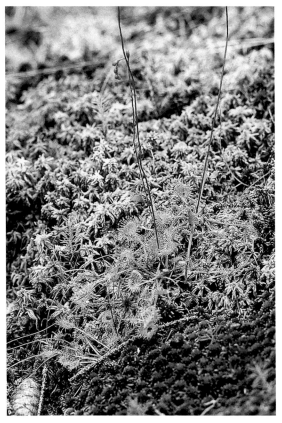

Roundleaf Sundew *(Drosera rotunifolia)*

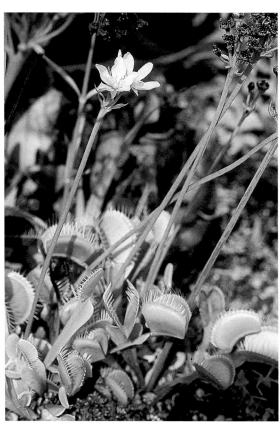

Venus's-Flytrap *(Dionaea muscipula)*

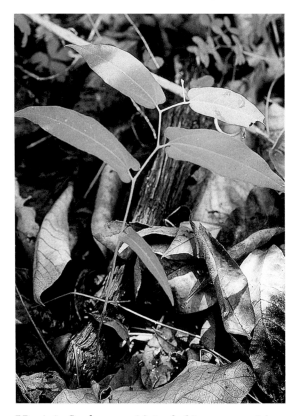

Virginia Snakeroot *(Aristolochia serpentaria)*

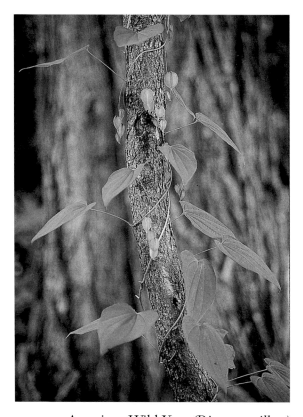

American Wild Yam *(Dioscorea villosa)*

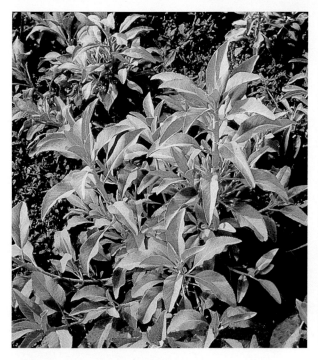

White Sage *(Salvia apiana)*

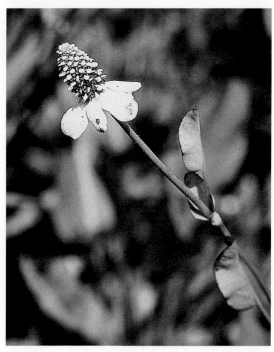

Yerba Mansa *(Anemopsis californica)*

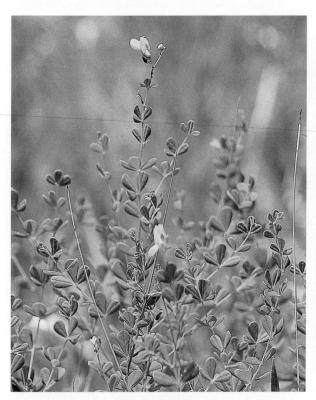

Wild Indigo *(Baptisia tinctoria)*

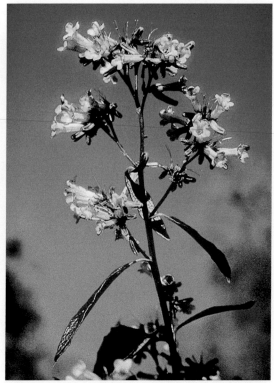

Yerba Santa *(Eriodictyon californicum)*

THE AMERICAN EXTRA PHARMACOPOEIA

DAVID WINSTON

In China the traditional pharmacopoeia of plant, mineral, and animal drugs is vast, containing over a thousand remedies; the same is true of India's Ayurvedic system of medicine. Other ancient and equally successful indigenous systems, such as the Ani Yvwiya (Cherokee) Nvwoti, Japan's Kampo, the Tibetan So-wa Rig-pa, and the Unani Tibb system, also use a large number of botanical drugs. Conversely, in the United States and Great Britain there is a trend toward relying on an ever dwindling materia medica. Possible reasons for this situation are many:

- The number of herbs available in the commercial marketplace dwindled as botanicals were dropped from official pharmacopoeias. In recent years the popularity of certain herbs has grown, but most herbal medicines are still obscure. The lack of sales means suppliers have little incentive to stock marginal herbs.

- The United States has no strong traditional culture and no ancient, time-tested system of medicine with accompanying herbal remedies. Two herbal systems that were practiced here, the Eclectic System of Medicine (1825–1939) and physiomedicalism (1850–1910), were almost entirely forgotten until recently.

- The scientific paradigm still reigns supreme! There is a strong tendency to rely on those few herbs that have been tested in the lab or petri dish. Purported active constituents indicate usefulness, rather than hundreds or thousands of years of successful empirical usage. Many Western practitioners are uncomfortable using herbs if research data do not confirm their traditional properties.

- Herb users (laypeople and professionals alike) often find it much easier to administer simply an astringent or a diuretic—assuming that herbs with the same generalized properties will have the same action. In truth, there are subtle differences among such herbs that often make one much more appropriate for a particular patient and symptom picture.

Our reliance on so small a pharmacopoeia can and has caused certain problems to develop. Many once-common herb species are now threatened or endangered, or are becoming increasingly scarce and costly. These include ginseng *(Panax quinquefolium)*, lady's slipper *(Cypripedium* spp.), slippery elm *(Ulmus fulva)*, goldenseal *(Hydrastis canadensis)*, gentian *(Gentiana* spp.), false unicorn root *(Chamaelirium luteum)*, and bethroot *(Trillium erectum)*. With the demand for these popular botanicals increasing and the supply shrinking, the chances of adulteration and/or spurious substitution increase.

TABLE 6	
COMMONLY ADULTERATED HERBS	
HERB	ADULTERANT
Black cohosh *(Cimicifuga racemosa)*	Baneberry *(Actaea* spp.)
Black haw *(Viburnum prunifolium)*	Striped maple *(Acer pensylvanicum)*
Echinacea *(E. angustifolia)*	Prairie dock *(Parthenium integrifolium)*
Goldenseal *(Hydrastis canadensis)*	Oregon grape root *(Mahonia aquifolium)*
Prickly ash *(Zanthoxylum clava-herculis)*	Bristly sarsaparilla *(Aralia spinosa)*
Sheep sorrel *(Rumex acetosella)*	Yellow dock leaf *(Rumex crispus)*
Siberian ginseng *(Eleutherococcus senticosus)*	*Periploca* or *Acanthopanax* spp.
Skullcap *(Scutellaria lateriflora)*	Germander *(Teucrium canadense)*
Slippery elm *(Ulmus fulva)*	Rice flour

As our materia medica shrinks, so do our options for treatment. The tendency of self-limitation creates practitioners who rely on the ten or twenty "most valuable herbs." The assumption is that this small number of botanicals is sufficient to cope with any disease or complaint.

This is all the more ironic when you realize that in the past, the average Cherokee layperson knew and used one to two hundred medicinal herbs, while a medicine person would be knowledgeable in more than eight hundred. How many of us can honestly say we are intimately familiar (taste, energy, usage, taxonomy, chemical constituents, and so on) with even one hundred herbs?

One way to correct this problem is to expand our locally available pharmacopoeias by the inclusion of unused but effective indigenous and introduced species. There are hundreds of such herbs available that have long histories of usage by peoples who depended on them for health and well-being. With a few exceptions, the plants on this list are little known and rarely used in this country; still, they are or once were commonly used throughout the world. Most species discussed are classified as adventurous, hardy weeds that are common throughout much of the United States and are abundant and easily procured while fresh and still potent. Many are considered noxious weeds. Millions of dollars are spent and thousands of pounds of toxic chemicals are applied yearly by farmers and lawn care providers in order to eradicate these helpful plants. The use of such herbs curbs their relentless spread, reduces the need to use polluting herbicides, and helps maintain sensitive ecosystems threatened by these aggressive foreign weeds. Creating and educating the public and practitioners about the American Extra Pharmacopoeia (AEP) will broaden our knowledge, enhance our clinical practices, and help create a system of planetary herbal medicine that is effective and ecologically sound.

THE AMERICAN EXTRA PHARMACOPOEIA

GROUND IVY

Latin name: *Glechoma hederacea*

Chinese name: Lian Qian Cao (*Glechoma longituba*)

Common names: Gill-over-the-ground, alehoof

Part used: Fresh or dried herb

Taste: Bitter

Energy: Cold and dry

Constituents: L-pinocamphone, L-menthone, L-pulegone, ∂ & ß pinene, limonene, ursolic acid

Action: Antiviral, cholagogue, expectorant

Dosage: *Tea*—Add 1 teaspoon of dried herb to 8 ounces of hot water. Steep, covered, for half an hour. Drink one 4-ounce cup three times per day. *Tincture*—1:2 fresh extract, 20–40 drops (1–2 ml), three times per day.

An aggressive garden and lawn weed, ground ivy has a long history of use throughout Europe and China. The Chinese use a closely related species (*Glechoma longituba*) to clear toxic heat for conditions such as jaundice and cystitis, and to help expel urinary and biliary stones. Recent research shows that the herb stimulates an increase in bile secretion and movement of the gallbladder sphincter. Ground ivy is also used topically to dispel blood stasis and for traumatic swellings such as sprains, bruises, and infections. European use parallels traditional Chinese medicine (TCM) usage as a liver/gallbladder and digestive herb, with additional activity based on the herb's antiviral and expectorant properties. It is effective for bronchitis, pneumonia, hot damp coughs, and chest colds.

JAPANESE KNOTWEED

Latin name: *Polygonum cuspidatum*

Chinese name: Hu Zhang

Part used: Dried root and leaf

Taste: Bitter

Energy: Cold and dry

Constituents: Anthraquinones and anthraglycosides, primarily emodin, rhein, chrysophenol, resveratrol, and tannins

Action: Astringent, antitumor, antibacterial, laxative, emmenagogue, expectorant

Dosage: *Tea*—Add 1 teaspoon of the dried root to 8 ounces of water. Decoct for ten minutes, or longer if you want to decrease the laxative effect. Steep for half an hour. Drink one 4-ounce cup of tea twice per day. *Tincture*—1:5, 40 percent alcohol, 20–30 drops (1–2 ml), twice per day.

The roots and leaves of this highly invasive weed are used in TCM to eliminate damp heat—dysentery, jaundice, appendicitis, hepatitis, and enteritis. It also promotes circulation of blood (*xue*), relieves pain, and is used orally and topically for snakebite, rheumatoid arthritis, burns, trauma injuries, abscesses, and boils. It has antibacterial and expectorant qualities, making it useful for bronchitis, pleurisy, and other damp-heat lung infections. Two constituents in Hu Zhang, rhein and emodin, have shown strong antitumor activity both in vitro and in vivo. A third ingredient, resveratrol, is a powerful antioxidant. This combination makes this herb a potential choice for cancer protocols. Excess amounts of the root can cause diarrhea and/or rebound constipation.

KUDZU

Latin name: *Pueraria lobata*

Chinese name: Gegen

Part used: Dried root, root starch, and flower

Taste: Sweet, pungent

Energy: Cold and moist

Constituents: Isoflavones, including puerarin, diadzein, and diadzin

Actions: Antihistamine, anti-inflammatory, antispasmodic, and demulcent

Dosage: *Tea*—Add 2 teaspoons of the dried root to 8 ounces of water. Decoct for thirty minutes. Steep for thirty minutes. Drink one 4-ounce cup three times per day. *Tincture*—1:5, 30 percent alcohol, 40–60 drops, three times per day (not appropriate for reducing alcohol cravings). *Capsule*—Two capsules twice per day.

Kudzu was introduced into the United States in the 1880s as an important and versatile economic plant. Later, in the 1930s, it was promoted as a way to control erosion. As a means of controlling and preventing erosion, the plant is indeed an incredible success. It is also successful in destroying native herbs, shrubs, and trees, and creating environmental havoc throughout the southeastern U.S.

The way to control this highly aggressive plant is to use it, a lot of it. Multiple parts of the plant can be used for medicine, food, animal fodder, and fiber. The root is used as a tea in TCM for colds and flu with fever, dry mouth, headaches, and muscle stiffness in the head and back. It is also useful for head colds, sinus congestion, and sinus headaches. Its antispasmodic actions make it effective for torticulis (wry neck), irritable bowel syndrome (IBS) with diarrhea, and ischaemic heart disease, especially angina. Recent research on kudzu found that the decoction of the root reduces alcohol cravings in Syrian golden hamsters, and has a similar effect in humans. In China the flowers were traditionally used for a related purpose—alcohol poisoning (hangovers).

Other parts of the plant have uses as well. The leaves can be eaten as fodder, especially by goats, and they are used as poultices for wounds. The root starch is used as a thickening agent for foods in Japan, as well as a medicine in the macrobiotic diet. Finally, the stems can be used to make fiber and can be woven into beautiful and durable baskets.

PURPLE LOOSESTRIFE

Latin name: *Lythrum salicaria*

Common name: Purple loosestrife

Part used: Dried flowering herb

Taste: Sour

Energy: Cool, dry, and moist

Constituents: Vitexin (a glucoside), salicarin, tannins, pectin

Action: Antibacterial, antiamoebic, astringent, demulcent, anti-inflammatory, anti-hemorraghic, antihistamine, antispasmodic

Dosage: *Tea*—Add 1–2 teaspoons of the dried herb to 8 ounces of hot water. Steep for one hour. Drink 1–3 cups of tea per day. *Tincture*—1:5 dry extract, 30 percent alcohol, 40–60 drops (2–3 ml) three to four times per day.

Originally planted as a perennial ornamental for its lovely purple-magenta flower spikes, purple loosestrife quickly wore out its welcome. It likes wetlands and now covers hundreds of thousands of acres, choking out native plants and the species of animals and insects that depended on them for food and habitat. Once commonly used in European herbal medicine, we need to utilize this weed again both for its valuable medicinal qualities and to reduce its invasive spread.

Upon first taking *Lythrum*, you will notice a pronounced astringency, later followed by a soothing demulcent quality. This combination of actions, along with others, makes this plant appropriate for diarrhea, bacterial or amoebic dysentery, enteritis, IBS, leaky gut syndrome,

and sore throats (as a gargle). Maude Grieve, in her book *A Modern Herbal,* says "that as an eye-wash Purple Loosestrife is superior to Eyebright for preserving the sight and curing sore eyes." Current European uses of this herb include the treatment of ophthalmic ulcers. The herb can also be used as a vaginal douche for leukorrhea and bacterial vaginosis, and as a nasal douche for nosebleeds. Topically the ointment is used for ulcers and sores; a poultice is soothing to bruises, abrasions, and irritated skin. The stems can be chewed for bleeding gums caused by pyorrhea and gingivitis.

SELF-HEAL

Latin name: *Prunella vulgaris*

Chinese name: Xia Ku Cao

Common name: Allheal, heal-all

Taste: Bitter, slightly pungent

Energy: Cold, slightly moistening

Part used: Dried flower spike and leaf

Constituents: Saponin (a triterpenoid), rutin, hyperoside, caffeic acid, d-camphor, and d-fenchone

Action: Antibacterial, antimutagenic, diuretic, hypotensive agent

Dosage: *Tea*—Add 1–2 teaspoons of the dried herb to 8 ounces of hot water. Steep for one hour. Drink 2–3 cups per day. *Tincture*—1:2 fresh extract, 30 percent alcohol, 40–60 drops, (2–3 ml), three times per day.

Self-heal is a small member of the Lamiaceae (Mint) family commonly found in lawns and waste areas. It has attractive spikes of purple flowers but is considered a nuisance weed. Once known as allheal, it is now little used in Europe and the United States but maintains a place in the Chinese materia medica. In TCM Xia Ku Cao is used to soften hardness (lumps, enlarged lymph nodes). It is also used for goiters, lipomas, mumps, mastitis, lymphosarcoma, and scrofula. In addition, it is used for pathological heat in the liver (liver fire rising). These conditions include liver fire headaches, acute conjunctivitis, hypertension, vertigo, and painful or light-sensitive eyes. Topically, self-heal is used for inflamed wounds that are red and painful to the touch as well as hot (fire poison)—boils, carbuncles, sties, and staph infections. Keewaydinoquay, an Anishnabe elder, says that self-heal is exceptionally effective as a compress for removing splinters of wood, metal, or glass.

SPICEBUSH

Latin name: *Lindera benzoin*

Cherokee name: Nodatsi

Common name: Spicewood

Part used: Dried bark, leaf, fruit

Taste: Pungent and sweet

Energy: Warm and dry

Constituents: Linderol, linderone, linderalactone

Action: Antiseptic, carminative, diaphoretic, emmenagogue, expectorant

Dosage: *Tea (bark/leaf)*—Add 1 teaspoon of the dried bark or leaf to 8 ounces of hot water. Steep (covered) for one hour. Drink 2–3 cups per day. *Tincture*—1:5 (dry) extract, 40 percent alcohol, 30–40 drops (1–2 ml), three times per day.

Spicebush is one of the most common understory shrubs throughout second- or third-growth eastern forests. Early in the spring it is covered with small yellow flowers, which perfume the air. Every part of spicebush is medicinal; the tea of this herb is used extensively for colds, flu, coughs, nausea, indigestion, croup, flatulence, and amenorrhea. The inhaled steam is used to clear clogged sinuses, and the decoction of the twigs makes a soothing bath for arthritic pain (some of the tea is also taken internally). A related species of spicebush, *L. strychnifolia*, is used in TCM for dysuria, fungal infections, asthma, dysmenorrhea, hernia pain, and diarrhea. Spicebush is also commonly used as a beverage tea, and the dried fruits can be used as a spice in baking.

SUMAC

Latin name: *Rhus glabra, R. copallina, R. typhina, R. aromatica*

Cherokee name: Qualagu

Common name: Staghorn sumac

Part used: Dried berry, bark

Taste: Sour

Energy: Cool, dry

Constituents: *Bark*—Gallic acid. B*erries*—Citric acid.

Action: Alterative (bark), antiseptic, astringent, diuretic

Dosage: *Tea (berry)*—Add 1 teaspoon of the dried fruit to 8 ounces of hot water. Steep for thirty minutes. Drink 2–4 cups per day. *Tea (bark)*—Add 1/2 teaspoon of the dried bark to 8 ounces of water. Decoct for fifteen minutes. Steep for one hour. Drink one 4-ounce cup twice per day. *Tincture (bark)*—1:5 dry extract, 30 percent alcohol, 10 percent vegetable glycerine, 20–30 drops (1–2 ml) three times per day. *Tincture* (berry)—1:5 dry extract, 30 percent alcohol, 10 percent vegetable glycerine, 40–60 (2–3 ml) three times per day.

Sumacs are small shrubby trees that bear highly visible clusters of bright red berries each autumn. Their toxic relative, poison sumac *(R. vernix)*, has white fruit and prefers swampy areas to the dry, open environment where other sumacs are found. Sumac berry tea is effective for urinary tract infections (it acidifies the urine), thrush, apthous stomatata, ulcerated mucous membranes, gingivitis, and some cases of bed-wetting (irritated bladder). The fruit tea can be taken hot or chilled as a refreshing beverage similar in taste to hibiscus or rose hips. The bark is a strong astringent (used for diarrhea and menorrhagia) that affects the female hormonal system. The Cherokee used the bark for alleviating menopausal discomfort (hot flashes, sweating) and as a galactogogue. Externally the berry or bark tea has been used as a wash for blisters, burns, and oozing sores.

The Eclectics used the bark of fragrant sumac *(R. aromatica)* for urinary incontinence, interstitial cystitis, and profuse clear urination associated with diabetes; some physicians felt it helped control diabetes as well.

REFERENCES

A Barefoot Doctors Manual. Seattle: Cloudburst Press, 1977.

Bensky, D., and A. Gamble. *Chinese Herbal Medicine Materia Medica.* Seattle: Eastland Press, 1986.

Bianchini, F., and F. Corbetta. *Health Plants of the World.* New York: Newsweek Books, 1975.

Boik, John. *Cancer & Natural Medicine.* Princeton, Minn.: Oregon Medical Press, 1996.

Chiej, R. *The MacDonald Encyclopedia of Medicinal Plants.* London: MacDonald, 1984.

Dastur, J. F. *Medicinal Plants of India & Pakistan.* Bombay: D. B. Taraporevala, 1970.

Duke, J. A., and E. S. Ayensu. *Medicinal Plants of China.* Algonac, Mich.: Reference Pub., 1985.

Felter, H. W., and J. U. Lloyd. *Kings American Dispensatory.* Vols. 1 and 2. Portland, Oreg.: Eclectic Med. Pub., 1983.

Fernald, M. L. *Grays Manual of Botany.* 8th ed. New York: American Book Co., 1950.

Foster, S., and Yue Chongxi. *Herbal Emissaries.* Rochester, Vt.: Healing Arts Press, 1992.

Garg, S. *Substitute and Adulterant Plants.* Delhi: Periodical Exports Book Agency, 1992.

Grieve, Mrs. Maude. *A Modern Herbal.* New York: Hafner, 1967.

Him Che Yeung. *Handbook of Chinese Herbs & Formulas.* Vol. 1. n.p.: author, 1985.

Hobbs, C. *Chinese Herbs Growing in the Western US.* Los Angeles: author, 1985.

———. *Medicinal Mushrooms.* Santa Cruz, Calif.: Botanica Press, 1995.

Hsu, Hong-Yen. *Oriental Materia Medica.* Long Beach, Calif.: OHAI, 1986.

Lad, Vasant, and David Frawley. *The Yoga of Herbs.* Santa Fe, N.M.: Lotus Press, 1986.

Li Ning-hon, ed. *Chinese Medicinal Herbs of Hong Kong.* Vols. 1–5. Hong Kong, 1983–1986.

Lou Zhicen. *Color Atlas of Chinese Traditinal Drugs.* Vol. 1. Beijing: Science Press, 1987.

Munz, Philip. *A California Flora.* Berkeley: University of California Press, 1962.

Radford, A., H. Ahles, and C. R. Bell. *Manual of the Vascular Flora of the Carolinas.* Chapel Hill: University of North Carolina Press, 1973.

Tsanusdi, Tawodi. Personal communication with author, 1980–1998.

U.S. Department of Agriculture. *Selected Weeds of the United States.* Agriculture Handbook 366. Washington, D.C.: Government Printing Office, 1976.

Xu Xiang Cai. *The Chinese Materia Medica.* Vol. 2 of *The English-Chinese Enyclopedia of Practical Traditional Chinese Medicine.* Beijing: Higher Education Press, 1990.

TABLE 7

THE AMERICAN EXTRA PHARMACOPOEIA

SYMBOLS		ABBREVIATIONS	
Δ	Common adventurous weeds	ADD	Attention Deficit Disorder
+	Easily cultivated	ADHD	Attention-Deficit Hyperactivity Disorder
∞	Locally abundant—use occasionally	BP	Blood pressure
#	China	BPH	Benign prostatic hyperplasia
√	Japan		
Ψ	Cherokee		
*	India		
φ	Eclectic		
X	Toxic		
Σ	European		

SYM	COMMON NAME	LATIN NAME	LOCAL NAME	PART USED	TASTE/ ENERGY	SUMMARY OF USES
#Δ	Abutilon	*Abutilon avicennae; A. indicum*	Dong Kui Zi	Seed	Sweet/cold/ moist	Demulcent, bulk laxative, anti-inflammatory
#Δ	Aster	*Aster tataricus*	Zi Wan	Root/ rhizome	Sweet/bitter/ warm	Expectorant, antibacterial, TB, bronchitis
ΔφΨ	Red aster	*Aster puniceus*	Purple-stem aster	Root/ rhizome	Acrid/bitter/ warm	Nervine, antispasmodic
ΔφΨ	Heart-leaved aster	*Aster cordifolius*		Root/ rhizome	Acrid/bitter	Diaphoretic
Σ+	Barberry	*Berberis vulgaris*		Root/bark	Bitter/cold/ dry	Topical, antibacterial, cholagogue

SYM	COMMON NAME	LATIN NAME	LOCAL NAME	PART USED	TASTE/ ENERGY	SUMMARY OF USES
#Δ	Beggarsticks	*Bidens pilosa*	Xian Feng Cao	Herb	Sweet/neutral	Febrifuge, lowers BP, dysentery, enteritis, BPH
Δ*	Bermuda grass	*Cynodon dactylon*	Dhub	Herb	Sour/neutral	Diuretic
Σ	Birch	*Betula* spp.		Bark/twigs	Neutral/dry	Betulinic acid (antitumor activity), prostatic inflammation
∞φ Ψ+	Bluebells	*Polemonium reptans*	Jacob's ladder	Root	Acrid/warm/ dry	Astringent, diaphoretic, pleurisy, pneumonia
#φΨ	Bugleweed	*Lycopus virginicus*	Ze Lan	Herb	Acrid/bitter/ warm	Sedative, mild narcotic, heart tonic, enteritis, anodyne, hemoptysis, hypothyroid
#Δφ	Bur marigold	*Bidens bipinnata*	Nian Shen Cao	Root/seed/ leaf	Bitter/warm	Emmenagogue, anti-inflammatory, expectorant, BPH
#+	Burnet	*Sanguisorba officinalis*	Di Yu	Root	Bitter/sour/ cool	Astringent, hemostatic, ulcers, menorrhagia
#Δ	Bur reed	*Scirpus sparganum stoloniferum* or *yagura*	San Leng	Rhizome	Acrid/bitter/ cold	Moves stagnant qi, relieves pain, uterine or abdominal cramps
ΔφΣ	Canadian fleabane	*Conyza canadensis*	Horseweed	Herb	Pungent/ bitter/ warm/dry	Antihemorrhagic, diuretic, carminative, hematuria, osteoar-thritis, diarrhea, dysentery
*#	Cassia	*Cassia tora*	Jue Ming Zi; Chakunda	Seed	Sweet/bitter/ cool	Lowers cholesterol, laxative, emollient, antihypertensive
#φ√	Catalpa	*Catalpa ovata*	Kisasage; Xin Ba Pi	Fruit	sweet/neutral	Diuretic, chronic bronchitis, nephritis

SYM	COMMON NAME	LATIN NAME	LOCAL NAME	PART USED	TASTE/ ENERGY	SUMMARY OF USES
#Δ	Cattail	*Typha latifolia*	Pu Huang	Pollen	Sweet/neutral	Hemostatic, diuretic, uterine bleeding, postpartum pain
Σ	Chaga	*Inonotus obliquus*	Clinker; polypore	Fungus	(Slightly) sweet/bitter/ warm	Immune potentiator, strong anticancer activity
φΔ	Chicory	*Cichorium intybus*	Blue sailers	Root	(Slightly) bitter/sweet/ moist	Liver and digestive tonic; source of fructo-oligosaccha-rides (FOS), which stimulate growth of healthy intestinal flora
#φX	Club moss *clavatum*	*Lycopodium*	Shen Jin Cao	Spores/ herb	Bitter/acrid/ warm	Relaxes muscles, clears meridians, rheumatic arthritis, urinary pain
Δ*Ψ	Cocklebur	*Xanthium strumarium*	Banokra	Herb/fruit	Acrid/bitter/ warm	Rhinitis, rheumatic arthritis, diaphoretic, sedative, lumbago
#+	Cockscomb	*Celosia cristata*	Ji Guan Hua	Flower/ seed	Sweet/cool	Astringent, trichomonas, uterine and rectal bleeding, hemorrhoids
ΔφΨ	Cow parsnip	*Heracleum lanatum*	Kanali	Root/seed	Acrid/warm	Petit mal epilepsy, antispasmodic, carminative
Δ#√	Dayflower	*Commelina communis*	Ya Zhi Cao; Tsuyu-kusa	Herb	Sweet/cool/ moist	Soothing diuretic, ulcers, sore throats, gastritis
Δ#X	Dodder	*Cuscuta* spp.	Tu Si Zi; Nu Watuyanuhi	Seed/herb	Acrid/sweet/ bitter/neutral/ cool	Kidney yang tonic, liver and bowel tonic, impotence, sciatica pain
Ψ∞	Dogwood	*Cornus florida*	Wousita	Bark	Bitter/cool/ dry	Malaria, muscle cramps, intermittent fevers

SYM	COMMON NAME	LATIN NAME	LOCAL NAME	PART USED	TASTE/ ENERGY	SUMMARY OF USES
#+	Dogwood	*Cornus officinalis*	Shan Zhu Yu	Berries	Sour/warm	Diuretic, impotence, uterine bleeding, lowers BP
#Δ	Duckweed	*Spirodela polyrhiza; Lemna minor*	Fu Ping	Herb	Acrid/cold	Cardiac tonic, diuretic, diaphoretic, edema
#*	Eclipta	*Eclipta alba*	Han Lian Cao; Bhringaraja	Herb	Sweet/sour/ cold	Liver/spleen congestion, balding, insomnia, alopecia, cirrhosis
#+	Euonymus	*Euonymus alata*	Gui Jian Yu	Twigs	Bitter/cold	Anodyne, emmenagogue, anthelmintic, lowers blood sugar levels
Δ#	Foxtail grass	*Alopecurus aequalis*	Gan Mai Niang	Herb	Sweet/ neutral	Diuretic, anti-inflammatory, chicken pox
#Ψ	Ganoderma	*Ganoderma tsugae*	Ling Zhi	Fungus	Sweet/warm	Immune stimulant, sedative, insomnia, asthma, debility, poor memory
φ+Ψ	Sweet goldenrod	*Solidago odora; S.* spp.	Unestala	Herb	Sweet/acrid/ warm	Diaphoretic, diuretic, sedative, lowers BP, cystitis
ΣΔ	Grape leaf	*Vitis vinifera*		Leaf	Sour/cool/ dry	Source of anthocyanin; flavanoids used for varicose veins, hemorrhoids, liver tonic
#+	Ground cherry	*Physalis alkekengi*	Suan Jiang	Root	Bitter/cold	Sedative, febrifuge
φΔ	Ground cherry	*Physalis subglabrata*		Fruit	Sour/cool	Diuretic, cardiac tonic
ΔφΨ	Hawkweed	*Hieracium venosum*	Ahwi Gali Gigageiuse	Root/leaf	Bitter/dry/ cool	Long history of use for snakebites, diarrhea, expectorant, vulnerary

SYM	COMMON NAME	LATIN NAME	LOCAL NAME	PART USED	TASTE/ ENERGY	SUMMARY OF USES
Ψφ	Hercules' club	*Aralia spinosa*	Ultsagitu; prickly elder	Berry/bark	Acrid/bitter/ warm	Anodyne—tooth-ache, moves qi, arthritic pain, paralysis, diaphoretic
Δ#	Honeysuckle	*Lonicera japonica*	Jin Yin Hua	Flower	Bitter/sweet/ cold/dry	Antibacterial, enteritis, anti-inflammatory, antipyretic, pneumo-nia, acute mastitis
Δ#	Honeysuckle	*Lonicera japonica*	Ren Dong Teng	Stem/leaf	(Slightly) sweet/bitter/ cold/dry	Appendicitis, infectious hepatitis, flu, rheumatic pain
∞φΨ	Indian-pipe	*Monotropa uniflora*		Root	Bitter/cold	Anodyne, antispas-modic, sedative, diaphoretic, fevers with pain, convulsions
Δ#	Indian strawberry	*Duchesnea indica*	She Mei	Herb	Bitter/sweet/ cold	Antipyretic, laryngitis, acute tonsilitis, coughs
Δ#	Knot grass	*Polygonum aviculare*	Bian Xu	Herb	Bitter/cool/ dry	Diuretic, chola-gogue, jaundice, urethritis, trichomonas, hemostatic
Δ#	Lespedeza	*Lespediza cuneata*	Ye Guan Men	Herb	Bitter/sweet/ cold	Expectorant, enuresis, anthelm-intic, traumatic injuries
ΔφΨ	Lion's-foot	*Prenanthes alba*	White lettuce	Root/leaf	Bitter/cool	Long history for rattlesnake bites, sedative, dysentery
ΔφΨ	Lion's-foot	*Prenanthes serpentaria*	Gall of the earth	Root/leaf	Bitter/cool	Long history for rattlesnake bites, sedative, dysentery
#Ψ	Lizard's-tail	*Saururus cernuus*	San Bai Cao	Herb	Acrid/sweet/ cold	Irritation and inflammation of GI tract and urinary tract

SYM	COMMON NAME	LATIN NAME	LOCAL NAME	PART USED	TASTE/ ENERGY	SUMMARY OF USES
#∞	Lopseed	*Phryma leptostachya*	Tou Gu Cao	Herb	Acrid/cool/ dry	Externally for ring-worm, insect bites, scabies
Δ+Ψ	Lyre-leaved sage	*Salvia lyrata*		Herb	Bitter/ pungent/ cool	Carminative, ulcers, colds, coughs, nervous exhaustion
#+	Mulberry	*Morus alba*	Sang Bai Pi	Root/bark	Sweet/cold /dry	Expectorant, diuretic, hyperten-sion, antiasthmatic
#+	Mulberry	*Morus alba*	Sang Shen	Fruit	Sweet/cool /moist	Anemia, tinnitus, vertigo
#+	Mulberry	*Morus alba*	Sang Ye	Leaf	Sweet/bitter /cold	Diaphoretic, anti-bacterial, colds, sore throats
#+	Mulberry	*Morus alba*	Sang Shi	Branch	Bitter/neutral/ dry	Antispasmodic, diuretic, joint pain, high blood pressure
Δ#*	Nut grass	*Cyperus rotundus*	Xiang Fu, Musta	Tuber	Acrid/bitter/ neutral	Carminative, anti-spasmodic, dysmen-orrhea, anodyne
Σ+	Olive leaf	*Olea europaea*		Leaf	Bitter/cold	Hypertension, anti-viral, diuretic
φΔΣ	Yellow oxalis	*Oxalis acetosella*	Sour grass	Herb	Sour/cool/ dry	Diuretic, UTI, extrenally for indolent ulcers
ΔφΣ	Oxeye daisy	*Chrysanthe-mum leucan-themum*		Herb	Sweet/ pungent/dry/ neutral	Stops excessive sweating, excessive mucous discharge
#Δ∞	Penny cress	*Thlaspi arvense*	Bai Jiang Cao	Herb	Bitter/acrid/ cold	Antibacterial, used for abscesses, erysipelas
#Δ√	Perilla	*Perilla frutescens*	Zi Su Ye	Herb	Acrid/warm/ dry	Diaphoretic, carmi-native, seafood poisoning, nausea
#+	Persimmon	*Diospyros* spp.	Shi Di	Calyx	Bitter/ neutral	Hiccups, hiatal hernia

SYM	COMMON NAME	LATIN NAME	LOCAL NAME	PART USED	TASTE/ ENERGY	SUMMARY OF USES
#+	Persimmon	*Diospyros* spp.		Unripe juice	Sour/dry	Hypertension
#*Δ	Puncture vine	*Tribulus terrestris*	Ci Ji Li; Gokshura	Fruit	Acrid/bitter/ neutral	Diuretic, lowers BP, dizziness, cystitis, builds kidney yang
Δ#*	Purslane	*Portulaca oleracea*	Ma Chi Xian; Bada Lunia	Herb	Sour/cool/ moist	Mild diuretic, liver tonic, mucous diarrhea with bleed- ing; seeds contain omega fatty acids
ΔΨφ	Ragweed	*Ambrosia trifida*	Ukwaste Luyetu	Herb	Bitter/acrid/ warm	Astringent, antisep- tic, styptic, vulner- ary, bitter tonic
ΔΨφ	Ragweed	*Ambrosia artemisiifolia*	Ukwaste Luyetu	Herb	Dry	Astringent, antisep- tic, styptic, vulner- ary, bitter tonic
Δ#	Reed	*Phragmites communis*	Lu Gen	Rhizome	Sweet/cold/ moist	Diuretic, cystitis, dissolves gallstones, seafood poisoning, vomiting
∞#+	Rose-of- Sharon	*Hibiscus syriacus*	Mu Jin Hua	Flower	Sweet/cool/ moist	Soothing demulcent to bladder, stomach, large intestine
Δ#	Rush	*Juncus effusus*	Deng Xin Cao	Pith	Sweet/cold/ moist	Febrifuge, diuretic, sore throats, urinary tract infections
#+	Sandwort	*Arenaria serpyllifolia*	Ling Ling Cao	Herb	Bitter/cool	Diuretic, febrifuge, coughs
#φΔ ΧΣ	Scarlet pimpernel	*Anagallis arvensis*	Jian Feng Hong	Herb	Bitter/cool	Poisonous bites, enlarged liver and spleen, edema
#Δφ	Smartweed	*Polygonum hydropiper- oides*	Shui Liao	Herb	Acrid/warm/ dry	Hemostatic, menor- rhagia, vomiting, bruises, dysentery
Ψφ	Sourwood	*Oxydendrum arboreum*	Udoqueya	Leaf	Sour/cool/ dry	Diuretic, antiseptic, benign prostrate enlargement, cystitis

SYM	COMMON NAME	LATIN NAME	LOCAL NAME	PART USED	TASTE/ ENERGY	SUMMARY OF USES
Ψ#	Sweet gum	*Liquidambar styraciflua*	Swamp maple	Fruit	Acrid/warm/ dry	Clears meridians, diuretic, rheumatic pain
Ψ#	Sweet gum	*Liquidambar styraciflua*	Swamp maple	Bark	Bitter/ neutral/dry	Astringent, diarrhea, dysentery, nervous stomach, menorrhagia
Ψ#	Sweet gum	*Liquidambar styraciflua*	Swamp maple	Gum resin	Acrid/warm/ dry	Angina, bedsores, expectorant, anti-inflammatory, topical herpes
ΔφΣ	Sweet melilot	*Melilotus officinalis*	Yellow clover	Herb	Sweet/bitter/ cold	Painful neuralgia, sciatica, colic, dysmenorrhea, ovarian pain
#+	Sweet wormwood	*Artemesia annua*	Qing Hao	Herb	Bitter/acrid/ cold	Antimalarial, febrifuge, antifungal, bitter tonic
Δ#Σ	Teasel	*Dipsacus* spp.	Xu Duan	Root	Bitter/warm/ dry	Antirheumatic, hemostatic, lower-back and joint pain, threatened abortion
ΔφΣ	Toadflax	*Linaria vulgaris*	Butter-and-eggs	Herb	Bitter/acrid/ salty	Raised bilyrubin levels, jaundice, splenic and hepatic hypertrophies
Δ#φX	Tree-of-heaven	*Ailanthus altissima*	Chun Pi	Bark	Bitter/cold/ dry	Febrifuge, astringent, antispasmodic, dysentery, cardiac palpitations
φ	Tulip tree	*Liriodendron tulipifera*	Yellow poplar; Tsiyu	Bark	Acrid/bitter/ warm	Diaphoretic, rheumatic pain, bitter tonic, fever with agitation
#Ψ	Turkey tails	*Trametes versicolor*	Coriolus versicolor	Fungus	Neutral/moist	Immune stimulant, antibiotic, tumor-inhibiting action
Δ*	Velvet Leaf	*Malva verticillata*	Velvet Leaf	Seed	Sweet/cold/ moist	Diuretic, bulk laxative

SYM	COMMON NAME	LATIN NAME	LOCAL NAME	PART USED	TASTE/ ENERGY	SUMMARY OF USES
#*	Water hyssop	*Bacopa monnieri*	Ba Ji Tian; Bhrami	Herb	Mild acrid/ warm	Builds kidney yang, low sperm count, impotence, ADHD, ADD, anxiety, back-ache, rheumatic pain, irregular menses
#	Water pennywort	*Hydrocotyle sibthorpioides*	Man Tian Xiang	Herb	Sweet/cool	Febrifuge, sore throats, coughs, cirrhosis of liver, jaundice
#Ψ	Water plantain	*Alisma plantago-aquatica*	Ze Xie	Tuber	Sweet/cold	Diuretic, lowers blood sugar and cholesterol levels, fatty liver
Ψφ	White ash	*Fraxinus americana*	Tsukanana	Bark	Bitter/acrid	Pelvic congestion, uterine fibroids
∞	White sage	*Salvia apiana*		Leaf	Pungent/cold/ dry	Benign prostatic hypertrophy, gargle—strep throat
#Δ	Whitlow grass	*Dabra nemorosa*	Ting Li Zi	Seed	Acrid/bitter/ cold	Expectorant, cardio-tonic, diuretic, asthma
#Δ	Whitlow grass	*Lepidium* spp.		Seed	Acrid/bitter/ cold	Expectorant, cardio-tonic, diuretic, asthma
#Δ	Wild radish	*Raphanus sativus*	Lai Fu Zi	Seed	Acrid/sweet/ neutral	Expectorant, carmin-ative, asthma, anti-fungal, increases hydrochloric acid production
Ψ+	Yellow root	*Xanthorhiza simplicissima*	Dalani Anai Yulti	Root	Bitter/cold/ dry	Antifungal, candidi-asis, thrush, liver and digestive tonic

FLOWER ESSENCES

❧

KATE GILDAY AND SHATOIYA DE LA TOUR

Let not the simplicity of this method deter you from its use, for you will find the further your researches advance, the greater you will realize the simplicity of all creation.

Edward Bach

WHAT ARE FLOWER ESSENCES?

Since the beginning of time, humans and flowers have had a deep relationship. Flowers are used to mark passages in human life; they are used as religious symbols and honored in many forms of art. There is even a "language of flowers" employed by Victorians and others. Is it any wonder that as we move to understand the nature of healing, we turn to the most beautiful in nature to heal us? As we begin to glimpse the connections among heart, body, mind, and soul, does it not follow that we would seek to find remedies that work on all these levels?

Through the remarkable work of Dr. Edward Bach (1886–1936), flower essences were brought to the attention of the modern world. A medical practitioner and spiritual seeker, Dr. Bach realized the healing potential waiting for us in the flowers. Flowers contain the most vital essence of the plant, its reproductive system, its life force. By connecting with that pure force through vibrational healing, we can raise our consciousness to those refined qualities inherent in nature, such as patience and love. While walking through a field, Dr. Bach saw the sunlight transforming and imparting (potentizing) the dew on a flower with the flower's vital energy. He realized that the four elements were working together to create a simple, healing remedy. He said, "The earth to nurture the plant, the air from which it feeds, the sun or fire to impart its power, and water to collect and be enriched with its beneficent healing."

For the next six years Dr. Bach and his colleagues devoted themselves to reproducing this simple method with many plants, to come up with thirty-eight remedies to ease the spirit as well as the body. These remedies come in the form of a concentrated liquid, taken in small doses under the tongue. Each remedy addresses an emotional issue and helps bring balance to that issue in the heart of the user. By bringing these issues to balance, we become closer to our divine self, healing on every level. Machelle Small Wright calls this healing the PEMS—physical, emotional, mental, and spiritual.

Dr. Bach's work opened up a whole new frontier for healers. Since his time more than fifty flower essence companies have been created, discovering new remedies from flowers all over the world. Many of these new essences relate to the challenges we face in a world more complex than Dr. Bach might ever have imagined.

Most important, at a time when mass consumption of plants worldwide for health reasons has begun to endanger different species, this method of healing uses a very small amount of plant material and does not greatly disturb the life of a plant (see Making a Flower Essence on page 58). As our relationships with plants evolve, and we come to understand how much healing can come from a small amount of plant, we will be able to use herbs more wisely. This will allow both humans and plants to prosper on our planet.

FLOWER ESSENCES OF AT-RISK WOODLAND PLANTS

Several years ago our family began making flower essences from the trees, shrubs, and forest-floor flowers found in the Northeast's woodlands. We felt guided to do this as a way of sharing the deep and gentle healing of the forest that we had become so familiar with. We now live and spend much of our time in the woods, where we have the opportunity to enjoy an ever-growing relationship with the trees, plants, and wildlife nurtured in this forest community.

Spending time in these eastern woodlands connects us with the spirit of the land and of our ancestors who lived so intimately with nature. As human beings, our connection with the forest community is ancient and profound. It is where we continue to return for inspiration and grounding, as well as for food, medicine, and shelter. Using the flower essences from these trees and plants can help bring you into the light and understanding of this timeless relationship. In the forest we walk in the footsteps of our ancestors. It is where we find and remember the sacred and all our relations.

Those who have used woodland essences have found them to hold not only the individual pattern and quality of each plant, but also the full, rich resonance of the forest. It has been a true delight to share the ancient pulse of healing and connection with others on their path of healing. The experience that led to the North American At-Risk Flower Essence Set came at the United Plant Savers conference on Sage Mountain in the summer of 1997. Gail Ulrich, flower essence practitioner and founder of the Blazing Star Herb School, and I presented a class on preparing flower essences (see Making a Flower Essence). We had been contemplating ways of using the UpS at-risk plants without damaging them, and were excited to try our new technique. Setting a clear crystal bowl filled with fresh springwater beneath the flowers and using a glass dropper, we gently released water, drop by drop, over the fully opened blossoms into the waiting bowl. Rosemary Gladstar's beautiful woodlands at Sage Mountain had several of the at-risk herbs planted among the trees, and to our delight we found American ginseng and goldenseal in bloom. The class prepared a flower essence of the ginseng during the workshop, and each participant went home with a bottle of the essence. While making the essence,

I felt a strong presence surrounding us and encouraging me to express my love for the green world in a new way—in return for all I had and continue to receive.

It was a natural step, then, for us to put together the North American At-Risk Flower Essence Set, which holds these nine essences: Black cohosh, blue cohosh, bloodroot, American ginseng, goldenseal, pink lady slipper, spikenard, red trillium, and wild ginger. These native plants are beautiful, and their essences are equally powerful. These old beings, who have offered humans deep healing as important botanical medicines for thousands of years, are now in a state of stress due to habitat destruction and overharvesting. Making flower essences is a way to use these plants as medicine without harming or interrupting their life cycles. No part of the plant is damaged in any way when making these beautiful flower essences. With the at-risk flower essences, we hope to share the strength, wisdom, and vibrational healing of some of these threatened woodland plants. The individual essences reflect the uniqueness of each plant, often mirroring the physical healing properties. The full set is similar to the community of plants growing together. Perhaps there are times when the flower essence of one of these plants could be used instead of a root preparation. As we attend to our spirits, our physical symptoms often clear. This is an area we would like to explore with other practitioners. Although our relationship with these plants goes back many years, using them as flower essences is new to us. We consider them research essences and would deeply appreciate learning how others use

and are touched by these essences. The North American At-Risk Flower Essence Set is available through Woodland Essence, 392 Tea Cup Street, Cold Brook, NY 13324.

BLACK COHOSH
(Cimicfuga racemosa)

Knowing and trusting in your inner strength and resources. Honesty and courage to deal with and heal past experiences of abuse and oppression. Releasing entanglements. Bright, strong sense of self-emergence.

BLUE COHOSH
(Caulophyllum thalictroides)

Gentle support for those feeling shy or awkward in their sexuality, especially during times of transition such as puberty, pregnancy, menopause, and midlife. Opens you to the mysteries and energy of your sexuality as sacred and life affirming. Graceful acceptance of the changes aging brings.

BLOODROOT
(Sanguinaria canadensis)

Trusting that you will be protected as you move forward in your evolution. Finding the courage and inner resources to heal old wounds and move from a place of despair and darkness to the light. Embracing your inner light.

AMERICAN GINSENG
(Panax quinquefolius)

Vitality, strength, and support when experiencing depletion or exhaustion of inner resources. Deeply healing. Releasing fear of expressing true self. Accepting personal power. Feeling whole and alive.

GOLDENSEAL
(Hydrastis canadensis)

Opening channels to allow free flow of energy. Releasing that which no longer serves, giving a sense of lightness and freedom. Cutting the cords that drain you, freeing up held energy. Clearing out the old to make room for the new. Energizing.

PINK LADY'S SLIPPER
(Cyripedium acaule)

Clarity and creative expression of inner purpose and true calling. Ability to express yourself more easily. Releasing shame. Understanding and delight in your sexuality, opening you to deeper levels of intimacy.

SPIKENARD
(Aralia racemosa)

Dancing gracefully through life's challenges as you let go of resistance. Present-moment awareness. Allowing the experience of the present to effortlessly guide you to the next moment. Calm, fluid motion.

TRILLIUM
(Trillium erectum)

Tender yet strong support during times of birth, death, and rebirth. Developing the courage and flexibility to flow with life's changes and cycles. Coming home to yourself. Peaceful centeredness, knowing that this is enough.

WILD GINGER
(Asarum canadense)

A simple, ancient guide inviting you to rekindle your connection with nature, the forest, and all beings, and reminding you that this is your birthright. Brings sense of being grounded and rooted.

MAKING A FLOWER ESSENCE

Perhaps there is a particular flower you have felt close to all your life. Perhaps there is an abundance of a certain flower in your backyard or a wild field near you that you feel has a certain message for you. A great way to connect with this energy is by making a flower essence of the plant. Making an essence is easy, but many makers of commercial remedies meditate and communicate with a flower for two or more years before ever attempting to create its essence. Clarity is essential in this type of work. Although every type of medicine making is a sacred act, it is especially important when creating vibrational medicine to be clear in your intent. Remember, energy follows intent, and the energy of the flower essence is where the healing begins.

You may want to prepare yourself with an herbal bath and meditation. All your tools should be sterilized and cleared energetically, through either prayer, smudging, laying on an amethyst crystal, or placing them under a new or full moon. There are a few different ways to make flower essences, but I offer the simplest here, the sun method, because it is the closest to Dr. Bach's original technique. You will need:

- A bottle of clean water (not distilled)
- A small, clear, glass bowl (a small Pyrex dessert cup is perfect)
- Scissors or chopsticks
- A good-quality brandy
- A pint bottle
- Two 1-ounce bottles with glass dropper caps

As in wildcrafting, you want to make sure that the area from which you're harvesting is as pristine as possible. Look for a good selection of the flowers you want, because you will be working with several different plants of the same type.

Without allowing your fingers to touch the inside of the bowl, fill it to the top with water. Gently carry the bowl from plant to plant and—using chopsticks, scissors, or even a leaf of the plant—pluck off flowers and place them on the surface of the water. Be careful that your fingers do not touch the blossoms. When the water's surface is covered, place the bowl on the ground next to the healing plant. Let it sit where it will get sun and no shadows for three to four hours.

After the allotted time, use a twig or leaf of the plant—or a chopstick—to brush the flowers off the top of the water. The water remaining in your bowl is the flower water. Take the pint bottle and fill it no more than halfway with this water, then fill it the rest of the way with brandy. This is called the mother water.

Now fill a 1-ounce bottle halfway with mother water and halfway with brandy. This is your stock bottle. Dosage bottles can then be made by putting 4 drops of a single remedy from a stock bottle into a 1-ounce bottle filled half with brandy and half with water. If you're combining remedies (using more than one stock bottle), put just 2 drops of each remedy into the dosage bottle.

To use a flower essence, apply 4 drops from the dosage bottle four times daily under your tongue; you can also mix them in a glass of water and drink. Store the stock bottles and make dosage bottles as needed. Flower essences should be kept in a cool, dark place.

REFERENCES

Barnard, Julian, and Martine Barnard. *The Healing Herbs of Edward Bach*. Bath, England: Ashgrove Press, 1997.

McIntyre, Anne. *Flower Power*. New York: Henry Holt, 1996.

Weeks, Nora. *The Medical Discoveries of Dr. Edward Bach, Physician*. New Canaan, Conn.: Keats Publishing, 1973.

ARNICA
Arnica spp.

BRIGITTE MARS

The first time I really got to know arnica was on a clear June morning in the early 1980s. I was on a trip collecting the vibrant golden flowers with two other herbalist friends, Sunny Mavor and Debra St. Claire. We packed up Debra's station wagon with the collection implements: gathering bags; knives and cutting boards; and olive oil and alcohol, so we could begin processing the freshly picked arnica as infused oil and liniment at the gathering site. Heading for the higher altitudes of the Rocky Mountains outside Nederland, Colorado, we found a large alpine area complete with beautiful meadow and woodland.

BOTANICAL FEATURES

Arnica is native to Europe, and it grows wild in North America from the high mountainous regions of southern California to Alaska and east into the Rockies of Colorado, Idaho, Montana, and Wyoming. It is, in fact, America's Pacific Northwest that features the most diverse group of arnica species on the planet. The plant is also known to grow in the high-altitude regions of Siberia. Arnica grows wild in alpine meadows, and can be found growing in rocky forest clearings. It hybridizes easily, and identifying the various species can be tedious. Be careful not to confuse it with senecio. In western North America *A. cordifolia* and *A. latifolia* predominate. Other North American species include *A. diversifolia*, *A. longifolia*, *A. mollis* (hairy arnica), and *A. parryi*. Alpine arnica (*A. alpina*, also known as *A. montana*) is also found growing in northern Alaska and British Columbia. In Europe *A. montana* is the official remedy. The word *arnica* is derived from the Greek *arnakis*, which means "lamb's skin"—a reference to the bracts of the plant and leaves, which are sometimes woolly feeling. Arnica is a member of the Asteraceae family. Common names include leopard's bane, sneezewort, mountain tobacco, mountain daisy, tumbler's cure all, wolf's bane, and "the flower of recovery."

Arnica is a hardy aromatic perennial, growing 6 inches to 2 feet high. It has large single (*A. cordifolia*) or several (*A. latifolia*) bright yellow daisylike flowers, 1 to 4 inches in diameter, that bloom during its second year and thereafter. In the first year the leaves are a basal rosette approximately $1\frac{1}{2}$ to $2\frac{3}{4}$ inches long. The leaves are hairy, oval shaped, light green, and opposite. A distinguishing characteristic from other yellow-flowered members of the Asteraceae family are the paired leaves on the stems. The *A. latifolia* leaf is lanceolate, the *A. cordifolia* heart shaped. The basal leaves are larger than the upper. Rubbing arnica leaves produces a sage-pine-like aroma. The rhizome creeps horizontally and sends up shoots from its nodes, producing arnica colonies.

HISTORICAL BACKGROUND

Arnica was widely used in German folk medicine in the sixteenth century. It was an official herb of the *United States Pharmacopoeia* from 1820 until 1851, with the flowers being official from 1851 to 1925. It was included in the *National Formulary* from 1926 until 1960. Sweden honored arnica in 1995, featuring the plant's image on a postage stamp.

MEDICINAL USES

The most-often-used arnica parts are the flowers with their hairy receptacles. The flowers are considered the safest part to use, although the receptacles can be prone to insect infestation and are sometimes removed. On occasion the leaves and rhizomes are used.

Arnica is an anticoagulant, anti-inflammatory, antiphlogistic, antiseptic, astringent, diaphoretic, diuretic, emollient, expectorant, immune stimulant, nerve stimulant, rubifacient, and vulnerary.

The plant has most often been used as a homeopathic remedy for the following conditions: angina, arteriosclerosis, catarrh, concussion, epilepsy, falls, fever, fracture, gout, inflammation, injury, jet lag and travel stress, pain, physical and mental shock, seasickness, postsurgical trauma, posttraumatic stress disorder (following exposure to violence, terror, death, disaster, hysteria), stroke, and whooping cough. It is also used for the aftereffects of concussion and stroke. Most effective immediately after a traumatic incident, it is often a staple in natural medicine first-aid kits. It is excellent for preventing bruising and swelling after invasive dental work, such as wisdom tooth extraction or root canal; the homeopathic remedy should be used a couple of days before the procedure, and continued every two to four hours afterward for several days. Arnica is also helpful in the aftermath of any trauma, to prevent postsurgical complications such as swelling and pain, and to speed recovery. When used to aid surgery, it is taken a few days before the event and continued for several days afterward. A friend of mine who is a plastic surgeon suggests his patients take homeopathic arnica before and after surgery to reduce the bruising that occurs from reconstruction.

Arnica is also widely used to treat overexertion during athletic activities. It is used internally as a homeopathic remedy for painful muscles, and is especially indicated when even the bed feels painful and the slightest touch aggravates the condition. It is indicated for any injury made worse by contact, cold, or dampness. The arnica personality tends to feel better when lying down.

As a flower essence, arnica is used to restore your life force after shock and trauma; it helps you feel grounded again after an event that leaves you disconnected, such as an accident.

Though arnica is used internally in tincture and tea forms, it is not considered a remedy for the novice and is best used under the counsel of a health professional. Always use caution when using arnica internally; it can irritate the kidneys, heart, stomach, and digestive tract. It has also been known to cause dizziness and trembling. It is best and most often used as a homeopathic remedy or topically. When using topically, apply it only to unbroken skin, because it can cause skin and mucous membrane irritation. Repeated applications tend to have the same undesirable effects. If tincture is to be applied to the skin, it is best diluted. If topical application causes rash, redness, or overheating of the joint, promptly discontinue its use.

Arnica is an aid to wound healing and, when used topically, helps bruising and muscle pain. It speeds the healing process and helps restore normal sleep. An arnica compress, poultice, liniment, salve, or oil can be used to treat back pain, bruises, chilblains, dislocations, phlebitis, rheumatic pain, sprains, and varicose veins. As mentioned previously, it should be used only on unbroken skin and not on open wounds. Arnica has been used topically to treat acne and cuperose skin conditions. It can be made into an effective gargle for laryngitis and sore throats and was treasured by opera singers to restore a failing voice. As a foot bath, arnica comforts sore feet. Arnica is often included in shampoos and conditioners as a hair growth stimulant and scalp tonic. The flower is made into an absolute that is used in perfumery.

Though it is not certain how arnica works, it is believed to increase the blood flow through affected capillaries, causing fluids that have escaped due to injury to be reabsorbed. Arnica improves coronary blood flow and aids in the reabsorption of fibrin, a blood protein produced by internal injuries. Arnica also stimulates macrophage activity, which helps digest congested blood and trapped fluids. It reduces swelling and pressure on the nerve endings, alleviating pain and stiffness. Arnica flavors are considered pungent, bitter, and sweet, while its temperature is considered hot. In magic arnica is associated with the element fire.

Important constituents of arnica include volatile oil (thymol), sesquiterpene lactones (arnicin, arnicolides, helenalin), flavonoids (eupafolin, patuletin, spinacetin), polysaccharides, mucilage, bitters, carotenoids, inulin, and tannin. The sesquiterpene lactone helenalin is most effective as an anti-inflammatory agent.

PREPARATION AND DOSAGE

The fresh herb is preferable for tinctures, while dry-wilted flowers are best for making oils, because they are less likely to cause rancidity. I have, however, made oils from fresh plants that I carefully chopped (not blended), using dry jars, knives, and cutting boards. These oils have kept well in the refrigerator for a couple of years.

PROPAGATION AND CULTIVATION

Arnica likes to germinate in a mixture of loam, peat, and sand. It can be propagated from seeds or by root division. When grown from seeds, it should be sown in a cold frame in the very early spring and planted outdoors in May. Be patient, because it is slow to germinate; it has been known to take as long as two years. It can be grown in a woodland garden, in a rock garden, or as a border plant. It likes sandy, rocky, acidic soil and will do best in a sunny location. It can sometimes become invasive, however. Use thinnings to make a salve, oil, or liniment. The bees will rejoice at this new addition to your garden.

HARVESTING

Arnica flowers are best harvested from mid-June to early July, when the plant is beginning to bloom. At very high altitudes, blooming may occur in July or August. Roots are harvested in autumn. Harvesting only flowers is the kindest environmentally. In some areas arnica is a protected plant and should not be harvested at all. In Europe, for example, native populations of arnica have diminished and now must be considered endangered. Herbalists are concerned that the same situation is occurring in the United States; overharvesting and habitat destruction are severely depleting sources of wild arnica.

UpS RECOMMENDATIONS

- No harvesting of *A. montana* is recommended at this time; the species is threatened in its entire range in Europe (see www.traffic.org/plants/species). Use cultivated resources whenever possible.

- Possible alternatives include yerba del lobo (*Helenium hoopesii*), calendula, comfrey (for musculoskeletal concerns), and yarrow (for bruising).

- Use all aerial parts rather than just the flowers.

- Limit any wild harvest of American sources.

On that beautiful day when we collected arnica, we also found osha, another at-risk plant. We were lucky enough to find uva-ursi and usnea as well, which we were able to harvest. My friends and I promised each other that though we had found this magical place, we would not come back to collect here.

63

BLACK COHOSH
Cimicifuga racemosa

❧

MATTHEW WOOD

Although black cohosh is not native quite as far west and north as my farm, it remains one of my favorite medicinal plants. It is characteristic of the "Big Woods" of eastern North America and the herbal tradition of the eastern woodland Indians. Within this tradition we find a large number of "female medicines," of which black cohosh is probably the archetypal representative. We also find plants associated with medicine animals or spirits, because of a resemblance to an animal. Black snakeroot, one of black cohosh's aliases, also scores here; the emerging flower spike resembles a snake, and the seedpods rattle like a rattlesnake. It is one of the Indian "snake medicines" considered to have a great deal of power, not just medicinal but also transformative and psychological. And finally, the physical properties of the plant suggest its established uses; black cohosh is thus a plant that illustrates the ancient doctrine of signatures, the idea that an herb "looks like what it treats."

Black cohosh was one of the many important and distinctive remedies that the pioneers learned about from the Native Americans. Members of all the important medical schools of the nineteenth century, including the allopaths, homeopaths, Eclectics, and physio-medicalists, used it. It has proven to be a widely useful medicine. It not only acts on important and common physical problems but also has properties that run in a deep psychological vein. Today it is still widely used, both by the more scientific phytotherapists and by the traditional community of herbalists drawing on established lore.

BOTANICAL FEATURES

Cimicifuga racemosa is a member of the Buttercup, or Ranunculaceae, family. This makes it a cousin of goldenseal, columbine, *Anemone pulsatilla*, and many other denizens of the field and wood. It is closely related to the genus *Actaea*. Indeed, it was originally classified as a member of that group and still appears, sometimes, in the older medical literature under the name *Actaea racemosa*. It is closely allied with two rare cousins, *C. americana* and *C. cordifolia*, which also grow in the eastern United States, and with *C. elata*, a native of the Pacific Northwest. The latter is similar to the Eurasian species, *C. foetida*, which is official in Chinese herbalism.

The botanical kinship of *Cimicifuga racemosa* to *Anemone pulsatilla* is notable since the former is the most important female remedy in eastern American Indian medicine, while the latter is the most important member of this class in European homeopathy. Both are used for PMS, scanty menses, cramps, problems dating to the onset of menstruation, irregular menses in teenage girls, fluid retention, menopausal problems, and eruptive diseases. There are also differences: Black cohosh is suited to a dark, brooding mentality, whereas *A. Pulsatilla* has a happy/sad, changeable, yielding disposition.

Black cohosh is native from the Atlantic seaboard to Oklahoma, northward as far as the lower Great Lakes, and down the Appalachian Highlands into Georgia and Alabama. It commonly grows on lightly wooded hillsides and slopes, especially in association with oak openings. *C. racemosa* and *C. americana* are also widely grown as shady ornamentals.

Black cohosh is a perennial that establishes a knotted cluster of roots and rhizomes from which a number of stalks shoot up, dividing into a crown of leaves 1 to 2 feet above the ground. The leaves are described in technical terms as large, alternate, and ternately compound; the leaflets, ovate-oblong, incisely serrate, and opposite. From the crown of leaves emerge spikes or racemes that rise 3 to 9 feet with a few leaves here and there and toward their ends are lined by long rows of small, round, creamy white flowers that look like tiny clouds. The flowers have a strange smell that makes you feel as if you're enclosed in a stuffy room. In technical terms the flowers are described as follows: sepals four or five in number, rounded, and white; petals from four to six, small, not so long as the sepals; stamens numerous and showy; anthers introrse and white; stigma sessile and lateral in the capsules when mature.

Several features of the plant suggest the traditional medicinal uses. The stems unravel like the tops of a fiddlehead fern in the spring, resembling a fetus; black cohosh was one of the most important birthing herbs in American Indian practice. As the spikes rise high above the ground, the flowers appear in a line, making a picture of the human spine. The wind, catching them, snaps them back and forth. To my eye this suggests the use of the plant for whiplash. I have had great success here. More generally, black cohosh is used to soothe painful muscles, what today would be called fibromyalgia, and back problems. This is a medicine plant that looks like and acts strongly on the spine. It is an important remedy in congestion of the cerebrospinal fluids, nervous spasm, and muscular pain. The dark, massed, fibrous root suggests the idea of congestion, as does the curious smell of the flower, which creates a contained, entrapped feeling. Both of these signatures point to the use of black cohosh by those suffering from dark, black, introspective, brooding, melancholic moods, and this usage has long been established in homeopathy. All of these signatures point to the main uses of the plant: as a female and pregnancy medicine; as a neurological and muscular remedy; in meningeal, cerebral, and spinal problems; and for a dark, brooding state of mind, particularly before the menses.

HISTORICAL BACKGROUND

The name *cohosh* seems to come from an Algonquian word associated with pregnancy. The two cohoshs, black and blue, have long been used as parturient remedies. Indian women were famous for the ease of their deliveries, and this was one of the herbs used, in the last few weeks, in small doses, to instill a successful parturition. It was also used for menstrual problems, especially for difficulties in young women, irregular periods, or problems dating to the onset of menstruation.

Another set of uses is indicated by the names *black snakeroot* and *rattle root*. J. I. Lightall, the great Indian medicine man, says of the latter name: "When the stalk is shaken the seeds will rattle, producing a sound like that of a rattlesnake, from which it takes the name of rattle root."[1] The stalk also looks like a snake when it first begins to grow.

Cimicifuga was one of the important "snake roots" used in American Indian medicine. The Indians considered it an important remedy for snakebite, though scientific medical authorities disparaged this usage. As usual, such critical comments were offered without proof or testing. The same remarks were made about its reputation as a treatment for smallpox. Here, however, we do find medical doctors who observed its positive effects; also, the Chinese *Cimicifuga* is used to bring out the rash from "toxic fevers."

The snake medicines of American Indian lore are a group of plants that resemble a snake in one fashion or another. Other examples would include *Aristolochia serpentaria* (Virginia snakeroot), *Eryngium yuccifolium* (rattlesnake master), *Polygala seneca* (Seneca snakeroot), and even the naturalized *Plantago major* (plantain, snakeweed). All these plants are used as snakebite remedies but also have deeper psychospiritual associations and uses. When a plant resembles an animal, it becomes the conduit for that animal. Snake medicine thus conveys the spirit of the snake.

What does this mean? I think we can safely draw analogies between the American Indian snake medicines and other traditions that use this animal as a psychospiritual symbol and see it as a real, active-in-life power. It would be safe to say that the Native American concept of snake medicine is similar to the concept of *kundalini* or serpent power in Ayurvedic medicine. The latter is seen as an energy that rises up the spine, actualizing the intellectual, psychological, and psychic faculties but also bringing with it a fierce, magnetic, seductive, sometimes fear-inspiring and nerve-disturbing power that is a challenge to live with and adjust to. When it actualizes the psychic faculties, serpent power allows greater insight and awareness but also brings the challenge of dealing with knowledge and power.

It is a striking feature of black cohosh—one that I've often observed in my own practice—that people who need this remedy are characteristically very aware on a psychic level. Many of their problems come from feeling entrapped, addicted, or abused in some relationship that exerts a psychic grip upon them. Last year, for instance, I saw a woman who with no prodding at all described herself as a "psychic/intuitive transmedium"—a pretty sophisticated and self-knowledgeable concept for a twenty-two-year-old. She had all the characteristic symptoms calling for black cohosh: neurological shocks of energy, spasms, involuntary (but not consciousness-diminishing) convulsions, menin-geal swelling, stiff upper and lower back, irregular periods (her problems beginning with puberty), and brooding and pensive states of mind before her period, which became better as soon as her flow began. Her physicians, with rather less inventiveness, diagnosed her as suffering from a "brain virus" that was "unnamed." She is now fully recovered and leading a normal life for the first time since puberty.

The use of black cohosh as a remedy for female and other disorders was picked up by the early settlers and pioneers. Benjamin Smith Barton first mentions the plant's use as a medicine among the Indians and settlers in 1801. It already saw widespread acceptance for veterinary use in cattle, so the white settlers had been learning from their own experiences with it for some time. Smith notes that it was highly esteemed by the Native people. Both conventional and unconventional physicians used and wrote about black cohosh in the 1820s and 1830s. It became official in the *United States Pharmacopoeia* in 1830 and was widely used by the middle of the century. *Cimicifuga* was the favorite remedy of Dr. John King, one of the founding fathers of Eclecticism. The American Medical Association reviewed it in 1848 and, after skeptically dismissing many traditional uses, concluded that it was a nervine sedative of the highest rank. In particular, it was defined carefully as fitting cases where the pulse was rapid and forceful ("hard or tense"—the old terminology is rather vague), indicating nervous irritation. It remained official in the *United States Pharmacopoeia* until 1936 and in the *National Formulary* until 1950. It is still well regarded in European phytotherapy, as well as in North American herbalism.

In 1856 *Cimicifuga* was given a homeopathic proving by Dr. C. J. Hemple, and it has continued to be used extensively in homeopathy, though not as much so as its cousin *Anemone pulsatilla*. The homeopathic and botanical uses of *Cimicifuga* are essentially in agreement.

Modern research on *Cimicifuga* has not advanced very far. It has been shown to contain cimicifugin (an amorphous resinous body), a volatile oil, sugars, tannins, phosphates, and sulfates. It contains small amounts of estrogenlike substances—not enough to substitute for the hormone, but evidently enough to have a stimulating effect on hormonal processes.

MEDICINAL USES

The majority of nineteenth-century physicians determined black cohosh's center of action to be the nervous system. More specifically, it was associated with the cerebrospinal system. From my own experience, I believe that it acts through the cerebrospinal fluid. This would explain why it is so strongly associated with the nerves, but also why it influences conditions associated with menstruation and the economy of liquids in the body. A characteristic symptom observed by so many women who respond to black cohosh is significant: Moods and neurological symptoms are better by the onset of menses.

Poetically generalizing, I believe (along with the medieval European authors) that the cerebrospinal fluids, which circulate in and out of the ventricles of the brain and down each nerve fiber, which they coat and soothe, are the vehicle of the soul or psyche, and that the strong action of this plant on people who describe themselves as psychics and transmediums (able to pick up on and feel other people's feelings) is appropriate. The psychically bound-up, congested psychological state of the black cohosh person is analogous to the bound-up cerebrospinal fluid. I have seen the one loosen up with the other so many times I can hardly count them.

Once we understand these affinities, we see how black cohosh is a remedy that acts strongly on the brain, meninges, spine, nerves, and muscles. It is specifically indicated in cases where there is brooding, a dark state of mind, or entrapment in romantic, sexual, or business affairs. Use it also to treat conditions where there are inequalities of the "charge on the nerves"—so that there are sensations of shocks and streamings through the nerves—and as a remedy for congestion and pain in the muscles and muscular attachments. A highly characteristic symptom is swelling and pain in the attachments of the trapezius muscle to the top of the shoulder blade, usually on both sides. This symptom is well known to most bodyworkers. Furthermore, black cohosh seems to directly associate with the fluid economy, so that the neurological and muscular symptoms are better by the onset of the period or worse from the cessation of the menstrual cycle at menopause. The tonifying effect of *Cimicifuga* in late pregnancy is probably associated with its relaxing effect on the nerves and muscles and the decongesting effect on the fluids.

Cimicifuga figures prominently as a remedy for fevers that affect the nerves and meninges. It has a history of successful use in cerebral meningitis and is beneficial in people who have headaches and pains lingering after such diseases. As noted above, it lessens the frequency and tension of the pulse. Finally, both the American and the Chinese *Cimicifuga* have a long history of use to lessen the severity of smallpox and skin rashes. (Coincidentally, homeopathic *Anemone pulsatilla* is also used to treat chicken pox.) This widely scattered testimony refutes the skepticism of nineteenth-century authors, who were only too willing to dismiss the wisdom of the American Indian medicine people and illiterate pioneers who had long turned to black cohosh for such complaints.

One very important modern use of black cohosh is as a hypotensive to relieve high blood pressure. Research on animals has shown that it has the effect of decreasing vasomotor tensions caused by clamping and unclamping the carotid arteries.[2] The explanation for this hypotensive effect is probably that black cohosh decongests the head and brings the nervous system as a whole into a state of relative balance, relieving local congestion and generalizing tensions. Many chiropractors feel that in a significant percentage of high blood pressure cases, the problem lies in cerebral congestion.

Case histories in my books *Seven Herbs, Plants as Teachers* (1986) and *The Book of Herbal Wisdom* (1997) illustrate most of these uses. Temple Hoyne, *Clinical Therapeutics* (1879–1880), gives a good selection of case histories from homeopathic literature. A comprehensive account of *Cimicifuga racemosa*, including some case histories, is given by J. U. and C. G. Lloyd in *Drugs and Medicines of North America*, Bulletin No. 30 (1931). J. I. Lightall (c. 1875) gives an account largely based on the Indian experience mixed with Eclectic indications.

PREPARATION AND DOSAGE

Black cohosh preparations are almost uniformly made from the dried root or rhizome. However, the fresh substance has a life, smell, and taste that the dried does not possess; you cannot boast of having really tasted or known this medicine until you've tried the fresh article. It tastes, somehow, like the deep, humus-laden forest floor from whence it comes. Black cohosh contains an appreciable amount of sugars, making the flavor pleasant if not exactly sweet.

The original method of preparation was tea. Dr. William Cook, the physiomedicalist, notes that black cohosh tea should always be prepared *as an infusion*—not by boiling, as is customary with most medicinal roots. "The usual direction for preparing this infusion is to boil the root; but boiling, or even the use of boiling water, damages it greatly. Nothing above a lukewarm temperature should be employed. The infusion represents most fully the nervine qualities of the article."[3] The infusion is made by pouring 2 to 3 cups of water on 1 ounce of the powdered dried or bruised fresh root. Of this, a wineglassful may be taken two or three times a day. The dried root or rhizome is also available in tablets and capsules.

A simple tincture can be made from the fresh or dried article. The former yields a product so far superior in taste and medicinal effect as to be almost incomparable, in my opinion, but the latter is the usual source. Cook gives the formula: Macerate 4 ounces of bruised black cohosh root or rhizome in 2 cups of 50 percent alcohol for ten days and filter.

The official extract, according to the *United States Pharmacopoeia* of 1870 and subsequent editions, is made from 16 troy ounces of powdered *Cimicifuga* extracted in 2 cups of 85 percent alcohol according to the usual procedures. The great Eclectic pharmacist John Uri Lloyd approved of this method.

Cimicifuga is generally not considered to have strong toxic properties, but it can be upsetting. Gastrointestinal discomfort can occur; large doses may cause vertigo, headache, nausea, impaired vision, vomiting, and impaired circulation.[4] I have seen aggravations occur from standard doses of the capsule or extract, but this is entirely avoided in small doses, which do the job certainly and slowly. Black cohosh often has serious structural changes to make in a person, and I believe this should be achieved slowly.

I personally use black cohosh in very small doses of the tincture: 1 to 3 drops, one to three times a day, for about six weeks. For menstrual problems, give the dose for two weeks before the period, for perhaps three cycles. J. I. Lightall gives the dose as 1 to 30 drops, with the average dosage being 5 to 10 drops of the tincture in water four times a day.[5]

"The combinations into which it may suitably enter are numerous, according to the end sought," remarks Dr. Cook. "With aralia hispida and fraxinus for dropsy, with cypripedium and scutellaria for neuralgic affections, with xanthoxylum or jeffersonia or the berries of phytolacca for rheumatism, with liriodendron and caulophylum in hysteria and other general spasms, etc."[6] These are mostly American Indian remedies and formulations. Pokeroot, prickly ash, and black cohosh, in equal parts, and in small doses, is an old remedy for rheumatic complaints.

A famous compound designed for the neurological effect is the B & B formula developed by Dr. John Christopher. Herbalist Terry Willard calls this "one of the most famous formulas" in Western herbalism. It consists of equal parts of blue vervain, black cohosh, blue cohosh, skullcap, and lobelia. Willard comments, "I have found this formula valuable for hiccups, ear infections, and medulla oblongata damage, and especially when medulla damage is caused by abuse of hallucinogenic drugs. It is also useful for asthma, whooping cough, and chorea."[7] *Chorea* is an old name for "spasm."

I once mixed up some B & B formula for an elderly woman who was using it to remove a tumor on the palate of her mouth. The first batch I made using black cohosh tinctured fresh, the second from the usual commercial extract made from the dried rhizome. A few weeks after leaving with the second formula, she came back to me very angry. She thought I was trying to rip her off. I didn't understand what she was talking about until she brought in the remnant of the first bottle to compare with the second bottle. The tastes were entirely different, and the commercial batch was not as good. Finally I realized that the difference was due to the substitution of black cohosh made from the dried article for that made from the fresh. This was the first time I became aware of the significant difference between these two forms of preparation.

PROPAGATION AND CULTIVATION

For technical information about propagation, I sought the help of horticulturist Heather McCargo, who passed on to me the following information. Black cohosh can easily be grown from seeds. It can also be propagated by breaking up the crown, but this is more tedious and does not yield as many plants. The seeds need to be stratified in a sequence of warm temperature, followed by cold for several months, and then warm again. The reason for this is to mimic the conditions of the central temperate region, where black cohosh grows wild, ripening its seeds in midsummer. It can be sown in the ground right then and will sprout the following spring. Farther north it does not ripen its seeds until August. This seems to be a limiting factor—causing it not to propagate naturally in the northern climes, since the seeds need warm, cold, warm stratification. If you do this artificially, the seeds will be ready to sprout in the spring.

Although *Cimicifuga* is native to woodlands, it is readily cultured in the sunlight, hence it can be grown fairly easily as a crop. This is important, since it is widely used in traditional and modern herbal medicine. This is one plant we should not be exterminating in the wild.

HARVESTING

The roots and rhizomes are dug in the fall, after the seeds have matured. Wash the dirt out of the fibrous, dense, compacted mass, then break apart the roots and rhizomes, spread them out, and slowly dry them in semishade. As mentioned above, the fresh article has more intense properties.

UpS RECOMMENDATIONS

- No wild harvest is recommended at this time.
- Purchase cultivated resources.
- Possible alternatives include yucca for musculoskeletal concerns; skullcap for headache relief, mood swings, and anxiety; and pulsatilla, motherwort, and chaste berries for general substitution.

NOTES

1. Lightall, *The Indian Folk Medicine Guide*, 47.

2. Mowrey, *Herbal Tonic Therapies*, 331.

3. Cook, *The Physio-Medical Dispensatory*, 344.

4. McGuffin, et al., *Botanical Safety Handbook*, 29.

5. Cook, *The Physio-Medical Dispensatory*, 344.

7. Willard, *Textbook of Modern Herbology*, 250.

REFERENCES

Cook, William. *The Physio-Medical Dispensatory*. 1st ed., 1869. Reprint, Portland, Oreg.: Eclectic Medical Publications, 1985.

Hoyne, Temple. *Clinical Therapeutics*. 2 vols. 1979–1980. Reprint, New Delhi: B. Jain Publisher, 1984.

Lightall, J. I. *The Indian Folk Medicine Guide*. c. 1875. Reprint, New York: Popular Library, 1973.

Lloyd, J. U., and C. G. Lloyd. *Drugs and Medicines of North America*. Bulletin No. 30, Reproduction Series No. 9. Part 2. Cincinnati: Lloyd Library of Botany, Pharmacy, and Materia Medica, 1931.

McGuffin, Michael, Christopher Hobbs, Roy Upton, and Alicia Goldberry. *Botanical Safety Handbook*. New York: CRC Press, 1997.

Mowrey, Daniel B. *Herbal Tonic Therapies*. New York: Wings Books, 1993.

Willard, Terry. *Textbook of Modern Herbology*. Calgary: Progressive Publishing, 1988.

Wood, Matthew. *Seven Herbs, Plants as Teachers*. Berkeley, Calif.: North Atlantic Books, 1986.

———. *The Book of Herbal Wisdom*. Berkeley, Calif.: North Atlantic Books, 1997.

BLOODROOT
Sanguinaria canadensis

PAM MONTGOMERY

My first encounter with bloodroot was in the woodlands of New York state. I was walking through the woods in the early spring and came across a small patch of exquisitely beautiful white flowers whose leaves were just beginning to form. I was so taken by these flowers that I stopped and sat down in order to observe them more closely. I had no idea what these stunning blooms could be. As I sat and looked at the delicate blossoms I was overcome with a deep peace. I closed my eyes and saw the Buddha sitting on a lotus blossom. This lovely little white flower reminded me of the many-petaled lotus. It wasn't how it looked, but more the energy that emanated from it that struck me. I called it the northeastern lotus until I discovered that its common name was bloodroot.

Years later, while studying plant spirit medicine with Eliot Cowan, I journeyed to the spirit of Bloodroot. I found myself deep in a forest glade where there were very bright lights, almost blinding to the eyes. This was where the spirit of Bloodroot lived. She appeared to me as a very kind older woman dressed in a shimmering silver gown. She looked almost like Glinda, the Good Witch of the North. She had what

seemed like a wand but it could also have been a walking stick. I asked her about the gifts that she offered to people. She said that her main gift was that of purity: She purified the blood, the emotions, and the spirit. She cautioned me to use her sparingly because her gift was so powerful. Her gift was to be used only in special cases. She then asked me if I wanted her to enter into me, to which, of course, I said yes. She touched me with her staff and I fell into an altered state of indescribable peace and clarity— purity of spirit.

BOTANICAL FEATURES

Bloodroot is a member of the Poppy family, which in Latin is known as the Papaveraceae. It is an herbaceous perennial native to North America. The solitary flowers are among the first to appear in early spring, doing so before the leaves have fully opened. They are 1 to 2 inches across with anywhere from seven to sixteen petals. The leaves are unique in appearance and provide an easy way to identify bloodroot. They begin by protectively wrapping themselves around the flower bud. Once opened, they are palmate in shape with deep lobes grooved out of each. The edges are scalloped. The leaves can reach 8 inches across at maturity, and the entire plant can grow from 6 to 14 inches in height. The rhizome—from which bloodroot received its common name—is the medicinal part of the plant. When cut, the horizontal rhizome exudes a reddish orange juice. Bloodroot grows in moist, deciduous woods and woodland slopes.

HISTORICAL BACKGROUND

Bloodroot's name comes from the fact that the root exudes a red juice similar to the color of human blood. Other common names are Indian paint, tetterwort, red puccoon, red root, coon root, snakebite, and sweet slumber. Many Native tribes used the juice of the root to decoratively paint their skin for ceremony. A bachelor of the Ponca tribe would use bloodroot as a love charm by rubbing the root on the palm of his hand and then shaking hands with the woman he wished to marry. After five or six days, if the charm was successful she would be willing to marry him.

The juice was also used to dye cloth and baskets. *Puccoon* is the Native name for bloodroot; *coon root* is the white man's distortion of this Native term. Bloodroot got the name *tetterwort* because it was used for skin infections, as well as ringworm, fungal growths, and warts. *Tetter* is an outdated term for blisterlike skin diseases such as herpes, ringworm, and eczema. The name *sweet slumber* likely comes from the fact that bloodroot is a member of the Poppy family and

contains protopine, an alkaloid also found in opium, thus giving it mild narcotic effects. I can find no references to bloodroot's use for snakebites in any of the literature; however, plants receive names for a reason. If you find yourself in the woods on a warm, sunny spring day and happen to surprise an eastern timber rattler sunning itself on a rock, don't ignore the bloodroot that may be growing within reach if you are bitten.

The Delaware Indians revered bloodroot, chewing a bit of root daily to maintain general good health. Like many Native tribes, they used it for conditions of the blood, feeling that it was purifying in such cases. Iroquois women used bloodroot for many of their "particular problems," as well as other problems associated with blood such as cuts, wounds, hemorrhages, and ulcers. Both the Potowatomi and Ojibwa squeezed the juice onto a lump of maple sugar, then let it melt in the mouth to treat sore throats much the way we use cough drops. N. R. Farnsworth notes, "Cherokee Indians employed extracts of this plant as a remedy for breast cancer as early as 1857, and it has been used empirically as a cancer remedy in Russia." At the same time that Native peoples were using bloodroot for cancer, Dr. Fells, a nineteenth-century physician, was successfully treating cancer patients. "Dr. Fells mixed bloodroot, flour, water, and zinc chloride together and applied this paste to cancers. Twenty-five breast cancers were treated in this manner at Middlesex Hospital in London, and this therapy was more successful than surgery" (Bolyard, 1981).

Bloodroot was listed in the *United States Pharmacopoeia* from 1820 to 1910, and in the

National Formulary from 1925 to 1965. It was classified as a stimulating expectorant, emetic, tonic, and alterative.

MEDICINAL AND OTHER USES

Sanguinaria canadensis received its Latin name from the word *sanguine*, which means "consisting of or relating to blood." Sanguinarine, the plant's predominant alkaloid (considered poisonous), can cause slight central nervous system depression and narcosis if taken internally. It also is known to disturb mitosis. At the same time, it has been found to have antimicrobial, anesthetic, and anticancer properties. Bloodroot is pharmacologically active, containing many other alkaloids, including alpha-allocryptopine, beta-allocryptopine, berberine, chelerythrine, chelilutine, chelirubine, coptisine, homochelidonine, oxysanguinarine, protopine, pseudochelerythrine, sanguidimerine, sanguilutine, and sanguirubine. The FDA has classified bloodroot as an unsafe herb. In large doses it causes burning in the stomach, paralysis, vomiting, faintness, vertigo, eye irritation, and, in James Duke's experience, "tunnel vision after chewing a small bite of rhizome." Regardless of its potentially toxic properties, Peter Good, in his *Materia Medica Botanica*, writes, "This plant is one of the most valuable medicinal articles of our country, and is already very generally introduced into practice. Few medical plants unite so many useful properties: but it requires to be administered with great care and skill, without which it may prove dangerous."

Bloodroot's medicinal use has been extensive.

Its most common use by Eclectic herbalists was in the treatment of bronchitis. It has stimulating properties and is expectorant, and at the same time has a relaxing action on the bronchial muscles. Its antispasmodic properties have made it useful as a cough remedy as well as an effective treatment for asthma, croup, and laryngitis. There are other indications of its use as an emmenagogue, in heart disease with weakness and palpitation of the heart, as a snuff for nasal polyps, and externally for various skin conditions including fungal growths, ulcers, and fleshy growths. It has fallen out of common use, most likely because of its potential toxic side effects, except as an escharotic salve for skin and breast cancers and as a useful plaque deterrent in mouth rinses and toothpastes. Even though bloodroot is primarily indicated for external use with cancer, I recall a conversation with Dr. Gary Glum (revivalist of the Essiac formula) during which he indicated that the original Ojibwa formula possibly contained bloodroot instead of turkey rhubarb root.

Several years ago I was in Montana with my friend Brooke Medicine Eagle. I showed her a patch of skin on my face that was red and had been so for quite some time. She encouraged me to put on it a salve called Compound X, which is known to have bloodroot as a main ingredient. Her brother had given it to her to use on a carcinoma on her nose. He had had much success himself using it on cows with ulcerations. Brooke told me she put this black salve on her nose and covered it with a Band-Aid. A week later she removed the Band-Aid; a black scab had formed over the application site. She removed the scab, put on more salve, and waited another week. When she removed the Band-Aid the second time, she found a small hole in her nose. She began to work at it and knead it. Eventually, a long, black, stringy substance came out of the hole in her nose. The carcinoma had shriveled. Within a couple weeks the hole closed, and only a tiny scar remained.

After hearing her story, I was game to try the salve. I applied it just as she had and left a Band-Aid on for a week. At the end of a week I took the Band-Aid off; a black scab had formed. I didn't touch the scab, letting it fall off by itself. New pink skin was forming. After the skin healed, I realized I had missed a patch. I applied salve there, using more this time. When the skin healed there was a small white scar. Apparently, I had actually burned my skin. Other than this scar my skin remained clear for some time, and then the patch of red skin gradually reappeared. In thinking back, I wonder about all the variables. Perhaps I should have applied a cell proliferant such as comfrey to help regenerate healthy cells, or maybe I should have kept the skin from sun exposure until it had healed completely. One thing I do know is that more is not always better.

In his book *Spontaneous Healing* Andrew Weil reports a more successful outcome to the use of bloodroot salve. "On the second day of applying the paste (to a pigmented mole that had been enlarging), the skin around the base of the mole became inflamed, an obvious immune reaction, and John said it was quite sore. On the third day, the mole turned pale and began to swell. On the fourth day, it fell off, leaving a perfectly circular wound that healed quickly."

More recently I have used bloodroot as one of the ingredients in mouth rinse that I make for myself. I have had a long history of bone loss and gum disease. I use the mouth rinse daily in a maintenance program to reduce plaque and strengthen gum tissue. Bloodroot is effective in vitro against oral bacteria that is known to cause plaque formation. It is a major ingredient in Viadent toothpaste and mouth rinse.

In veterinary medicine, bloodroot leaf is used to destroy botfly larvae on horses.

Bloodroot flowers are made into a flower essence by Kate Gilday of Woodland Essence. See her description of this flower's gifts on page 57.

Bloodroot's other uses are primarily as a dye plant and for body painting. Using bloodroot as a dye works best on wool and silk. You can obtain a range of colors, depending on whether you use a mordant or not. To obtain an orange color use no mordant at all; a mordant of alum and cream of tartar leaves a rust color; tin creates a reddish pink shade. For best results use the root of bloodroot fresh-harvested in the fall.

The Native American custom of painting the body with bloodroot is being resurrected these days, too. Many young people are turning to body painting as an outward expression that is much less permanent than tattooing. My most recent experience with this art form was with Nance Dean, an apprentice of mine, in 1999. She had chosen bloodroot as her plant ally for the duration of the apprentice program. At our closing ceremony each apprentice presented his or her plant ally. Nance's presentation included elaborate decoration of her skin with the fresh juice of the bloodroot rhizome. She proceeded to paint everyone's skin, leaving us looking more like an aboriginal tribe than middle-class white Americans.

PREPARATION AND DOSAGE

Bloodroot can be prepared in many ways. Traditionally, it was decocted by placing 1 teaspoon of dried rhizome in 1 cup of cold water and bringing it to a boil. Then it was left to steep for ten minutes. Drink 1 teaspoon three to six times a day. Bloodroot may be tinctured by using the spring or fall fresh-harvested rhizome. Chop the rhizome and add it to 50 percent dilute grain alcohol. An average dosage of tincture is 1 to 2 ml (1 ml equals approximately 25 drops) three times a day.

There are many cautions against using large doses of bloodroot. One woman friend of mine reported nausea and spaced-out feelings after ingesting one dropperful (30 drops) of bloodroot tincture. My recommendation would be to stay on the low end of the dosage range (10 drops three times per day in a little water) until you determine your sensitivity to the herb.

Bloodroot can also be dried and powdered. Taken as a dried powder, an average dosage is 10 to 30 grains (a grain is 0.002083 ounce). Bloodroot may be made into an oil by slow heat extraction in olive oil. Melt beeswax in the oil to bring the mixture to a salve consistency. As an escharotic salve, bloodroot powder is blended with lard to make a thick paste for external application. The proportions are approximately 1 ounce of powdered root to 3 ounces of lard.

The fresh root poultice may be directly applied to skin eruptions and cancerous lesions.

PROPAGATION AND CULTIVATION

Bloodroot is hardy to Zone 3 and likes a soil temperature of 60–70 degrees for best germination. It prefers partial shade but can grow in full sun. Ideally, the soil will be a moist, well-drained, rich, sandy loam. You can easily cultivate bloodroot from seeds, but it must be planted fresh; you thus need to watch vigilantly for seed maturity (usually midsummer to fall). If you do let the seeds dry out, the germination rate decreases significantly. Germination is usually in the spring after one or two seasons. Richo Cech of Horizon Herbs reports, "The seed has an eliasome [fatty protruberence] which attracts ants to carry it away to their nests. Then, the ants remove the eliasome and discard the [still viable] seed, which then has a chance to grow at some distance from its mother." Propagation of bloodroot can also be accomplished by rhizome division. Break off the side shoots and replant immediately to avoid root rot. Plant the bud facing upward $1/2$ inch deep. Covering with well-decayed leaf mulch enhances growth.

HARVESTING

Harvest bloodroot rhizomes and roots in fall after the leaf has died back, or in very early spring at the onset of leaf emergence. Bloodroot should be laid out to dry on screens in a well-ventilated and very dry room where absolutely no moisture can get back into the plant material after the drying process has begun. Bloodroot is highly susceptible to rot and will deteriorate quickly if not dried in a timely manner and then stored in an airtight container. Do not cut the rhizome and root into pieces for drying; leave them whole. The precious juices exude profusely from the plant when it is cut.

UpS RECOMMENDATIONS

- Use cultivated resources only.

- As an alternative, celandine may be used. Also, for respiratory issues, skin conditions, and antimicrobial action, rosemary is a good substitute.

The lush carpets of bloodroot that once existed in the Northeast are vanishing. You still find occasional large stands, such as in the Adirondack Park of New York state. I really don't know why the plant is disappearing. I doubt that it is from overharvest, since bloodroot is an herb used with caution; only the experienced herbalist feels comfortable with its application. Even though it is used in commercial dental products, it is still not commonplace because of discrepancies in clinical trials. Could this be one of our native plants that is being lost to a population explosion or perhaps environmental pollutants? Only further investigation can answer this question. Thankfully, in the right conditions bloodroot does well under cultivation, and it makes a beautiful garden flower, too. In order to allow our wild populations to reestablish themselves, avoid plants from wild sources.

I recall my first encounter with bloodroot years ago and the breathtaking beauty of its flower. I was so hungry for flowers after the long, cold winter. Now I anxiously await bloodroot's arrival each spring, and the promise of renewal that it brings.

REFERENCES

Bolyard, Judith L. *Medicinal Plants and Home Remedies of Appalachia*. Springfield, Ill.: Charles C. Thomas, 1981.

Duke, James A. *Handbook of Medicinal Herbs*. Boca Raton, Fla.: CRC Press, 1985.

Elliott, Doug. *Wild Roots: A Forager's Guide to the Edible and Medicinal Roots, Tubers, Corms, and Rhizomes of North America*. Rochester, Vt.: Healing Arts Press, 1995.

Good, Peter. *Materia Medica Botanica*. Vol. 1. Elizabethtown, N.J.: author.

Grieve, Mrs. Maude. *A Modern Herbal*. Vol. 1. New York: Dover Publishing, 1971.

Hoffmann, David. *Therapeutic Herbalism*. Correspondence course. Sebastopol, Calif.: author.

Kowalchik, Hylton, et al. *Rodale's Illustrated Encyclopedia of Herbs*. Emmaus, Penn.: Rodale Press, 1987.

Lawrence Review. Nov. 1986.

Leung, Albert, and Steven Foster. *Encyclopedia of Common Natural Ingredients Used in Food, Drugs, and Cosmetics*, 2d ed. Glen Rock, N.J.: John Wiley and Sons, 1995.

Lloydia 3 (2). Jan. 1970.

Moerman, Daniel. *Geraniums for the Iroquois*. Algonac, Mich.: Reference Publications, 1981.

Weil, Andrew. *Spontaneous Healing*. New York: Alfred A. Knopf, 1995.

BLUE COHOSH
Caulophyllum thalictroides

RICHO CECH

Big weather was on the way. The high white clouds of an eastern Ohio spring gave way to a steely overcast. The radio was full of storm reports. Twisters had already touched down in a few surrounding counties, and flood warnings had been issued for Meigs County, where the newly formed United Plant Savers board was sequestered for a three-day seminal gathering. I personally hoped that the floods would detain us longer in this rich botanical paradise, but kept a wary eye out for funnel clouds.

From my vantage point on the porch of the cabin, I watched as the first rain of the afternoon, carried by skittish winds, effaced all reflections from the surface of the overfull pond. The geese with goslings had taken cover, and the catfish and carp no longer rolled in the shallows but waited in the deeps. Herbalists came hurrying back out of the woods, where many had disappeared for a short botanical break from our discussions.

We gathered around a small fire in the main room of the cabin and got back to work. Then somebody noticed that one of our members was missing. Who had been with her in the woods? Where had she last been seen? Someone went

to check the outhouse and the kitchen. A gale of wind shook the cabin with window-rattling force, followed by a conversation-stopping roll of thunder. Soon the reports came back. She had last been seen up on the ridge trail, and as far as we could tell, she had not come down. Suspending all thoughts of the meeting, we donned our boots and went back up into the woods.

When botanizing among the hills and hollows of our eastern hardwood forests, stopping here to appreciate a trillium, walking beneath the spreading branches of a tulip poplar, observing the seeding habits of goldenseal and bloodroot, it is delightfully easy to go on for miles without really taking account of the lay of the land. Clear trails give way to deer trails, which lead to denser forest or drop down into creekbeds. One "holler" looks like the next. Not wanting to add my name to the list of the lost, I kept careful track of where my footsteps were leading and tried to maintain visual contact with the others who were headed in the same direction, combing the woods. Our calls weren't carrying far, being nearly drowned out by the sound of rain against turgid leaves. Where could she have gone? We reached the spot where she had last been seen and split up from there, some going up the ridge, some milling around, the rest going down the trail.

I passed the paw paw patch, the plants' big dog-tongue leaves dripping a bit disconsolately, and headed down toward Ramp Holler. Although concerned about our lost comrade, I was beginning to feel the thrill of being out in the woods in a storm, and at this moment realized that I was alone. There was a flash of light and a simultaneous clap of thunder, which brought me to my knees. A sassafras tree on the slope disappeared into a thousand pieces of smoldering punk. Giving a silent prayer that this was not where our lost soul had chosen to weather out the storm, I got back on my feet and hightailed it for lower ground.

The path was overrun with water. I glimpsed a broken bloodroot, looking like the red end of a dismembered finger, eroding from the bank where a small switchback led down toward the creek bottoms. The path was brown with mud. Then, like diving into a deep pool, I found myself down among the blue cohosh at the base of the deep draw, sheltered from the storm. It was as if these plants had been waiting for me. They grew everywhere here, awake, their distinct three-lobed leaves beautifully raised to the water filtering down out of the sky, holding silent dominion. And they were letting me in.

Walking carefully now to avoid treading on any plants, I found a rocky outcrop, sat down on the moss, closed my eyes, and felt my heart return to a slow *thrub-drub*. Is it possible for plants to speak to humans? Or to somehow purify and reflect our own thoughts? At this

moment I knew, very simply, that everything was all right. Our lost comrade would be found. The storm would play itself out, and the searchers would straggle in from the woods. Paul would stoke up the little fire in the cabin by the pond. We would all be together again, and there would be tea.

Not being one for rain gear, I had worn two denim jackets, which were quickly absorbing water as I sat on the rock. Their pockets were stuffed with my damp little treasures: broken arrowheads, a half-used packet of pea seeds, matches, fencing staples, a collection of lint going back to sometime before my hair had any gray in it. I fished out a piece of a tobacco plug, which had been twisted the year before from leaves grown and cured in Oregon. It was hard for me to find a spot below the blue cohosh that was not covered with some kind of delicate growth, such as ramps or violets, but I pulled back some moss and nestled the tobacco down into the forest loam. This was my offering, giving thanks to the plants for being there, a prayer of hope for all lost humans.

BOTANICAL FEATURES

Shy of people and traffic, blue cohosh inhabits the low ravines and hollows of northern Appalachia. When conditions are ideal, this plant can spread in large thigh-high patches that shade the deep, loamy soil of the forest with soft foliage. Growing from a perennial crown, the plant unfolds in early spring as a forked stalk bearing purplish, three-lobed leaves. As the plant matures, the leaves take on a soothing and characteristic blue-green color. The inconspicuous brown, green, and yellow flower is star shaped, and sometimes by a quirk of nature appears immediately as the plant emerges in the spring. The flower gives way to several pea-sized seeds (drupes), dark blue, which appear in clusters above the foliage of the plant. They ripen in August. These seeds are the most significant identifying characteristic of the plant, and have led to the common name *blueberry*. The plant collapses with late-summer drought or certainly by the first frosts, contributing more organic loam to the soil, which will nourish it again come spring. When the stalks of blue cohosh die back, they leave craterlike stem scars on the rhizome, which are to the trained eye characteristic identifying features.

HISTORICAL BACKGROUND

Prior to the time of European settlement Native Americans knew the uses of blue cohosh, and employed it commonly. The roots were dug, washed, and made into a tea while still fresh or dried for later use. The herb was taken to treat "fits and hysterics," to alleviate inflammation of the womb and menstrual cramping, and to facilitate childbirth.

Peter Smith was a traveling preacher who learned much from the Natives and wrote one of the earliest treatises on the use of native medicinal plants, called *The Indian Doctor's Dispensatory* (1812). He writes, "When a woman finds that she is in labor, let her drink [blue cohosh root tea] . . . having her help at hand—if it is not her time, she will probably get easy and be well; but if it is her time, expect the delivery will be facilitated with much safety."

The Eclectic physicians used this herb in small quantities during the course of a pregnancy, due to its unique ability to both decrease the activity of premature contractions (antiabortifacient effect) and improve the quality of contractions during labor. In the nineteenth century, pharmacist John Uri Lloyd and Dr. Harvey Felter considered blue cohosh "one of our oldest Eclectic remedies."

MEDICINAL USES

Traditional uses of blue cohosh hold true to this day. The herb has a profound normalizing effect on the uterus, stemming excessive menstruation or bringing on a delayed period, as need dictates. It will promote regular menstrual discharge while lessening the severity of cramping. Most important, it is a superior *partus preparator* that may be used during overterm pregnancies and during childbirth to ease delivery, lessen pain in labor, reduce the incidence of false labor pains, increase the effectiveness of contractions (speed dilation), and afford rapid recovery after birth.

Blue cohosh stimulates the pituitary gland to signal increased production of a substance known as oxytocin, a hormone that stimulates labor, increases the force of contractions, and helps contract the uterine muscle after delivery of the placenta. In prescribing blue cohosh, most modern herbalists have taken a conservative approach, suggesting that it should not be used during early pregnancy due to the possible (though unlikely) risk of miscarriage. Certainly blue cohosh may be safely employed during menstruation, in the last week or two before birth, and during labor.

PREPARATION AND DOSAGE

When broken apart, the dried root gives off an acrid dust that can be quite unpleasant when inhaled, so it is advisable to wear a protective mask during grinding. Chewing on the fresh root is also not advised, because it can cause temporary discomfort of the mucous membranes of mouth and throat.

Mrs. Maude Grieve describes the preparation of the dried root powder for tea: "Decoction or infusion. 1 oz of root to 1 pint of boiling water macerated for $1/_2$ hour. Dose, 2 to 4 fluid ounces three or four times a day."

At the Herb Pharm Analytical Laboratory, an unpublished chromatographic study designed to test the efficacy of fresh root extraction in comparison to extraction of the dried root was performed. The purpose of this experiment was to compare the relative strength of fresh and dried plant extracts of blue cohosh, with an eye toward making the most efficient use of available active constituents. The constituents measured in this analysis were the alkaloids aporphine and magnoflorine; the saponin caulosaponin; triterpenes; and steroids. The alcohol contents of each extract were equilibrated at 70 percent. On the basis of the dry weight, the same amount of root went into each extraction. The results showed that for all parameters tested, the fresh extract contained more of the active constituents than the extract of dried root. In other words, some of the active chemistry of the root is lost during the drying process. Both extracts were a light yellowish brown color. The fresh extract tasted slightly more bitter, and the dried extract was earthier in flavor. Still, for therapeutic purposes the extracts of both the dried and the fresh root make useful preparations. Speaking purely from a plant-protection stance, it is probably wiser to use the roots in their fresh (undried) form because they are more potent. The optimum dosage of any given preparation must be determined from experience and altered according to the potency of the medicine, the sensitivity of the individual being treated, the severity of the problem, and the degree of activity desired.

PROPAGATION AND CULTIVATION

Blue cohosh prefers low ground, deep shade, and a moist, loamy soil. The plant grows best under the shade of mixed hardwoods and as part of a community consisting of the plants that normally accompany it in the wild, such as bloodroot, black cohosh, ginseng, goldenseal, ramps, and violets. Creating a diverse cropping system—that is, interspersing beds of the main crop with plantings of natural companion species—helps the plants sequester the soil bacteria and fungi that assist in nutrient assimilation and protect them from insects, parasites, and disease organisms.

My experience with propagating by root division has been mixed. Moving the entire dormant roots (intact in a ball of soil) a short distance gives reliable results, as long as the correct environmental requirements are met and the transplant is done quickly and without much trauma. Long transport times for bare rootstock should be avoided, because the rootlets tend to mold, which reduces vigor and decreases survival rate. The rhizome may be divided into two or more pieces. Fall transplanting of pieces of the rhizome that contain at least one nascent bud will almost always produce a plant the following spring. Pieces of rhizome that do not show a visible bud are less likely to produce a plant in the first year, but may emerge as a healthy new plant in the second. Spring transplants generally lie dormant until the following spring. The new plants are usually quite tiny in the first year of growth, but given the right conditions they will get much larger in their second year. After three years of growth the roots may be large enough to harvest, but the longer the plants stay in the ground, the bigger they get.

Dry-stored seeds are not viable. Fresh seeds can be sown immediately in permanent, shaded beds, or stored through the winter months in the refrigerator (put them in a plastic bag with moist peat moss), then sown outdoors in the spring. The seeds may begin to produce rootlets in the refrigerator, but this is not a cause for alarm. Fresh seeds can also be sown in pots or flats and kept moist and shaded until germination. Once seedlings emerge, they are grown out in the original container or in a nursery bed for a full summer season, then transplanted in the fall to permanent, shaded beds.

In the wild the natural process of regeneration via seeds will be encouraged if you take fresh, mature seeds from the plants and push them into the surrounding soil about $1/2$ inch deep. Areas where blue cohosh has been harvested are prime replanting grounds. Each seed puts down a 4-inch root system during its first year of growth, then produces an aerial sprout in its second spring, about eighteen months after planting. This is a long time. The adaptive advantage of this two-phase germination is that the rooted seed emerges vigorously early in the spring, prior to the emergence of many other herbaceous plants that would otherwise shade it.

HARVESTING

Fresh blue cohosh roots can be dug in the fall or early winter, after the plant has disseminated its seeds and after the stems begin to die back. The root consists of a horizontal rhizome and many matted rootlets. Traditionally, the whole root is taken up; in a dense stand, where the roots of several plants are intertwined, there is a tendency to remove many plants simultaneously. If you're harvesting like this, it is important to remember to leave behind a generous quantity of entire roots interspersed throughout the digging area, in order to assure regeneration. Unlike goldenseal, the plant does not readily regenerate from root hairs or small pieces of the rhizome left in the disturbed soil after digging. Instead of harvesting entire roots—which kills the plant—it is possible to expose the rhizome, breaking off a portion from behind the pre-emergent bud, leaving the younger portion of the rhizome intact with rootlets and bud attached. Then return soil around the remaining rhizome; the plant will continue to grow the following year.

UpS RECOMMENDATIONS

• Some limited wild harvest is permissible.

• Motherwort is a possible alternative to blue cohosh.

Given the difficulties involved with propagation of this timid plant, the increasing popularity of herbal medicine in general, and the very specific and limited wild habitat required for its healthy growth, it is difficult to predict a rosy future for blue cohosh. Probably the most significant gains can be made in the areas of wild cultivation and very conscientious wildcrafting—the kind in which, as Paul Strauss says, "Harvesting and planting are one and the same." The deep woodland coves where blue cohosh holds silent court are themselves precious jewels. These places beg respect. It is up to us to learn to hear the voice of the plants, and treat every wild place like our own irreplaceable garden.

REFERENCES

Felter, Harvey Wickes, M.D., and John Uri Lloyd. *King's American Dispensatory*. Vol. 1. 1898. Reprint, Portland, Oreg.: Eclectic Medical Publications, 1983.

Grieve, Mrs. Maude. *A Modern Herbal*. Vol 1. 1931. Reprint, New York: Dover, 1971.

Hamel, Paul B., and Mary U. Chiltoskey. *Cherokee Plants and Their Uses*. Sylva, N.C.: Herald Publishing, 1975.

Smith, Peter. *The Indian Doctor's Dispensatory*. Bulletin No. 2. Cincinnati: Lloyd Library of Botany, Pharmacy, and Materia Medica, 1812.

Amarquaye, Ambrose, and Richard A. Cech. "Comparative Study on Blue Cohosh." Williams, Oreg.: Herb Pharm Analytical Laboratory (Ed Smith, director), 1998.

CALAMUS ROOT
Acorus calamus

DON BABINEAU

Calamus is a reedlike aquatic plant inhabiting small streams, mountain bogs, edges of ponds, lakes, and creeks—wherever marshy conditions exist. In upstate New York I have found calamus growing along slow-moving, clear-water streams that wind through deep, muddy soil. The underlying meshlike root system of this plant helps maintain the muddy banks, securing its special aquatic environment. Cattails and other reeds may share such a bog, as may several types of willow and the marsh marigold (*Caltha palustris*).

BOTANICAL FEATURES

Calamus, or sweet flag, is a perennial herb with an extensive root system made up of segmented rhizomes from which small white rootlets spread into the soil. The leaves of the plant grow directly out of the rhizomes, extending 3 to 4 feet in height. The tall leaves are slightly sword shaped, resembling those of the cattail. Another plant with which it may be confused is blue flag (*Iris versicolor*), also known as poison flag. Take special care in making a positive identification if you are harvesting calamus. Fortunately, the unique and aromatic smell of crushed calamus leaves is a sure way of identifying this wetland plant. The leaf scars on the rhizome indicate the plant's growth in previous years. The flower heads emerge from a triangular stem about 12 to 18 inches from the ground. These heads are shaped like a finger, jutting upward at a slight angle. The tiny flowers covering the head are yellow. In my experiences growing calamus in our garden and finding it in several wetland areas, I have seen the unusual flowers each summer. However, a number of reference books suggest that these flowers may be rare and that, in North America, the production of seeds is questionable. It is thought that the insects necessary for pollinating the sweet-scented flowers are not present here. It would be interesting to attempt to hand-pollinate these flowers to produce berries and seeds.

HISTORICAL BACKGROUND

Calamus is diverse in its range. Because of its medicinal uses, it has been cultivated in many parts of the world. Its native range seems to be northern India and China, where its use goes back to ancient times. It has been naturalized in Asia Minor, Russia, Southeast Asia, and in several European countries. It seems to be indigenous to North America. Calamus may have migrated here with early tribes moving across the land bridge from Siberia, or it may have arrived here even earlier through some natural process. When the first explorers came to North America, calamus was growing abundantly.

Mongolians thought of calamus as both a natural water purifier and a medicine. As they traveled, they planted it for medicine to treat their horses as well as their armies. In 1574 the famous Viennese botanist Clusius obtained roots from Asia Minor. He cultivated the roots in Vienna, Austria, and spread them to other botanists in western Europe. Calamus became naturalized in Germany and has been collected there through the years, up to the present time. It was also introduced into England around 1600, by botanist and herbalist John Gerard, and was quickly naturalized in the Thames marshes. The plant harvested in India is preferred by many people for its stronger and sweeter flavor. In North America calamus is found throughout the United States, from Canada south to the Gulf of Mexico and westward, locally, into Montana and Oregon.

The historical uses of calamus range from medicine to thatching material in English cottages. In addition, the mature leaves were strewn on the floors of cottages and churches to sweeten the air with their fragrance. Cardinal Wolsey, a contemporary of Henry VIII of England, was reportedly charged with the crime of extravagance for using calamus rushes on all of his floors. Apparently, calamus had to be shipped in from a great distance at a substantial cost.

MEDICINAL USES

There are many common medicinal uses for calamus. It has been used to help people stop smoking; they just chew a bit of the dried root when the desire for a cigarette occurs. It is said to have the ability to clear the mind and stimulate the nervous system so that those taking it can stay awake to study or drive long distances. Calamus extract diluted in bathwater is useful for nervous and exhausted conditions. Chewing the root in large quantities is said to have a hallucinogenic effect, so take care how much root you chew!

Calamus root has also been used as an aromatic bitter to improve appetite and digestion, and is often combined with gentian (*Gentiana* spp.). It has also been used as a mild tonic in the treatment of certain stomach disorders. To treat nervous complaints and mild headaches, the powdered root may be made into an infusion and drunk.

Native American use was extensive throughout the plant's natural range. It was taken both fresh and dried, often as a tea, for many ailments. The Iroquois prepared it as a gargle for sore throats, as an emetic for women with epilepsy, and as drops for earaches. It was used similarly in many tribes. The compounded root was also used to treat burns as a wash or poultice, and was taken internally to help cure colds. The Mohegan considered calamus a panacea and chewed small amounts to ensure good health.

The root has also been candied and taken to sweeten the breath. Where I live in blackfly country, calamus is used to repel insects by rubbing the crushed leaves on exposed skin.

PROPAGATION AND CULTIVATION

Propagation and cultivation of calamus are accomplished mainly through root division and are best done in the springtime, giving the plants a full season to establish themselves. Remember that the plant's natural environment is the edges of wetlands; it can, however, be grown in the garden or field. In the garden it needs daily watering and deep, rich soil. Field conditions are rich soil kept moist year-round. This is a wonderful plant for gardeners to cultivate, with its beautiful leaves and flowers as well as its aromatic presence. Try to locate existing populations of calamus and study how it grows.

At this point calamus suffers from a century of overharvesting and a lack of suitable natural ecosystems. Due to such overharvest, the sites where you might expect to find calamus are often missing this beautiful plant. To replant the root, first obtain fresh, good-quality rootstock. Try to re-create the natural conditions where it grows as closely as possible. Plant on a cloudy day and keep the roots moist. Calamus is very easy to grow and enjoys full sun or partial shade.

HARVESTING

Calamus root is harvested in early spring or late autumn, when the plant's constituents are stored in the roots. It is best to harvest roots that are no more than two to three years old; older roots can become hollow. In collecting any rhizome it is possible to harvest with care, ensuring continued growth, by taking only part of the rootstock. Commercial collection in large cultivated beds is done by cutting sizable squares of root, cleaning them in large baths, and then sorting the plant material.

To collect by hand, you need only a pail, shovel, and boots. A sunny day is also recommended. Good-quality fresh root is reddish or greenish white in color, is 4 to 6 inches in length, and has a firm, spongy texture, a sweet aromatic odor, and a pungent, slightly bitter taste. After you gather the roots and rhizomes, they should be cleaned and either chopped for fresh extract preparation, or kept whole and dried in a warm, dry area, using screens or well-ventilated baskets. Once the roots are thoroughly dry, they may be stored in glass jars away from sun and heat for future use. The roots should not be peeled, because the aromatic oils are present in the root bark.

UpS RECOMMENDATIONS

- Some limited wild harvest is permissible. Use calamus only when really necessary and substitute other herbs whenever possible.

- Possible alternatives are centaury (*Centaurium* spp.), wormwood, and blue vervain. Dill and fennel are good for carminative, antispasmodic effects.

Calamus is an easy plant to propagate and could be spread to many new locations with little effort. It could help restore balance in our wetland environments. As amateur naturalists, we enjoy seeing calamus shoot up in the spring and feel deep satisfaction in knowing one more plant ally. The joy of gardening or caretaking these wild plants without necessarily harvesting for personal use is a very important consideration. Caretaking this or any other endangered plant can and will lead to the healing of our own spirits.

REFERENCES

Cech, Richo. *Horizon Herbs, Strictly Medicinal Growing Guide and 1998 Growing Catalog.* Williams, Oreg.: author, 1998.

Elliott, Doug. *Wild Roots: A Forager's Guide to the Edible and Medicinal Roots, Tubers, Corms, and Rhizomes of North America.* Rochester, Vt.: Healing Arts Press, 1995.

Foster, Steven, and James A. Duke. *Peterson's Field Guide: Eastern/Central Medicinal Plants.* Boston: Houghton Mifflin, 1990.

Grieve, Mrs. Maude. *A Modern Herbal.* Vol. 2. 1931. Reprint, New York: Dover, 1971.

Harding, A. R. *Ginseng and Other Medicinal Plants.* Rev. ed. Columbus, Ohio: author, 1972.

Hutchins, Alma R. *Indian Herbology of North America.* Windsor, Ont.: Merco Publishers, 1973.

McGuffin, Michael, Christopher Hobbs, Roy Upton, and Alicia Goldberry. *Botanical Safety Handbook.* New York: CRC Press, 1997.

Moerman, Daniel. *Medicinal Plants of Native America.* Vols. 1 and 2. Technical Reports No. 17. Ann Arbor: University of Michigan Museum of Anthropology, 1986.

Weiss, Rudolph Fritz, M.D. *Herbal Medicine.* Beaconsfield, U.K.: Beaconsfield Publishers, 1988.

CASCARA SAGRADA
Rhamnus purshiana

RICHO CECH

My neighbor Louie leaned on the fence, bending down the top wire, a wire already seriously stretched by the daily escape of our buck goat, which nobody except myself was willing to tackle and bring back to pasture. Not that the rest of my family was *afraid* of the goat; simply that he stank with an eye-smarting fragrance that only a doe goat in heat could admire, and only a staunch believer in social life after garlic could possibly withstand for long. But Louie paid no attention to the vestigial aroma of goat grease that exuded from the fence and (probably) from my soiled blue jeans. His good eye followed me from under the sun-scorched brow, in turns pleading and plotting, because there was something he wanted, and he was ready to use any persuasion available to get it (and given the daily marauding of my goats into his pasture, he figured he just might have some bargaining power).

You see, there were chittam (otherwise known as cascara sagrada or *Rhamnus purshiana*) trees on my land, trees that yield a bark much in demand by pharmaceutical companies for the manufacture of a cathartic extract. It makes you go. In fact, the going joke among West Coast woodspeople—a joke that has been funny for sev-

eral centuries—is to offhandedly mispronounce *chittam* as *shit 'em*. But I digress. The reason Louie wanted permission to cut the bark off my trees was that all the trees on *his* side of the fence were already denuded of bark, from root to tip. I could see several white skeletons from my vantage point, and I was darned if the trees on my land would be similarly fated. So Louie went home, hitching his pants and limping across the pasture, disgruntled, leaving me to reflect on how to keep a goat in and, when I grew tired of that, on conservation and how to harvest without taking the life of the tree (or plant). I was somewhere in the middle of a long learning process. The answer for chittam is that if you cut the tree off with a tall stump, it will coppice (resprout from the stump), producing multiple trunks that bear usable bark again in a few years. Old Louie must not have known this, because he simply stripped the trees standing, and they died.

BOTANICAL FEATURES

Cascara sagrada is native to the western coast of North America and the Rocky Mountains. It prefers the moist soils of river valleys, stream drainages, and ravines. This is a midsized deciduous tree. The bark is gray or whitish and warty; it tends to harbor lichens. In the spring the tree unfolds its prominently veined leaves, then forms the cup-shaped greenish flowers that give way to the blackish fruits. The trees are good for climbing, as my children proved many a time throughout their early years. Chittam does not mind harboring treehouses, either.

HISTORICAL BACKGROUND

Native American uses of cascara sagrada centered on its effectiveness as an emetic purgative (fresh fruit, leaves, and bark) and laxative (assumedly the cured bark or very small amounts of the uncured bark). A review of the ethnographic literature demonstrates familiarity with the tree by the Cowlitz, Green River, Klallam, Lummi, Makah, Auileute, Quinalt, Skagit, Squaxin, and Swinomish tribes. In addition, the practice among the Skagit tribes—who used the bark as an antidiarrheal—demonstrates a more complete understanding of the herb. Here we see an application based on its gastrointestinal tonifying effect, paralleling the Chinese and European use of another anthraquinone-type laxative known as rhubarb root. Since these early times the herb was rediscovered by the Spanish colonists and by the Eclectic physicians, finally coming into general usage as a fluid extract, a form of administration originally introduced by the Parke, Davis pharmaceutical company. It is currently one of the very few herbal drugs still afforded over-the-counter status by the U.S. Food and Drug Administration.

MEDICINAL USES

Cascara sagrada is a bitter tonic, slightly stimulating to the liver and with a noticeable laxative effect. The classic indications are indigestion and constipation. Because the straining that sometimes accompanies constipation can cause hemorrhoids, cascara sagrada is also commonly listed as a treatment to help reduce hemorrhoids. The herb takes awhile to have an effect. As with other anthraquinone laxatives, the medicine is taken at night, generally producing an effect in the morning of the next day. If digestion is very slow, the response may be delayed for up to another twenty-four hours. Given this delayed action, it is very important to take the recommended dosage and then wait. The tendency, born of ignorance, to take a dose, wait an hour with no results, then take another dose or even (horror) *another* will eventually be answered by an unpleasantly explosive session, a sort of bathroom version of the Battle of the Bulge. Believe me, you do not want to do this. Taken in reasonable doses, cascara sagrada is nongriping and safe. It stands to reason, however, that this medicine should not be taken in cases of intestinal blockage, nor should any laxative be taken long-term on a daily basis, lest dependency develop.

PREPARATION AND DOSAGE

The cured bark can be taken straight as a powder, cold infusion, tea, or tincture. In all cases it is best to grind the bark to a coarse powder before proceeding. This can be accomplished by breaking the bark into small pieces and grinding in an electric coffee grinder or blender. Using a commercial hammer mill, you can easily pulverize large quantities. The dosage of plain powder is $1/3$ gram, taken straight and chased with water, or packed in a capsule and swallowed. The tea is made by steeping 1 teaspoon of the cured, ground bark in 1 cup of hot water.

The tincture is made by combining 1 part by weight (in grams) of cured, powdered bark with 5 parts of liquid (in ml). This liquid, which is known as the menstruum, consists of 75 percent distilled water and 25 percent grain alcohol (190 proof). Using this recipe, 100 grams of the powdered bark would be added to 500 ml of menstruum, which is in turn composed of 375 ml distilled water and 125 ml grain alcohol. Add the menstruum over the ground bark in a jar, then tightly cap the jar and shake it. Store it in a cool, dark place, shaking daily for at least three weeks, after which you pour off the herb and liquid through cheesecloth, thoroughly squeezing into a bowl. The remaining bark, now divested of its medicinal virtues, may be composted. Pour the dark liquid back into a jar, allow it to sit overnight, and then filter it by pouring it slowly through at least four layers of clean cheesecloth in order to remove any remaining particulate matter. The resulting finished tincture should be stored in an amber glass bottle, in a cool place and out of the light. The dosage is 30 to 60 drops.

Cold infusion is a useful technique for preparing an effective tea. Make a "tea bag" from $1/4$ ounce of the cured, powdered bark by wrapping it in cheesecloth or another light fabric and suspending it in 2 cups of cold water. The bag should be just under the surface of the water; let it steep for twelve hours. In the case of cascara sagrada, which is generally taken at night, a cold infusion started in the morning is ready to take before bed. Simply remove the tea bag and drink the tea before retiring. The dosage is $1/2$ to 1 cup. The tea should not be stored, but made fresh each time it is required.

The correct dosage of any cascara sagrada preparation is dependent on individual body weight, personal sensitivity, and the degree of activity required. It is best to begin with a low dosage, adjusting it according to the degree of response. If the herb is to be used over a period of time, reduce the dosage gradually until, by means of this tonification of the gastrointestinal tract coupled with appropriate dietary improvements, the herb is no longer needed.

PROPAGATION AND CULTIVATION

The seeds of cascara sagrada are contained in blackish drupes that are distributed by birds or by falling to the ground when fully ripe. It is fairly common to find young seedlings downslope from a tree, where the fruits or seeds fall and wash into the ground during autumn rains, germinating in the spring. These seedlings can be dug up, potted, allowed to grow in pots until they are sufficiently strong, then transplanted to the landscape as desired.

For home or nursery propagation, the seeds should be obtained fresh in the fall and kept refrigerated until planting. They have a short life span and should be used within a year of harvest. A mass of 28 seeds is 1 gram. They are colored light tan, elegantly rounded on the dorsal surface, and wedge shaped and ridged on the ventral surface, allowing three seeds to fit snugly in a berry. They sport a yellowish nipple at the hilum, and upon breaking reveal a pea green endosperm. The seeds have a naturally low germination rate of 15 to 20 percent, even when ideal conditions are met. Sow the seeds $\frac{1}{4}$ inch deep in an outdoor nursery bed in the fall, midwinter, or very early spring for germination as the soils warm. Alternately, a two-month conditioning in the refrigerator (store the seeds in damp sand or damp peat moss) will give some results. Grow out the seedlings for one year in the nursery bed or in gallon pots, then transplant to the landscape. Cascara sagrada will grow in most temperate locations, but prefers coastal climates. The tree prefers moist soils and full sun to partial shade.

HARVESTING

Correct harvesting of cascara sagrada will help maintain populations in their native habitats. For home use, only a small amount of tree bark will ever be required, and this can be sustainably acquired without much damage to the tree by cutting a single limb and barking it with a knife. Actually, a curve-bladed knife such as those used to cut roofing or linoleum works particularly well for this. The bark should be cut when the sap is up, in the spring, when it peels easily from the wood beneath. To harvest commercial quantities, the tree is cut down, leaving a 4-foot stump. Then the fallen tree (but *not* the stump) can be barked, and the stump will usually resprout. I might add that although the new sprouts that arise from the stump can attain harvestable size within three to five years, the form of the tree is never so pleasant after it is cut back in this way, and the shade it produces is not so spreading or inviting. The fallen tree can be further cut up into firewood, and it also makes very durable and rot-resistant fence posts. In the Oregon coast mountains, where cascara sagrada was once quite prolific, many trees have been lost by harvesters who systematically removed the bark from standing trees. Because they resist deterioration, the many stark, bone white skeletons are a sad testament to unconscious wild-harvesting.

After stripping, the bark is generally chopped into smaller pieces, dried in the shade, and stored in loosely woven burlap bags. Because burlap is usually treated with fungicides, any bags of uncertain history must be thoroughly washed with soap and dried in the sun before use. The bags of dried bark are cured in a shady place with good ventilation for at least a year. If you omit this process, the herb will produce unpleasant intestinal griping or even emesis. For home use, the pieces of dried bark may be cured in a paper or cloth bag for a full year before use. All bags of stored bark must be dated to indicate when the curing process will be complete.

UpS RECOMMENDATIONS

- Some limited wild harvesting is permissible, but only when necessary.

- Possible substitutes are senna, prunes, cassia, cultivated turkey rhubarb, buckthorn, and other *Rhamnus* species.

It is estimated that more than 3 million pounds of cascara sagrada bark are harvested annually. There is an increasing awareness among wildcrafters that in order to assure a sustainable supply of the bark, proper harvesting practices must be maintained. Although many localities have been picked out, the plant's range is wide and includes much inaccessible land. There is little danger of this tree becoming extinct, but it behooves us to bring it back into areas where it was once abundant. Chittam is a small tree, and it is not overly vigorous or conspicuous. If I were to invest it with personality, the word *meek* would come to mind—but this is a meek tree that carries a unique power. By conserving cascara sagrada and by stewarding the land where it grows and prospers, we empower ourselves as well.

REFERENCES

Felter, Harvey Wickes, M.D., and John Uri Lloyd. *King's American Dispensatory*. Vol.1. 1898. Reprint, Portland, Oreg.: Eclectic Medical Publications, 1983.

Gunther, Erna. *Ethnobotany of Western Washington*. Rev. ed. Seattle: University of Washington Press, 1973.

Willard, Terry. *Edible and Medicinal Plants of the Rocky Mountains and Neighbouring Territories*. Calgary: Mountain Rose Books, 1992.

ECHINACEA
Echinacea spp.

STEVEN FOSTER

The year 1980 marked my first summer in Arkansas. What a summer it was! I had spent the previous year in California, where I had moved at age twenty-one from my home in Maine. That year was the hottest summer on record in Arkansas. In June alone we had twenty-five days in a row with temperatures over 100. By July even the oak trees were wilting. Still, one roadside wildflower seemed to survive the drought better than any other. It caught my eye—echinacea.

Ed Smith, known to his friends as Herbal Ed and the founder of Herb Pharm, first introduced me to echinacea as an herbal medicine back in the mid-1970s when I took a class from him in Boston. At that time he ran his business out of a fishing tackle box. His passion for herbal medicine was infectious. Ed had with him a tincture of echinacea made by Alfred Vogel's Swiss company Bioforce, which has sold herbal products since the late 1930s. It was the first echinacea product I had tasted. Ed inspired me to dig deeper into the history and use of this plant.

I was already focused on the botany, cultivation, and historical uses of herbs from the four years spent at the herb department of the Sabbathday Lake Shaker Community in Maine, where I began my career in 1974 at age seventeen. Echinacea did not grow in Maine and at that point was a relatively uncommon garden perennial. I paid little attention to it then. It, like hundreds of other herbs, was to my mind little more than an historical footnote. So when I got to Arkansas in 1980, it caught my eye. Not only did it survive the drought, but it was one of the state's most beautiful wildflowers.

I soon learned that echinacea was a group of plants, not just one type. *Echinacea* is a genus of nine species found exclusively in North America. Arkansas happens to be near the center of the genus's geographical range, with five of the nine species native to the state. A friend of mine, the late Richard Davis, a botanist who worked for Arkansas's Natural Heritage Program, came to visit me at my remote home in Izard County, Arkansas. His job was to look for locations of rare plants in Arkansas. We decided to search for *E. paradoxa*, a species endemic to the Ozarks that had not been collected since the mid-1940s. We went to a location historically known for the plant, and found it. My interest was piqued.

One of the reasons I decided to settle in the Ozarks was the area's flora. I love the plants here. In the Ozarks our flora is dominated by the eastern deciduous forest, a mix of oak, hickories, and other hardwoods. On north-facing slopes we find important American medicinal plants such as ginseng (*Panax quinquefolius*), goldenseal (*Hydrastis canadensis*), and black cohosh (*Cimicifuga racemosa*). We have elements of the Southwest, such as Ashe's juniper, prickly pear cactus, and yucca. The southern pine forests from the West Gulf Coastal Plain also contribute to the Ozarks' plant collection. Since the Ozark region is an ancient landmass not flooded or glaciated for more than two hundred million years—about the time that flowering plants first appeared on earth—these hills have many endemic plants (species that occur only in the Ozarks, not elsewhere). Our dry limestone hillsides also have lots of glades—open, miniature prairielike habitats that harbor dozens of species associated with the Great Plains. The Ozarks were a great place for a fledgling herbalist to settle.

My interest in echinacea grew. For more than twenty-five years, I have collected herb books, and I became fascinated by the writings of the Cincinnati pharmacist John Uri Lloyd (1849–1934). My friend Ed Smith, who shared a passion for old books, sent me a photocopy of a Lloyd publication called *A Treatise on Echinacea*, published in 1921. This gave me the historical foundation to pursue a major study of echinacea. In 1984 that study resulted in a little thirty-one-page book I wrote called *Echinacea Exalted! The Botany, Culture, History and Medicinal Uses of the Purple Coneflowers*.

While I have worked with many plants over the past quarter century, the main group that I have studied is the *Echinacea* genus. My interest in this genus turned to concern when in the early 1980s I observed dramatic declines in roadside populations of echinacea, particularly in Missouri, where it was heavily wildcrafted for the commercial herb trade. Concern led to action. In 1983 and 1984 I wrote letters to conservation agencies and officials in midwestern states where the plant was being harvested. No one was seriously interested in protecting echinacea. It was not endangered, nor was it on rare-plant lists in these states. Budgets were minuscule for plant conservation and it was a low priority. I also wrote to Dr. Ronald K. McGregor, now professor emeritus at the University of Kansas. Dr. McGregor was at that time the last botanist to have monographed the genus. I wrote to him about my conservation concerns and he responded with a thoughtful letter. One comment struck me. Dr. McGregor wrote, "If Echinacea had a little fur and cute little black eyes, one could elicit a little attention."

Indeed conservation resources around the world focus much more on animals than on plants, despite the fact that plant-species loss is far greater than loss of animal life. Echinacea poses some special conservation concerns. Three of the genus's nine—*E. angustifolia, E. pallida, and E. purpurea*—are commercially traded on world markets as the herbal medicine known as phytomedicine or the herbal dietary supplement echinacea. In the wholesale herb market *E. angustifolia* is traded as Kansas snakeroot. I discovered that the commercial supply of Kansas snakeroot, however, did not just involve *E. angustifolia*. Other species of echinacea were being thrown into mixed lots of the herb, including *E. angustifolia, E. pallida, E. atrorubens, E. paradoxa*, and *E. simulata*. To my mind the conservation problem in the 1980s was not that *E. angustifolia* was being harvested, but that other species with relatively narrow ranges—such *as E. atrorubens, E. simulata*, and *E. paradoxa*—were being harvested as *E. angustifolia*. This conscious or unconscious misidentification was at the root of real conservation concerns.

BOTANICAL FEATURES

Current taxonomic concepts of the genus *Echinacea* by botanists include nine species and two varieties. *Echinacea* is a member of the Aster family (Asteraceae or Compositae). *E. angustifolia* grows from 6 to 20 inches tall. The long, narrow, lance-shaped leaves have stiff hairs. The purple ray flowers are relatively short—usually about $^3/_4$ inch to $1^3/_8$ inches long. The species grows on dry prairies from Minnesota to Texas, to western Oklahoma, Kansas, Nebraska, and Iowa; the Dakotas; eastern Colorado, Wyoming, and Montana; and extreme southern Saskatchewan and Manitoba. *E. angustifolia* var. *strigosa* is somewhat smaller and more branched; it has strigose rather than tuberculate-hirsute or hispid hairs. It grows from north-central Texas through central Oklahoma.

Echinacea pallida is a larger plant than *E. angustifolia*, growing to 4 feet in height, with flower petals up to 4 inches long. In flower it is easily distinguished by its white pollen (all other echinaceas have yellow pollen). It is found on glades and rocky prairies from northeastern Texas, eastern Oklahoma, and Kansas; north to Iowa and Wisconsin; and east to Indiana.

Echinacea purpurea, the common purple coneflower, is the most familiar species, because it is commonly grown as a perennial in herb and flower gardens. It has been grown in Europe since 1699. Unlike most echinaceas, it has oval, toothed leaves (most echinaceas have untoothed, narrow, lance-shaped leaves). The tips of the spines on the flowers are bright orange. It is the only echinacea with a fibrous root; all others have taproots. It is the most widespread, though not the most common, species. It grows in open woods, prairies, and thickets from Louisiana, the northeastern tip of Texas, and eastern Oklahoma, north through Ohio, Michigan, and eastward. The entire world's commercial supply of *E. purpurea* is commercially cultivated, not wildcrafted. This alone makes it the best echinacea species. There is no negative conservation impact associated with *E. purpurea*.

Echinacea atrorubens, a relatively rare endemic of the eastern edge of Oklahoma and Kansas, has been threatened in recent years due to collection of its roots as *E. angustifolia*. It grows up to 4 feet high; its stems are light green and nearly without hairs. The flowers have strongly curved petals. It grows on prairies in a very narrow range, from Houston, Texas; to Ardmore, Oklahoma; and north to the Topeka, Kansas, area. It is a species at risk from overharvest.

Echinacea paradoxa has yellow rather than purple ray flowers, hence the species name *paradoxa*. It grows to 4 feet high and also has light green, mostly smooth (without hairs) stems and leaves. It is found on bald knobs and rocky prairies in the Ozarks, in seventeen counties in Missouri and five in Arkansas. It has recently been found in two northeastern Oklahoma counties. Its root, too, has been harvested and sold as *E. angustifolia*. It is at risk from overharvest.

Echinacea sanguinea (sometimes called *E. pallida* var. *sanguinea*) is the southernmost species of echinacea, occurring in open sandy fields and open pine woods within southwestern Arkansas, southeastern Oklahoma, western Louisiana, and eastern Texas. The flower head is nearly hemispherical, and it has slender stems and narrow, dark red, rarely white, ray flowers. Little is known about the plant or its chemistry. Digging of the species has been observed. Its conservation status is not known.

Echinacea simulata was first described and named by Dr. McGregor in 1968. It is closely related to *E. pallida* but has yellow rather than white pollen. Once thought to be endemic to the Ozarks, it is now believed that the echinacea growing east of the Mississippi, once thought to be *E. pallida*, is really *E. simulata*. This was observed by Kathy McKeown, a biologist working on echinacea genetic diversity resources. In the summer of 1998 she traveled more than 20,000 miles in the United States observing echinacea in the wild—the most extensive fieldwork ever conducted on echinacea.

Finally, *Echinacea tennesseensis* and *E. laevigata* deserve a special note. *E. tennesseensis*, found in about a half-dozen populations in Tennessee, was believed to be extinct but rediscovered in 1968. It has upturned rather than drooping pet-

als. On June 6, 1979, the U.S. Fish and Wildlife Service officially listed it as an endangered species. *E. laevigata* (smooth coneflower) is very similar to *E. purpurea* but has a taproot, is relatively smooth (without hairs), and has special flower features that distinguish it from *E. purpurea*. It is by far the rarest species of echinacea. Just over twenty populations are known in the wild with fewer than six thousand individual plants—only 2 percent as many plants known in the wild as the endangered *E. tennesseensis*. *E. laevigata* became a federally listed endangered species on November 9, 1992. It is an Appalachian species found in open woods in Virginia, the Carolinas, and Georgia.

HISTORICAL BACKGROUND

The founder of the world's first ethnobotanical laboratory, Melvin R. Gilmore, noted the importance of echinacea to native groups of the Missouri River region. "This plant was universally used as an antidote for snake bite and other venomous bites and stings and poisonous conditions. Echinacea seems to have been used as a remedy for more ailments than any other plant."

In an 1887 article Eclectic physician John King introduced *E. angustifolia* to the medical profession. The first echinacea product was introduced into American pharmacy in 1895 by John Uri Lloyd, a Cincinnati pharmacist and cofounder of Lloyd Brothers Pharmacists, Inc. Within a few years, the Lloyds' echinacea preparations became their best-selling products (out of more than three hundred) made from American plants, outselling the second-best seller by more than three to one. By 1895 echinacea was also used by homeopathic physicians in Germany. Over the next thirty years the demand increased, while shortages were prevalent in Europe. Consequently, in the late 1930s commercial cultivation of *E. purpurea* began in Germany, introducing echinacea products to a wide European audience for the first time.

MEDICINAL USES

The primary modern use of echinacea preparations is as nonspecific immunostimulants. Echinacea is used to enhance or stimulate the body's own resistance against infections, especially in the prevention of colds and flu and to reduce severity and duration of symptoms. If taken at the onset of symptoms, in small, frequent doses—every two to three hours for the first two days—it often helps mobilize the body's own resistance to the condition. Based on present knowledge, the immunostimulatory activity of alcoholic and water-soluble extracts depends upon the combined action of several constituents, rather than one plant constituent. The lipophilic alkylamides and caffeic acid derivative known as ascichoric acid contribute to the activity of alcoholic extracts. Polysaccharides, glycoproteins, and cichoric acid are active constituents in the expressed juice of *E. purpurea* as well as orally administered powdered whole herb.

PREPARATION AND DOSAGE

Echinacea products include those from the aboveground parts and roots of *E. angustifolia*, *E. pallida*, and *E. purpurea*. These include (among other product forms) tablets, capsules, flextabs, and liquids such as tinctures, glycerites, extracts, and the expressed juice of the fresh flowering *E. purpurea* plant, on which most research has been done. A dose of 60 drops of *E. purpurea* root tincture three times a day is equivalent to 1 gram of the dried root three times a day. Rather than being used continuously (like vitamin C) to prevent colds, echinacea is used as needed at the onset of symptoms or in early stages of infection, usually for two weeks, followed by a resting period of one week. This is based on theory, rather than clinical studies. Many new products are calibrated to contain the equivalent of 900 to 1000 mg of the root (or herb) per daily dose.

PROPAGATION AND CULTIVATION

Echinacea purpurea has been cultivated as a hardy, showy, perennial garden ornamental since the early 1700s, in both North America and Europe. It is easily grown from seeds, is drought tolerant, will grow in full sun or partial shade, and thrives on neglect. *E. pallida* is commonly planted in prairie restoration projects, meadow lawn plantings, and sometimes in herb gardens. *E. angustifolia* is the most difficult echinacea species to grow.

Commercial growers of *Echinacea purpurea* often direct-sow seeds to a depth of about 1/4 inch, keeping the soil moist until emergence (generally in about two weeks). If the *E. purpurea* seeds are from a wild source (not cultivated material), a period of cold, moist stratification at 43 degrees for thirty days is recommended. Echinacea seeds are embryo dormant, and a period of cold, moist stratification greatly increases the speed and frequency of germination. Seeds can be placed in a mix of sand and peat, set outdoors (covered with a mesh screen to keep critters out), and left over the winter. For *E. pallida* seeds thirty to sixty days of stratification is sufficient. For *E. angustifolia* sixty to ninety days of cold, moist stratification is recommended. A study published in 1994 by researchers at South Dakota State University found that a two-week prechill treatment combined with ethephon and continuous light, followed by a two-week germination period in light (sixteen hours per day) at 77 degrees, could induce better than 95 percent seed germination in *E. angustifolia*, which is significantly higher than with any method previously known. Once established, echinaceas thrive with little care. If grown from seeds, expect flowers in the second or third year. When other plants succumb to droughty conditions, echinaceas will withstand the dry weather with little attention. They do well in any average, well-drained garden soil and prefer a slightly alkaline to neutral pH. Good drainage is essential. Echinaceas do not favor highly enriched, wet soils. Full sun is preferable, though *E. purpurea* does well under dappled shade. Yields of up to a ton of dried root and tops per acre can be expected.

HARVESTING

The roots of echinacea species are ideally harvested when vegetative growth is dormant, preferably in the fall (when moisture content is generally lower than in the spring). In practice, however, wildcrafters usually harvest the roots during May through August, when the plants are in flower. Since the plants put up a purple flag denoting their location, it is easy to find the roots during this period. This practice contributes to conservation concerns, since flowering plants are not able to develop and set seeds. *E. pallida* and *E. angustifolia* have taproots, some traveling to a depth of more than 4 feet.

The root is dug with a sharp, narrow spade. Since the soils in which it grows in the wild are often hard and rocky, only 4 to 8 inches of the root and its crown are normally taken. It has been observed that as much as 30 percent of these broken roots will regrow from the broken taproot left in the ground (even when cut to depths of as much as 8 inches). *Echinacea purpurea* roots are often harvested in the fall of their second or third year of growth. Vegetative growth is harvested when the plant is in full bloom. The entire commercial supply of *E. purpurea* is cultivated.

UPS RECOMMENDATIONS

- Use only cultivated resources.
- Possible alternatives include marsh mallow, boneset, and astragalus. Spilanthes nicely replaces the herb's antibacterial, antiviral, immunostimulating, and antifungal effects. Burdock is antibacterial for bacteria classified as gram-positive, and thyme has antibacterial, antifungal, and antiviral properties; both of these herbs are also good alternatives.

The future of echinacea, from both a conservation and a cultivation perspective, is surprisingly bright. Finally, conservation groups and state legislatures have begun to pay attention to echinacea conservation concerns. Harvest is now protected in several states. In 1999 the state of Montana passed legislation (Senate Bill 178) placing legal restrictions on the harvest of *E. angustifolia* on public lands in the state. While the legislation is geared toward the echinacea harvest, it restricts the harvest of all medicinal plants. In the spring of 1999 the North Dakota legislature passed a bill (HB 1200) that makes digging echinacea (without written permission of the landowner) a Class A misdemeanor, subject to court restitution to the landowner or the state, with civil penalties of up to $10,000, along with forfeiture of any vehicle or other property used to take or transport echinacea. The bill was declared an emergency measure. This legislation responded to an emotional reaction to the taking of echinacea rather than sound scientific data on the actual impact of echinacea harvest in these two states. If states are willing to make it a crime to harvest a plant, they should also be willing to fund research on the plants' basic biology. In addition to conservation legislation, *E. angustifolia* and *E. pallida* are now cultivated on a significant commercial scale. In the next five years increasing amounts of these two species will be supplied by cultivation rather than wildcrafting. Given the current attention paid to the use, cultivation, propagation, and conservation of echinacea, the future of the genus is positive. However, the persistent problem of harvest of rare or endemic species such as *E. paradoxa*, *E. atrorubens*, *E. simulata*, and *E. sanguinea* as *E. angustifolia* has not been addressed and puts these species at continued risk for the future.

REFERENCES

Bauer R., and H. Wagner, "Echinacea species as potential immunostimulatory drugs." In *Economic and Medicinal Plant Research*, Vol. 5, edited by H. Wagner and N. R. Farnsworth. New York: Academic Press, 1991.

Feghahati, S. M. J., and R. N. Reese. "Ethylene-, light-, and prechill-enhanced germination of Echinacea angustifolia seeds." *Journal of American Horticultural Science* 119 (4): 853–58, (1994).

Foster, Steven. *Echinacea Exalted! The Botany, Culture, History and Medicinal Uses of the Purple Coneflower*. Drury, Mo: Ozark Beneficial Plant Project, New Life Farm, 1984.

———. *Echinacea: Nature's Immune Enhancer*. Rochester, Vt.: Healing Arts Press, 1991.

———. *Echinacea: The Purple Coneflowers*. Botanical Series No. 301, 2d ed. Austin, Tex.: American Botanical Council, 1996.

———. *Medicinal Herbs—An Illustrated Guide*. Loveland, Colo.: Interweave Press, 1998.

Gilmore, M. "Uses of plants by Indians of the Missouri River region." In *33rd Annual Report of the Bureau of American Ethnology*. 1919. Washington, D.C.: Smithsonian Institution. Reprint, Lincoln: University of Nebraska Press, 1977.

King, J.. "Echinacea angustifolia." *Eclectic Medical Journal* 42 (1887): 209–10.

Lloyd, John Uri. *A Treatise on Echinacea*. Drug Treatise No. 30. Cincinnati: Lloyd Brothers, Pharmacists, 1924.

McGregor, R. L. "The taxonomy of the genus Echinacea (Compositae)." *University of Kansas Science Bulletin* 48 (1968): 113–42.

EYEBRIGHT
Euphrasia officinalis

SARA KATZ

I first met eyebright on an overcast June afternoon in 1991 while hiking with our friends Gianni and Aline in the Perugia region of the northern Italian Alps. They, like many other families in the region, make their living gathering arnica, artemesia, gentian, monkshood (aconite), and valerian in those majestic mountains, just as their ancestors did for centuries before them.

While Gianni and Aline were pointing out one herb after another during our climb along the steep, rocky outcrops that day, I found myself being drawn to a cluster of charming little plants with lilac-colored flowers that grew in pockets scattered throughout the subalpine terrain. What a thrill it was to find that this was eyebright, a plant that I had often seen provide relief from the symptoms of winter colds thousands of miles away back home in Oregon.

BOTANICAL FEATURES

Eyebright, classified as *Euphrasia officinalis* by Linnaeus, is a member of the Figwort family, or Scrophulariaceae. There has been a good deal of debate within the botanical community over whether *E. officinalis* is in fact one quite variable species or whether it is numerous species, including *E. rostkoviana*, *E. stricta*, and *E. montana*. The one characteristic that groups these plants together is that they bear glandular hairs on their calyxes. Despite the fact that all of these closely related plants vary slightly in their botanical features, they are nonetheless quite similar biochemically and can be used interchangeably.

Eyebright is an annual that flowers from July to September and has branched, erect, square, downy stems ranging from 2 to 8 inches high. Its deeply cut leaves are crenate-serrate, $1/4$ to $1/2$ inches long, sometimes ovoid, sometimes pointed and narrow, with spikes of opposite, small ($1/2$ inch), white or pale lilac-pink flowers in the axils of the upper leaves. The upper lips of the flowers are about $1/2$ inch in length and have purple veins. The lower lip has three lobes and a bright yellow spot where it enters the throat of the flower.

The various Eyebright species tolerate a very wide range of soil types and conditions in their native habitatat. Some, for example, can be found in marshes, woods, and clearings from sea level up to 9,000 feet, where the soil conditions are both moist and of poor quality. Others, however, can be found in such dry conditions as heaths and dry pastures, especially where there is chalky soil.

This elegant little plant, indigenous to the British Isles and eastern Europe, is also found in North America in the White Mountains of New England and near Lake Superior. According to herbalist David Winston, "Eyebright grows in central to northern Maine, northern Vermont and New Hampshire, and sparsely in northern New York. It is most prolific in coastal Maine, Nova Scotia, Labrador, and Newfoundland. I have had reports of Eyebright growing at higher elevation in the upper Catskills but have yet to see it."

HISTORICAL BACKGROUND

The botanical name for eyebright, *Euphrasia*, comes from the Greek prefix *eu*, meaning "good" or "well," and is thought to have derived from Euphrosyne, the name of one of the three Graces in Greek mythology who was known for her joy and mirth. It is further believed that this name was given to the plant due to its value in preserving eyesight and in so doing, "bringing gladness into the life of the sufferer."

In European history the use of eyebright goes back centuries. Evidence of its use as an eye medicine, for example, dates back to the medical literature of the twelfth century, when it appeared in the works of the pioneering naturalist St. Hildegard von Bingen. Later, in the seventeenth century, the herbalist Nicholas Culpeper claimed that if eyebright's use was to

become more widespread it would "half spoil the spectacle-maker's trade." In fact, apothecaries of old knew the plant as ocularia and othalmica, both referring to its beneficial effect on the eyes.

According to an old European teaching called the doctrine of signatures, the use of plants for specific medicinal purposes was associated with each plant's resemblance to a particular body part. In the case of eyebright the purple veins and yellow spots on the flower somewhat resemble bloodshot eyes; the plant was thus thought to be curative for the eyes.

According to Maude Grieve, in Iceland the juiced plant is used, and in Scotland the Highlanders make a "tea" of the herb by steeping it in hot milk, straining it, and brushing it onto weak or inflamed eyes with a feather.

MEDICINAL USES

Eyebright is useful in a variety of conditions that require the drying up of runny, watery discharges from the eyes, nose, and bronchial passages, particularly when there is heat, pain, burning, and sneezing present. It has a mild stimulating, and astringent action that constricts the blood vessels of the nasal passages and the conjunctival (lachrymal) mucous membranes, helping dispel mucus and other exudates that result from inflammation. In homeopathy the characteristic symptom calling for the use of eyebright is acrid (biting) discharges, either thin and watery or thick and yellow. According to the Eclectic physicians (a group of medical doctors in the United States who used herbal medicine extensively in the early twentieth century), using eyebright can help prevent eye disorders that sometimes proceed measles.

Taken internally as a tea or tincture, eyebright is useful for a wet cough and hoarseness; for earache and headache associated with a cold; for congestion of the frontal sinus, such as in hay fever; for functional disturbances of vision that are of muscular and nervous origin (twitchy, achy, or burning eyes, for instance); for sniffles in children; and to dispel catarrh (free discharge resulting from inflamed mucous membranes). It should be noted that due to its astringent and drying qualities, eyebright would not be the herb of choice in cases of dry sinuses, throat, and nasal passages.

The well-strained tea can also be used as an eyewash or as a compress for eye fatigue, conjunctivitis, sties, and other congestive conditions of the eyes with profuse tearing. It is also useful as a nasal douche for nasal catarrh, head colds, and sinusitis.

Eyebright poultices have been used to aid wound healing, and the dried herb has been used as an ingredient in British herbal tobacco, which Mrs. Grieve notes as being "smoked most usefully for chronic bronchial colds." Personally, I would not recommend smoking an herbal blend while you suffer from a bronchial cold, though it is probably an effective way to get the warmed herbal goodies into the bronchial passages.

PREPARATION AND DOSAGE

In preparing teas, tinctures, eyewashes, compresses, and poultices for the various conditions described above, it is often useful to combine the whole plant (fresh or dried eyebright) with fennel seeds and/or goldenseal, which complement its stimulating, astringent, and tonic affects on the mucous membranes.

To make a tincture, steep 1 part of cut-up, dried eyebright in 5 parts of vodka. Cover and shake thoroughly, continuing to shake at least once daily for two weeks. After this time, filter the mixture through several layers of cheesecloth. It may now be used or stored in a closed container in a dark cupboard. For respiratory problems, take from 15 to 40 drops every three to four hours, although in acute cases it is better to take 10 to15 drops every hour or two. For very young infants, quick relief is often achieved by giving 5 or 10 drops of the tincture, dropped into 4 ounces of water, giving a teaspoonful every fifteen minutes. As for the tea, in most conditions drink $1/_2$ to 1 cup three or four times per day.

To make an infusion (tea) that can be used for an eyewash, nasal douche, or compress, bring a cup of distilled water to a boil, turn off the heat, and add 1 teaspoon of dried eyebright (or 3 teaspoons of fresh eyebright if you have it). Steep for half an hour, then strain through several layers of cheesecloth or cotton cloth to remove all particles.

To use eyebright as an eyewash, fill an eye cup with the cooled, well-strained tea and rinse your eyes with it one to three times. Then close your eyes and relax for five or ten minutes. While many pharmaceutical ophthalmic preparations of eyebright are dropped directly into the eyes, be cautious about applying the tea or other nonsterile solution directly into your eyes.

To use eyebright as a compress, soak a folded piece of cotton cloth or puffed cotton in the cooled tea and place gently on closed eyelids. Lie back and relax for ten to twenty minutes, refreshing the cotton with more tea every five minutes.

Inflammation of the eye can lead to serious problems. If symptoms of eye irritation, infection, or injury are severe or persist for more than a few days, especially if there is a fever, promptly seek qualified health care.

PROPAGATION AND CULTIVATION

Although eyebright self-propagates by seeds and grows in a variety of climatic conditions, it is by nature a "wild plant," difficult to cultivate in the garden. In fact, I know of no one who has succeeded at doing so. The reason is thought to be that eyebright is a semiparasitic plant, needing to grow among certain grasses from which it gets its nourishment. Viewed from above the ground, eyebright does not have the appearance of a parasitic plant in that it has normal flowers and bright green leaves; parasitic plants are usually devoid of the green color of chlorophyll. Below ground, however, the suckers from eyebright's roots entangle themselves among the roots of the surrounding grasses, forming tiny nodules which come into contact with and absorb nutrients from the grass rootlets. The grasses are not seriously affected, because the absorptive cells from eyebright's nodules do not penetrate deeply into the grass rootlets, and because eyebright—an annual that dies off each winter—does not cause a permanent nutrient drain on the grasses.

Eyebright continues to be collected only from the wild, and is therefore at great risk of being overharvested. Some other plants that share similarly mild astringent properties and that can thus be used in its stead are sage, green tea (especially in the form of compresses), Chinese coptis, red clover, and yarrow. Hopefully someday a green-thumbed person will figure out how to cultivate this lovely healing plant so we can once again, in good conscience, freely avail ourselves of eyebright's special curative properties.

UpS RECOMMENDATIONS

- Use only cultivated resources, if you can find them.

- Good substitutes are sage, horseradish, green tea, Chinese coptis, red clover, and yarrow. Ambrosia may be used as an astringent and antihistamine for eyes, throat, ears, and sinuses.

Thinking back to my herb walk years ago in the Italian Alps, I reflect on the fact that people had collected wild plants in those ancient collecting grounds for centuries, doing so in a conscientious way that ensured the plants' continued abundance. Through careful pruning of the aerial parts of existing plants, the replanting of remaining rootlets and crowns, and the scattering of seeds, the herbs that provided livelihood and medicine for centuries continued to thrive. With the current popularity and ever increasing demand for eyebright, however, there is now concern that continued harvesting could lead to the plants' eventual depletion. It is of utmost importance that any collecting of wild medicinal plants be done with reverence for the plants and in a knowledgeable, respectful, and sustainable manner. Only this way can we ensure that the plants and the medicinal gifts we receive from them will continue to be there for generations and centuries to come.

REFERENCES

Clymer, R. S., M.D. *Nature's Healing Agents*. 1905. Reprint, Philadelphia: Dorrance, 1963.

Ellingwood, Finley. *American Materia Medica, Therapeutics and Pharmacognosy*. 1898. Reprint, Portland, Oreg.: Eclectic Medical Publications, 1983.

Felter, Harvey Wickes, M.D. *Eclectic Materia Medica, Pharmacology and Therapeutics*. 1922. Reprint, Portland, Oreg.: Eclectic Medical Publications, 1983.

Felter, Harvey Wickes, M.D., and John Uri Lloyd. *King's American Dispensatory*. Vol. 1. 1898. Reprint, Portland, Oreg.: Eclectic Medical Publications, 1983.

Flüch, Hans. *Medicinal Plants and Their Uses*. New York: W. Foulsham, 1976.

Grieve, Mrs. Maude. *A Modern Herbal*. 1931. Reprint, New York: Dover, 1971.

Kutz-Chereaux, A. W., M.D., ed. *Naturae Medicina and Naturopathic Dispensatory*. Yellow Springs, Ohio: American Naturopathic Physicians and Surgeons Association, 1953.

Locke, Frederick J., M.D. *Eclectic Materia Medica*. Cincinnati: John M. Scudder's Sons, 1895.

Newall, C. A., L. A. Anderson, and J. D. Phillipson. *Herbal Medicines: A Guide for Health Care Professionals*. London: Pharmaceutical Press, 1966.

Priest A. W., and L. R. Priest. *Herbal Medication*. London: L. N. Fowler,1982.

Scudder, John M., M.D. *Specific Medication*. Cincinnati: Scudder Bros., 1913.

Stuart, Malcom. *Encyclopedia of Herbs and Herbalism*. New York: Grosset and Dunlap, 1979.

Stary and Jirasek. *Herbs*. Translated from the Czech, by F. J. Evans. London: Hamlyn Press, 1973.

Thompson, W. *Healing Plants*. London: McGraw-Hill, 1978.

Tyler, Varro E. *The New Honest Herbal*. Philadelphia: George F. Stickley, 1987.

Weiss, Rudolph Fritz, M.D. *Herbal Medicine*. Beaconsfield, U.K.: Beaconsfield Publishers, 1988.

Wichtl, Max. *Herbal Drugs*. English ed. Stuttgart: MedPharm, 1994.

AMERICAN GINSENG
Panax quinquefolius

KATHI KEVILLE

A twenty-five-hundred-year-old Chinese myth from Sheni Province tells of villagers hearing a loud voice calling to them from underneath a plant. When they dug up the root, it was shaped like a man, so they named it *jen-shen* or "man root." (Westerners who later heard the name pronounced it *JIN-seng*.) Said to be a manifestation of *tu ching*, or "spirit of the ground," this root became the object of spiritual quests by Chinese people, who would recite an ancient chant before digging it.

Chinese Prayer to Jen-Shen

Great Spirit! Do not go away
I have come with a clean heart
My soul is unstained
It is purged of sin and wicked design
Remain here, O Greatest of Spirits

Likewise, Native Americans considered North American ginseng to possess magical, as well as healing, properties. The Iroquois know it as *garent-oquen*, or "man's thighs and legs separated." Warriors carried it as a talisman and used it for rejuvenation. The Cherokee named ginseng "little man" and used it to increase the potency of herbal formulas.

The Chinese consider their ginseng *(Panax ginseng)* more warming and stimulating than American ginseng, but they do prefer the American species for certain conditions. Many Western herbalists use the two interchangeably. There are several other species, including Japanese ginseng *(P. japonicus)* and a small dwarf American ginseng *(P. trifolius)*. Red ginseng is Chinese ginseng soaked in other herbs and steamed and pressed to produce a translucent red root. The popular Siberian ginseng *(Eleutherococcus sentiocosus)* is in the Ginseng family—Araliaceae—and shares many of *Panax*'s attributes, so it's often confused with true ginseng.

BOTANICAL FEATURES

I must admit that I have been captivated by ginseng's presence. I always feel reluctant to pull it from the ground, even in my own garden. But then I become excited as the pudgy, human-shaped root emerges. This white taproot, which can measure up to several inches in width in older roots, twists into the shape of elongated, dancing legs, with side roots providing arms.

However, don't be surprised to find roots with more than two "legs" or "arms." If you count the number of little bulges along the "neck" or the stem, rising from the root crown, you can determine the age of that particular root.

The plant itself is a foot or two tall, with the largest specimens spanning about a foot across. However, they are very sparse, with a main stem supporting a few side stems, each bearing a cluster of paper-thin leaves. In fact, when you encounter a ginseng plant, it may not stop you in your tracks unless it is bearing the vivid, bright red berries that appear in late summer or fall. These berries are about $1/2$ inch in diameter and contain two hard seeds inside. Eat one and the warm, bitter taste of ginseng root fills your mouth. The berries are preceded by small yellowish green flowers in May or June.

HISTORICAL BACKGROUND

Wars have been fought over ginseng, and emperors have monopolized the right to harvest it. Although I often hear claims that Chinese ginseng is superior, the Chinese themselves have imported large amounts of American ginseng since 1718, when the Jesuits of Canada first initiated trade with China. 'Seng hunting in the United States started out as a lucrative business run by fur traders, who frequented the same areas where it grew. By the 1770s an average of 140,000 tons of ginseng roots were exported from North America every year. The year 1824 set a new record, with more than 600,000 tons of roots exported. The first successful U.S. ginseng crop, reported in an 1895 New York paper, sparked interest in cultivating ginseng; the U.S. Department of Agriculture printed a bulletin on its cultivation. In 1902 a *Special Crops* publication began networking growers. Six years later A. R. Harding discussed its cultivation in *Ginseng and Other Medicinal Plants*.

Sadly, you're not likely to stumble upon wild ginseng. At one time it grew abundantly in the shade of North America's eastern hardwood forests from Québec to Georgia and west to Oklahoma and Minnesota, but no more. I imagine that few, if any, of the early 'seng traders considered the impact that collecting millions of tons of wild roots from the American wilderness made. Unfortunately, they did not adopt careful harvesting practices like those of the Ojibwa Indians, who lived on Lake Superior. These Natives harvested ginseng only after the berries turned red so they could replant the seeds and help replace the plants they took. To the 'seng hunters, thoguh, ginseng must have seemed an infinite resource, so they filled their bags with roots and their pockets with money as they depleted the woods of ginseng.

The impact was severe. Today ginseng is considered threatened or endangered in Kentucky, Tennessee, Virginia, and Illinois. The Convention on International Trade in Endangered Species (CITES), the U.S. Fish and Wildlife Service, and the U.S. Department of Agriculture regulate its trade in every state. A permit is required to dig roots, and even then the practice is restricted to the months of August through November in many states. A federal permit is needed to export either cultivated or wild ginseng. However, with prices topping $600 a pound for wild roots, there is a large black market for ginseng. More than 14,500 pounds of supposed wild roots found their way to Asia in 1992.

MEDICINAL USE

Ginseng has long been considered a panacea, as implied by its botanical name *Panax:* the word *pan* is Latin for "all," and *akos* means "remedy." The plant is used to treat many different disorders because it regulates many physiological functions. For this reason Russian researcher I. I. Brekhman dubbed it an "adaptogen." Ginseng does indeed help the body adapt, producing different effects depending on what an individual needs. For example, it can either sedate or stimulate the central nervous system.

Hundreds of studies have been done on ginseng, although relatively few used human volunteers. Still, they do show ginseng's ability to increase mental and physical efficiency and general resistance to stress and disease. For example, nurses on the night shift in a London hospital experienced better endurance and concentration when they took ginseng. Rorschach tests show that ginseng improves psychological function as well. It is no surprise that the Chinese Academy of Medical Science in Beijing found that the compounds in ginseng called ginsenosides increase protein synthesis and neurotransmitter activity in the brain. Ginseng also helps regulate the heart, to keep it pumping at a healthy rate, and it increases the amount of oxygen reaching the lungs, brain, and muscles as well as its utilization. Many menopausal women report that ginseng helps reduce the number of their hot flashes. Ginseng also encourages better functioning in people who have liver problems, and seems to help protect the liver from damage in the first place. When volunteers took 3 grams of ginseng with alcohol, their resulting blood alcohol level was one-third to one-half lower than that of a control group. Studies also show that ginseng improves the tolerance of carbohydrate in diabetics. In addition to all of the above, it increases natural immunity, specifically increasing the number of infection-fighting natural killer cells and white blood cells, and possibly even fending off some types of cancer.

Few problems result from using ginseng, although large doses—more than what is suggested for medicine—have been reported to cause depression, insomnia, nervousness, and high blood pressure. Also, be cautious combining this herb with pharmaceutical drugs, especially antipsychotics, stimulants, antidepressants, and narcotic relaxants; it's possible that ginseng makes them more or less potent. Problems may even result from drinking lots of coffee. Although ginseng is used to maximize energy, it works best to stabilize and regulate the system and offer a boost when you're feeling worn out. It won't turn you into Superman or Wonder Woman. The Chinese generally combine it with other herbs. It is best to not take ginseng in the evening unless you want to stay awake at night.

PREPARATION AND DOSAGE

Ginseng is available as a tea, as a tincture, or in capsules (generally 300 to 5,000 mg). Most of ginseng's medicinal properties are attributed to compounds called ginsenosides. Some products are standardized to assure that they contain at least 2 percent ginsenosides. Your general health, your constitution, and the condition you are treating all influence the recommended dose. However, a generic amount to take daily is 1 to 3 capsules, a few cups of tea, or 1 to 4 dropperfuls. A wide spectrum of products in varying strengths is available, so read the recommendations on the label. There are also elixirs, syrups, candies, soft drinks, toffee—even ginseng ice cream and chewing gum! Ginseng is expensive, so most of these products contain relatively little of the root. The Chinese add small amounts of chopped ginseng root to soups and stews.

To make tea, add 1 teaspoon of sliced or powdered root for every cup of water and gently simmer for twenty to thirty minutes. Then take it off the heat and steep for another fifteen minutes. When it's cool enough, strain and drink. To use a whole root to make tea, first soak it overnight in water to make it soft enough to slice. The taste does not appeal to everyone, but it is very good cooked with a thin slice of ginger.

PROPAGATION AND CULTIVATION

Ginseng doesn't grow wild in the western United States where I live, so my first experience with the plant was in my garden. I was encouraged because old-timers told me that the mountain town in which I then resided, Camptonville, was home to a ginseng farm for the Eli Lilly drug company around the turn of the twentieth century. Indeed, ginseng likes

mountain weather, especially the solid winter freezes that give it a needed rest during the cold season. Ginseng plants that I gave to herbalists in warmer climates—even herb growers with green thumbs—never fared well.

As with other plants in my garden that hale from other climates, I look to ginseng's natural habitat to learn what growing conditions it prefers. I alter my soil to mimic the rich, well-drained, humusy, and more alkaline soil of the Midwest. (The best pH is 5 to 6.) An automatic mister provides some resemblance to the humid air and summer rain where it grows wild.

My first fifty ginseng rootlets grew very well—that is, until I took a two-week trip. I came home to find all but six plants eaten by gophers. (And yes, that summer the farm had some of the healthiest gophers ever seen.) I planted the next crop in a wooden box with a chicken-wire bottom (the heavy wire type with small holes), and that did the trick. Some sunlight encourages root growth, but too much can kill it. Since ginseng likes about 70 percent shade, I choose the diffused light in the forest; shade cloth will also prevent the sun from frying the leaves.

If you're going to grow ginseng from seeds rather than rootlets, you must first carefully score the tough, outer shells of the seeds with a razor. Then stratify the seeds in wet sand in a freezer for eight months to mimic winter. Although they cost less than rootlets, seeds require patience; they can take more than a year to germinate. Most people like to get a head start on ginseng by planting two-year-old rootlets. Plant them about 2 feet apart.

I should warn you that ginseng is susceptible

not only to gophers, but also to snails, insects such as pill bugs, various diseases, and even a careless foot. Since ginseng relies on a thin main stalk, it is easily damaged. Other predators are poachers—people who make their living collecting medicinal roots from the wild, and, in some cases, from other people's land! Most commercial growers unfortunately turn to pesticides and herbicides to protect their investment.

However, it is relatively simple to organically grow your own small plot of ginseng—certainly enough for your family and friends—almost anywhere. It is amazing what can be done with compost and an automatic sprinkler system. I've seen one small commercial operation that cultivated ginseng under the shade of the piñon pine and sagebrush in Nevada's high desert! You can even cultivate it in a gallon pot. Give ginseng growing a try and experience its magic for yourself.

HARVESTING

It takes five to six years before a ginseng root is mature enough to harvest, but it is not considered fully grown until it's twenty or so years old. Generally, the older and larger the root, the more valuable it is. When you are ready to harvest your ginseng roots, carefully dig and wash them. The best-quality roots are usually sold whole. Store ginseng in a dry, airtight container. The ginsenosides in it have been shown to be fairly stable, but they do break down after a couple of years. You can also preserve fresh roots by completely submerging them in a 40 percent alcohol such as vodka.

UpS RECOMMENDATIONS

- No wild harvest is recommended.
- Purchase cultivated roots only. Even woods-grown plants are suspect.
- Use Chinese ginseng (*Panax ginseng*), Siberian ginseng, astragalus, and ashwagandha as possible substitutes.

REFERENCES

Bensky, D., and A. Gamble. *Chinese Herbal Medicine: Materia Medica.* Seattle, Wash.: Eastland Press, 1986.

Dörling, E., et al. "Do ginsenosides influence the performance? Results of a double blind study." *Notabene Medici* 10 (5): 241–46 (1980).

Forgo, I., et al. "Effect of a standardized ginseng extract on general health, reactive capacity and pulmonary function." In *Proceedings of the Third International Ginseng Symposium.* Seoul: Korean Research Institute, 1980.

Hallstrom, C., et al. "Effects of ginseng on the performance of nurses on night duty." *Comparative Medicine Journal* 6 (1982): 277–82.

Liu, J., et al. "Stimulating effect of saponin from *Panax ginseng* on immune function of lymphocytes in the elderly." *Mechanisms of Aging and Development* 10 (1995): 43–53.

Pritts, Kim Derek. *Ginseng: How to Find, Grow, and Use America's Forest Gold.* Mechanicsburg, Penn.: Stackpole Books, 1995.

Quiroga, H. A., et al. "The effect of *Panax ginseng* extract on cerebrovascular deficits." *Orientacion Medica* 1202 (1979): 86–87.

Rosenfield, M. S., et al. "Evaluation of the efficacy of a standardized ginseng extract in patients with psychophysical asthenia and neurological disorders." *La Semana Medica* 173 (1989): 148–54.

Sandburg, F. "Vitality and senility—effects of ginsenosides on performance." *Svensk Farmeceitisk Tidskrift* 84 (1980): 499–502.

Zuin, M. "Effects of . . . ginseng combined with trace elements and multivitamins against hepatoxin-induced chronic liver disease in the elderly." *Journal of Internal Medical Research* 15 (1987): 276–81.

GOLDENSEAL
Hydrastis canadensis

MARK BLUMENTHAL

Goldenseal is the rhizome and rootlets of *Hydrastis canadensis*. In commerce the herb typically ranks as one of the most widely used herbs in the North American market and is second only to wild American ginseng *(Panax quinquefolius)* in commercial importance in the native North American medicinal plant trade. Its sales are typically highest in natural food store outlets, rather than in mass-market retail stores. Nevertheless, goldenseal products are found consistently ranked among the top dozen herbs sold in both classes of trade. In 1997 goldenseal sales ranked fourth in the natural food trade, at 6 percent of total herb sales; 1998 sales were ranked seventh, at 4 percent of total sales, the drop being due in part to the rise of St.-John's-wort *(Hypericum perforatum).*[1] In mainstream stores goldenseal sales in 1998 were bundled with echinacea (as both individual and combination products), ranking fifth at $69.7 million total, with the majority of this figure presumably being due to the heightened popularity of echinacea.[2]

Some herbal experts find this popularity a bit of an anomaly, since most of the top-selling herbs sold in the United States in the past few years have seen their popularity jump due to reports of the scientific and clinical studies suggesting and/or confirming their health benefits. The market data indicates that goldenseal stands as an exception to this trend of the better-researched herbs enjoying the top sales positions in the mainstream market: There have been no clinical studies published on goldenseal in more than sixty years. Thus, goldenseal stands in distinct contrast to some of its popular Native American medicinal plant cousins, which have received significant attention from scientists in Europe: black cohosh root *(Cimicifuga racemosa)*, echinacea herb and root *(Echinacea* spp.), and saw palmetto berries *(Serenoa repens)*. The reasons for its popularity are rooted primarily in the high regard it has maintained in American folklore and herbalism.

Although often called a root, goldenseal is actually a rhizome, an underground lateral stem. The name *goldenseal* derives from the seal-like scars on the rhizome, which are yellow or golden in color.[3] Other common names for goldenseal include orange root, yellow puccoon, ground raspberry, eye-balm, and eye-root, the latter two names referring to its use as a collirium or eyewash. Goldenseal's traditional use as a dye plant is evidenced by the following common names: Indian paint, yellow paint, Indian dye, golden root, Indian turmeric, wild turmeric, curcuma (kurkuma), Ohio curcuma, wild curcuma, jaundice root, and yellow eye, although the increasing scarcity and high price of the root precludes its use as a dyestuff today. (Note that goldenseal has no botanical relationship with the common spice and medicinal plant turmeric, *Curcuma longa*.) Fortunately for herbalists and the general public, the herb used in commerce goes almost exclusively by the name *goldenseal*, which, along with the little-used *yellow puccoon*, are the only names generally agreed upon by the American Herbal Products Association in its book of acceptable common names for the most popular herbs, *Herbs of Commerce*.[4]

The Latin name *Hydrastis* was based on the work of the eighteenth-century botanist Linnaeus, who originally published the genus as *Hydrophyllum* (waterleaf) in the *Species Plantarum* (1753 edition), based on the erroneous classification of the plant in the family Hydrophyllaceae due to observation of the leaves only.[5] In the tenth (1759) edition of *System Naturale* Linnaeus corrected this mistake by renaming the genus *Hydrastis*, based on the misconception that the plant grew in "bog meadows" (he's been supplied with a flowering specimen by John Ellis, who had called it by this name). During this time a colored picture of goldenseal was also published as *Warneria* in honor of Richard Warner;[6] the name was later changed to *Warnera* but it did not persist in the botanical literature.

BOTANICAL FEATURES

Goldenseal is a member of the Buttercup family (Ranunculaceae) and is found in deciduous woodlands in eastern North America, from Vermont to Georgia, Alabama, west to Arkansas, and back up to Minnesota. The plant is a hairy perennial 6 to12 inches high, usually containing two leaves on a forked branch, one leaf being larger than the other. Each leaf is rounded with five to seven double-toothed lobes,[7] although herbalist and raconteur Doug Elliott writes that there are five to nine lobes.[8] The plant produces a single flower in April through May, with greenish white stamens in clusters, often protected by one of the immature leaves. The berries resemble a raspberry,[9] hence the occasionally used common name *ground raspberry*.[10] Elliott writes that other young forest plants can resemble immature goldenseal, so when he wants to ensure that one is goldenseal, he checks it out by removing an inch or two of soil at the base of the stem to find the bright yellow color of the root, which extends up to the stem base. In a stand of goldenseal plants, he adds, there are often many immature, sterile plants with only one leaf. He states that three years are needed for the goldenseal plant to be able to flower and reproduce.[11]

HISTORICAL BACKGROUND

The earliest accounts of the native medicinal plants of North America did not mention the therapeutic values of goldenseal. The first documented account of the plant dates to a 1782 speech by Hugh Martin to the American Philosophical Society, published a year later in the society's *Transactions* under the title "An Account of some of the Principal Dyes employed by the North American Indians."[12] Benjamin Smith Barton was the first to bring it to the attention of the medical profession in a brief note in 1798, crediting the Cherokee with its use; in an 1804 publication he gives more attention to goldenseal.[13] In 1828 Rafinesque claimed that the Cherokee used the root for cancer, but that other remedies were considered better for this purpose. He wrote that other Indians used it as a stimulant. However, its principal use was described as being for skin disease and sore or inflamed eyes. These latter applications eventually made their way into popular usage.[14] Some tribes reportedly used goldenseal for gonorrhea.[15] One of the most authoritative summaries of Native American usage is found in the recent compilation by Moerman, who notes that the Iroquois used the root for its antidiarrheal and carminative properties, as an ear and eye medicine, as an emetic, for fevers, as a gastrointestinal aid, for heart and liver trouble, for tuberculosis, and as a stimulant. Other Iroquois uses of goldenseal include whooping cough, pulmonary problems such as pneumonia and tuberculosis, and scrofula (tubercular nodes on the neck). Moerman notes that the Cherokee used goldenseal for cancer, as a tonic and wash for local inflammations, to improve appetite, and for general debility and dyspepsia. The Micmac used a root preparation for chapped lips.[16]

MEDICINAL USES

ECLECTIC MEDICAL USES

The most extensive monograph on goldenseal in the classic literature was written more than one hundred years ago by the famous Eclectic pharmacist John Uri Lloyd and his mycologist brother, Curtiss Gates Lloyd, in 1884–1885. It compiled all the chemistry, botany, and therapeutic information known at that time in more than a hundred pages of text and drawings. In contrast, the most recent comprehensive review was written by medical herbalist Paul Bergner.[17]

Probably the most detailed account of clinical uses for goldenseal and its preparations is found in *King's American Dispensatory* (eighteenth edition, third revision) by the famous Eclectic physician Harvey Wickes Felter and John Uri Lloyd. Per *King's*, goldenseal was employed for the following indications by the Eclectics:

> Indicated in catarrhal states of the mucous membranes, when unaccompanied with acute inflammation. An apparent exception to this is in acute otitis media, in which it is said to act better than in chronic conditions; gastric irritability; irritation of parts with feeble circulation; muscular tenderness and soreness, worse under pressure or on motion; passive hemorrhages from uterus and other pelvic tissues; skin diseases depending on a gastric abnormality, indicating hydrastis.

King's also relates the use of goldenseal for "convalesence from diseases having excessive mucoid discharges, or where hemorrhage has played an important part." Also noted is its use as a bitter tonic in specific types of subacute and chronic inflammation of the stomach or atonic gastric conditions,[18] including atonic dyspepsia associated with alcoholism.[19]

Almost thirty years later, Felter (in the 1983 reprint of his classic 1922 text) notes the following about goldenseal: "Hydrastis is one of our most efficient topical medicines when applied in disorders of the mucous membranes; and is occasionally of service upon the skin. It is most important perhaps in ophthalmic practice, being a thoroughly effective subastringent and soothing agent in acute and subacute catarrhal and follicular conjunctivitis."[20] He also calls goldenseal "among the most successful remedies for catarrhs of the nose and throat."

For other internal uses, Felter claims that goldenseal is one of the most effective bitter tonics, increasing appetite and enhancing digestion. He also claims that goldenseal controls "passive hemorrhage" but is not suited for "copious active hemorrhages, as gastric and postpartum bleeding in which small quantities of blood are passed at a time and are recurrent in form."[21] He notes the herb's use in menstrual disorders, being relatively slow acting but producing permanent effects.

Hobbs writes that this enthusiastic use by the Eclectics helped goldenseal cross over into use by regular (conventional) physicians, as evidenced by inclusion in the *United States Pharmacopoeia* and *National Formulary* (see below). Actually, however, inclusion of goldenseal (at least initially in 1830 and again in 1860) in the *Pharmacopoeia* preceded the growth of the Eclectic movement, which reached its zenith at the end of the nineteenth and into the early twentieth century. Hobbs notes that King in the 1860s "was more critical than previous authors, and omitted some of what he considered to be overblown claims for the plant."[22] About 130 years later medical botanist Paul Bergner writes that some of the contemporary uses for goldenseal, especially to treat colds and flus, are not well founded. In his experiences both selling herbs at the retail level and seeing patients in a clinic, he writes, "Not even 10% of the goldenseal use in the U.S. is clinically appropriate. When someone pops large amounts of goldenseal 'for a cold,' especially in its early stages, they are wasting both their money and an endangered [*sic*; it is officially threatened] plant."[23]

MODERN USES

The *British Herbal Compendium* notes antihemorrhagic, choleretic, and antimicrobial actions of goldenseal to be used for the following indications: menorrhagia, atonic dyspepsia, gastritis, plus mucosal inflammations and, topically, in eyewashes.[24] One account notes that goldenseal extract was used in some Russian hospitals, administered to women for excess bleeding and the disturbances and pain of monthly periods.[25] Hydrastine hydrochloride, the salt form of hydrastine, an alkaloid in goldenseal, has been used to control uterine bleeding.[26]

CHEMISTRY AND PHARMACOLOGY

The primary active compounds in goldenseal are the isoquinoline alkaloids berberine, hydrastine, canadine, and candaline.[27] From the perspective of quality control using chemical assays, the tenth edition of the *French Pharmacopoeia* stipulates that the root and rhizome material must contain not less than 2.5 percent hydrastine compared to the dry weight of the material.[28]

Although goldenseal and other plants containing berberine and related alkaloids are relatively safe, there are certain cautions that apply. Goldenseal is often contraindicated in pregnancy,[29] due to the uterine contraction activity demonstrated by the alkaloids.[30] It is also contraindicated for those with high blood pressure.[31]

One of the primary effects noted for the action of berberine in goldenseal when used internally (and in some other substitute plants; see below) is its antimicrobial action against numerous digestive pathogens. This microbial action has sometimes been referred to inappropriately as "antibiotic" activity; however, medical authorities usually define an *antibiotic agent* as "one derived from fungal molds, not from higher plants." The list of pathogens that have been shown to be affected by goldenseal and/or berberine (by either in-vitro studies or animal research) include eighteen varieties of bacteria (such as *E. coli, Salmonella paratyphi, Salmonella typhimurium, Shigella boydii, Staphylococcus aureus,* and *Staphylococcus pyrogens*), fungi (such as *Candida albicans*), and parasites (such as *Giardia lamblia, Leishmania donovani,* and *Trichomonas vaginalis*).[32] In support of the antimicrobial ac-

tivity, some authorities note that berberine is bacteriostatic at low doses and a bacteriocide in higher doses.[33]

Regarding the antimicrobial action, the herbalist Bergner writes, "It is my opinion that goldenseal acts as an 'antibiotic' to the mucous membranes not by killing germs directly, but by increasing the flow of healthy mucus, which contains its own innate antibiotic factors—IgA antibodies. This effect is unnecessary in the early stages of a cold or flu, when mucus is already flowing freely."[34] This immunoglobulin activity has been suggested in recent research in which goldenseal extract (produced by the Eclectic Institute, Sandy, Oregon) showed some increase in a specific type of immune marker (IgM) in rats after about two weeks of treatment.[35] The implications of this research for humans remain to be confirmed scientifically.

Although modern controlled clinical studies on goldenseal are lacking, there have been some published on alkaloid berberine. Caution must be exercised whenever we attempt to extrapolate the results of studies conducted on one isolated plant constituent to the activity of the entire herbal material, but in the case of berberine and goldenseal such a projection can be instructive. Clinical studies on berberine have confirmed the ability to be effective in cases of acute diarrhea.[36] Studies on berberine have raised questions as to its oral absorption[37] and thus its systemic effects. As noted by Professor Varro E. Tyler, dean and distinguished professor of pharmacognosy emeritus at Purdue University, "berberine is not absorbed from the GI tract. Consequently, all effects of the principal alkaloids of the herb are local in character when administered orally. These include topical applications or effects within the digestive system. It can be effective there. The so-called systemic effects were either obtained by in-vitro studies or by *injecting* the alkaloid(s) in small animals. These include anticancer, anti-elasolytic, vasodilation, and other similar activities."[38] Thus, despite the oral use of goldenseal for the prevention or treatment of traveler's diarrhea and related conditions—although these are rational uses given the empirical literature and modern scientific studies on berberine—goldenseal's activity is really topical in nature.

Other clinical research on berberine supports these activities: stimulating bile and bilirubin secretion, improving symptoms of chronic cholecystitis, and normalizing elevated tyramine levels in people with cirrhosis of the liver.[39]

PREPARATION AND DOSAGE

The current thinking among herbalists is that internal use of Goldenseal may be beneficial in relatively small doses: 10 to 15 drops of a tincture (usually 1:5 or 1:10) or a fluid extract (1:1) in water.[40] (Note that this may yield a range of five to ten times the amount of goldenseal alkaloids.) Bergner states that it may take a few days to a week for the herb to produce its benefits.[41] The *British Herbal Compendium* suggests a three-times-daily dose of the dried rhizome and root at 0.5 to 1.0 gram; tincture (1:10, 60 percent ethanol), 2 to 4 ml; fluid extract (1:1, 60 percent ethanol), 0.3 to 1 ml.[42]

PROPAGATION AND CULTIVATION

It is most difficult to grow goldenseal from seeds. Like the modern cultivated American ginseng *(Panax quinquefolius)* industry, the increasing number of commercial growing operations propagate by breaking a rhizome into several pieces and planting them about 8 inches apart in the fall. Well-drained soil that's rich in humus and approximates the natural growing conditions is necessary. As with the wild plants, about 60 to 75 percent shade conditions must be created using lath cloth. Some accounts estimate that thirty-two plants can be grown in a square yard, producing about 2 pounds (dry) in three years.[43] There has been rapidly growing interest in producing goldenseal on a commercially sustainable basis. Horticulturist Jeanine Davis at the North Carolina State University's Mountain Horticultural Crop Research and Extension Center has been studying the optimum agronomics of goldenseal.[44] This study was funded partly under a grant from the herb companies Nature's Way, Gaia, and QBI—which, before the recent Convention on Trade in Endangered Species (CITES) classification of goldenseal as threatened, saw the need to develop sustainable harvesting techniques and, eventually, a viable commercially cultivated goldenseal harvest. Another herb company, Frontier Herbs, has initiated a "Save the goldenseal" campaign to help increase industry and consumer awareness about the conservation issues related to this plant. Frontier, like some other herb companies, has dedicated itself to move to sustainably harvested goldenseal as the sole source of the root in its products. Herbs for Kids uses only substitute herbs (see below) in its products in order to help reduce commercial pressure on goldenseal.

Toward this end Michael McGuffin, president of the American Herbal Products Association (AHPA, the leading herbal industry trade group), has written that AHPA has conducted an industry tonnage survey on goldenseal to determine the levels to which recent cultivation attempts have been successful at producing a viable alternative to the wild-harvested product.[45] The AHPA survey reported a total estimate of 265,000 pounds of dried root. For the sake of comparison, McGuffin cites statistics from early in the twentieth century: 200,000 to 300,000 pounds in 1908, according to a U.S. government publication; 200,000 to 400,000 pounds, according to a 1927 Canadian publication and one from 1949 by the U.S. government. McGuffin reports that in addition to the dried root harvest noted above, an *additional* 62,000 pounds of fresh goldenseal root was harvested as stock for goldenseal "gardens"—small plots of the herb planted either in partially cleared forest areas or under artificial shade to be grown for commercial sale. The survey reports that the average time for harvest is 3.6 to 3.8 years from the planting of the roots. The total commercially grown goldenseal crop in the 1998 harvest was about 6,400 pounds (about 2.4 percent); projections for the following four years are about 35,000 pounds per year, with a peak projection of 82,000 pounds in the fall of 2000. Thus, the total projected harvest from commercial sources is estimated to be 15 to 30 percent.[46]

HARVESTING

The sustainability of the native populations of goldenseal has become an issue of mounting interest to members of the herbal industry as well as conservation biologists and federal and international regulators. As is the case with virtually any root crop, especially one that is relatively difficult to cultivate in a commercial setting, the harvesting of the plant's root requires that the plant be killed in order to obtain the medicinally valuable component. Concern about possible harm to native goldenseal stands by habitat destruction (not necessarily overharvesting) were mentioned as far back as a hundred years ago.[47] In light of increasing concern over the perceived scarcity of goldenseal populations in eastern North America, the herb has been listed as Appendix II (threatened plant) by CITES. This action occurred at the biannual CITES convention in Zimbabwe, proposed by members of the U.S. Fish and Wildlife Service.[48]

According to some accounts, demand for goldenseal has been increasing in recent years, with collections from the wild growing nearly 600 percent from 1989 to 1994. Efforts to preserve the root are increasing. Of the twenty-seven states in which goldenseal grows, seventeen have declared it imperiled or uncommon based on categories developed by The Nature Conservancy in 1995. The plant is considered threatened in Canada. In the United States the Monongahela National Forest in eastern West Virginia has not issued permits for collection in response to a survey by its own biologist, which found that goldenseal was rarer than American ginseng.[49]

Out of consideration for the dwindling supplies of wild goldenseal, some authors and herbal industry leaders have begun to recommend the substitution of other berberine-rich plants. These include barberry root *(Berberis aquifolium)*, goldthread *(Coptis* spp.), Oregon grape *(Mahonia aquifolium)*, and yerba mansa *(Anemopsis californica)*. Due to the rising cost of goldenseal over the past decade, it is possible that some of the commercial material sold as goldenseal may have been adulterated and/or substituted with goldthread root from either India or China. [Editor's Note: Goldthread, Oregon grape, and yerba mansa are herbs currently on the UpS To-Watch List as potentially at risk.]

UpS RECOMMENDATIONS

- Possible alternatives include barberry, cultivated Oregon grape, cultivated yerba mansa, and other cultivated *Berberis* species.

- Use only cultivated goldenseal if possible.

Probably one of the most interesting uses of goldenseal root relates not to its purported medicinal effects but to its claimed ability to mask a positive result in urinalysis used in testing for illicit drugs. It is probable that a significant but undetermined amount of goldenseal consumption in the late 1980s and early 1990s can be attributed to the modern myth circulated among users of various recreational drugs that the ingestion of this root will help mask a positive result in urine testing. However, as at least one unlucky Indiana man discovered after being arrested for allegedly using marijuana and cocaine after he had taken goldenseal to beat the tests, this doesn't work, at least not for him! The misconception of goldenseal's masking of drug tests has been traced by botanical expert Steven Foster to a novel by John Uri Lloyd, *Stringtown on the Pike* (Dodd Mead, 1900), in which a man is accused of poisoning his uncle with strychnine, which had been found in the dead man's stomach based on alkaloid color reagent tests.[50] As it turns out, supposedly hydrastine from goldenseal, when mixed with morphine, produces the same test result. The dead man was fond of drinking stomach bitters, which, among various other ingredients, contained goldenseal, an obviously good candidate for inclusion in such a mixture. Because Lloyd was a man of such renown in pharmacy and plant chemistry, his goldenseal reaction became the subject of letters and articles in subsequent journals. This, writes Foster, is the reason this myth crept into the modern herbal conventional wisdom. But there is no real basis in fact to confirm such action by goldenseal. In fact, Foster cites a study published in 1975 in which subjects were given 120 mg of codeine over a six-day period; they were also given 15.6 grams of goldenseal for the final 2.5 days before their urine was tested. Not surprisingly, no difference was noticed in the urine samples, leading to the conclusion that goldenseal does *not* mask the presence of opiates.[51]

In addition to the drug-masking myth just noted, another myth driving goldenseal sales is the general misconception that it is an antibiotic. As already explained, goldenseal's activity is antimicrobial, not antibiotic, and the antimicrobial activity is really based on topical use, including ingestion, since the absorption of the alkaloids is in question. Thus, to really support the use of goldenseal for internal use, users should be aware of its potential to check or kill gastrointestinal pathogens; other touted benefits are subject to question.

There is a compelling need for some group to fund clinical research to determine the scientifically verifiable benefits of goldenseal. At the AHPA– and United Plant Savers–sponsored meeting on goldenseal sustainability in Anaheim, California, in 1997, where most of the members of the goldenseal industry were present (the major sellers of goldenseal and those representing collectors, processors, and exporters), I suggested that the industry develop a fund to finance at least one clinical study measuring the ability of goldenseal to alleviate symptoms of colds and flus, measuring potential immunostimulant activity, and/or determining related benefits.[52] When you consider the fact that this precious botanical resource is already recognized by wildlife biologists as threatened, as well as the charge by some leading herbalists that much of the common usage of goldenseal is inappropriate, it becomes all the more imperative for those in the supply side of the industry and/or the federal government to finance much-needed scientific research to document scientifically the potential benefits of one of America's leading botanical medicines.

The editors of this volume have asked that the contributors add a note about some personal experience they have had with the herb about which they are writing. Although I usually prefer not to write in the first person, to honor the request I offer the following anecdote: Several years ago I received a letter from a man who called himself "an herbalist," writing to me in response to an article I had written previously in a leading natural products industry trade magazine in which I lamented the lack of research on goldenseal in more than sixty years. Aside from a few ad hominem attacks on me, the letter writer claimed that there was significant science to support claims for goldenseal. I quickly wrote him back, asking if this were true, then why did he not cite such research in his letter? He responded with copies of information from the 1920s from Eclectic medical literature (some of which is cited above), plus some old research on berberine, not goldenseal root. When I pointed out to him that he had actually reinforced my initial position on the lack of research, he begrudgingly conceded his allegations, agreed with my lamentation, and thanked me for making an issue out of this in the first place. Since then we have become cordial acquaintances. I point this out as an example to my brothers and sisters who love herbs, especially those native to North America, and who would like to see more widespread acceptance of their potential benefits, not to mention their conservation—a primary objective of the United Plant Savers. While I sympathize with those who want to see more personal and professional use of native American herbs, the fact remains that ultimately they must undergo some clinical studies. This is a perfect area for the federal government to invest research funds. By the way,

I always take goldenseal root capsules with me while traveling to developing countries in order to help prevent and/or treat traveler's diarrhea. Based on the known pharmacology of some of the ingredients, plus my own experience, I do believe this is at least one rational and legitimate use for goldenseal.

NOTES

1. Brevoort, "The booming U.S. botanical market."

2. Blumenthal, "Herb market levels after five years of boom."

3. Lloyd and Lloyd, *Drugs and Medicines of North America*, Vol. 1.

4. Foster, *Herbs of Commerce.*

5. Hobbs, "Goldenseal in early American botany."

6. Foster, "Goldenseal masking of drug tests."

7. Foster and Duke, *Peterson's Field Guide: Eastern/ Central Medicinal Plants.*

8. Elliott, *Wild Roots: A Forager's Guide to the Edible and Medicinal Roots, Tubers, Corms, and Rhizomes of North America.*

9. Foster and Duke, *Peterson's Field Guide: Eastern/ Central Medicinal Plants.*

10. Lloyd, *Origin and History of All the Pharmacopeial Vegetable Drugs.*

11. Elliott, *Wild Roots: A Forager's Guide to the Edible and Medicinal Roots, Tubers, Corms, and Rhizomes of North America.*

12. Lloyd, *Origin and History of All the Pharmacopeial Vegetable Drugs.*

13. Ibid.

14. Ibid.

15. Ibid.

16. Moerman, *Native American Ethnobotany.*

17. Bergner, *The Healing Power of Echinacea and Goldenseal.*

18. Felter and Lloyd, *King's American Dispensatory.*

19. Ellingwood, *American Materia Medica, Therapeutics and Pharmacology.*

20. Felter, *The Eclectic Materia Medica, Pharmacology and Therapeutics.*

21. Ibid.

22. Hobbs, "Goldenseal in early American botany."

23. Bergner, "Goldenseal and the common cold."

24. Bradley, *The British Herbal Compendium*, Vol. 1.

25. Hutchins, *Indian Herbology of North America.*

26. Trease and Evans, *Pharmacognosy.*

27. Leone et al., "HPLC determination of the major alkaloids extracted from *Hydrastis canadensis* L."

28. Bradley, *The British Herbal Compendium.*

29. Ibid.

30. Newell, Anderson, and Phillipson, *Herbal Medicines: A Guide for Health-care Professionals.*

31. Ibid.

32. Bergner, "Goldenseal and the common cold"; Bergner, *The Healing Power of Echinacea and Goldenseal*; Newell, Anderson, and Phillipson, *Herbal Medicines: A Guide for Health-care Professionals.*

33. Bruneton, *Pharmacognosy, Phytochemistry, Medicinal Plants.*

34. Bergner, "Goldenseal and the common cold."

35. Rehman et al., "Increased production of antigen-specific immunoglobulins G and M following in vivo treatment with the medicinal plants *Echinacea angustifolia* and *Hydrastis canadensis.*"

36. Newell, Anderson, and Phillipson, *Herbal Medicines: A Guide for Health-care Professionals*; Snow, "Hydrastis canadensis L. (Ranunculaceae)."

37. Bhide, Chavan, and Dutta, "Absorption, distribution, and excretion of berberine."

38. Tyler, personal communication to Ginger Webb, American Botanical Council.

39. Newell, Anderson, and Phillipson, *Herbal Medicines: A Guide for Health-care Professionals.*

40. Bergner, "Goldenseal and the common cold."

41. Ibid.

42. Bradley, *The British Herbal Compendium*, Vol. 1.

43. Grieve, *A Modern Herbal.*

44. Davis, *Advances in Goldenseal Cultivation.*

45. McGuffin, "AHPA Goldenseal survey measures increased agricultural production."

46. Ibid.

47. Lloyd and Lloyd, *Drugs and Medicines of North America.*

48. Bannerman, "Goldenseal in world trade: Pressure and potentials."

49. Concannon and DeMeo, "Goldenseal: Facing a hidden crisis."

50. Foster, "Goldenseal masking of drug tests."

51. Ibid.

52. Liebmann et al., "Industry and organizations form partnership for goldenseal conservation."

REFERENCES

Anonymous. "Suspected cocaine dealer enters guilty plea." *Lafayette (Ind.) Journal and Courier,* 1 June 1995.

Bannerman, J. E. "Goldenseal in world trade: Pressure and potentials." *HerbalGram* 41 (1997): 51–52.

Bergner, Paul. *The Healing Power of Echinacea and Goldenseal and Other Immune System Herbs.* Rocklin, Calif.: Prima Publishing, 1997.

———. "Goldenseal and the common cold: The antibiotic myth." *Medical Herbalism* 8 (4): 1, 4–6 (1996–1997).

———. "Goldenseal substitutes." *Medical Herbalism* 8 (4): 6–10 (1996–1997).

Bhide, M. B., S. R. Chavan, N. K. Dutta. "Absorption, distribution, and excretion of berberine." *Indian Journal of Medical Research* 57 (1969): 2128–31.

Blumenthal, M. "Herb market levels after five years of boom: 1999 sales in mainstream markets up only 11% in first half of 1999 after 55% increase in 1998." *HerbalGram* 47 (1999): 64–65.

Bradley, P. R. *The British Herbal Compendium.* Vol. 1. Bournemouth, U.K.: British Herbal Medicine Association, 1992.

Bruneton, J. *Pharmacognosy, Phytochemistry, Medicinal Plants.* New York: Lavoisier, 1995.

Brevoort, P. "The booming U.S. botanical market—A new overview." *HerbalGram* 44 (1998): 33–48.

Concannon, J. A., and T. E. DeMeo. "Goldenseal: Facing a hidden crisis." *Endangered Species Bulletin.* 22 (6): 10–12 (Nov/Dec. 1997).

Davis, J. *Advances in Goldenseal Cultivation.* Fletcher: North Carolina Cooperative Extension Service, 1996.

Ellingwood, Finley. *American Materia Medica, Therapeutics and Pharmacology.* 1898. Reprint, Portland, Oreg.: Eclectic Medical Publications, 1983.

Elliott, Doug. *Wild Roots: A Forager's Guide to the Edible and Medicinal Roots, Tubers, Corms, and Rhizomes of North America.* Rochester, Vt.: Healing Arts Press, 1995.

Evans, W. C. *Trease and Evans's Pharmacognosy,* 14th ed. London: W. B. Saunders Co., Ltd., 1989.

Felter, Harvey Wickes, M.D. *Eclectic Materia Medica, Pharmacology and Therapeutics.* 1922. Reprint, Portland, Oreg.: Eclectic Medical Publications, 1983.

Felter, Harvey Wickes, M.D., and John Uri Lloyd. *King's American Dispensatory.* Vol. 2. 1898. Reprint, Sandy, Oreg.: Eclectic Medical Publications, 1983.

Foster, Steven. *Goldenseal, Hydrastis canadensis.* Botanical Booklet Series No. 309. Austin, Tex.: American Botanical Council, 1996.

———. *Herbs of Commerce*. Austin, Tex.: American Herbal Products Association, 1992.

———. "Goldenseal masking of drug tests: From fiction to fallacy: An historical anomaly." *HerbalGram* 21 (1989): 7, 35.

Foster Steven, and James A. Duke. *Peterson's Field Guide: Eastern/Central Medicinal Plants*. Boston: Houghton Mifflin, 1990.

Grieve, Mrs. Maude. *A Modern Herbal*. Vol. 1. 1931. Reprint, New York: Dover, 1971.

Hobbs. Christopher. "Goldenseal in early American medical botany." *Pharmacy in History* 32 (2): 79–82 (1990).

Hutchins, A. R. *Indian Herbology of North America*. Windsor, Ont.: Merco Publishers, 1973.

Leone, M. G., M. F. Cometa, M. Palmery, L. Saso. "HPLC determination of the major alkaloids extracted from *Hydrastis canadensis* L." *Phytotherapy Research* 10 (1996): 45–46.

Liebmann, R., R. Cech, S. Goodman, F. Hathaway, T. Hayes, A. Lockard, M. Maruca, C. Robbins. "Industry and organizations form partnership for goldenseal conservation." *HerbalGram* 44 (1998): 58–59.

Lloyd, John Uri. *Origin and History of All the Pharmacopeial Vegetable Drugs*. Cincinnati: Caxton Press, 1929.

Lloyd, John Uri, and C. G. Lloyd. *Drugs and Medicines of North America*. Vol. 1—Ranunculaceae. Cincinnati: authors, 1884–1885.

Millspaugh, Charles. *American Medicinal Plants, an Illustrated and Descriptive Guide to the American Plants Used as Homeopathic Remedies*. 1884–1885. Reprint, New York: Dover, 1974.

McGuffin, Michael. "AHPA goldenseal survey measures increased agricultural production." *HerbalGram* 46 (1999): 66–67.

Moerman, Daniel. *Native American Ethnobotany*. Portland, Oreg.: Timber Press, 1998.

Newall, C. A., L. A. Anderson, and J. D. Phillipson. *Herbal Medicines: A Guide for Health-care Professionals*. London: Pharmaceutical Press, 1996.

Pharmacopée Française, 10th ed. Paris: La Commission Nationale de Pharmacopée, 1994.

Rehman, J., J. M. Dillow, S. M. Carter, J. Chou, B. Le, A. S. Maisel. "Increased production of antigen-specific immunoglobulins G and M following in vivo treatment with the medicinal plants *Echinacea angustifolia* and *Hydrastis canadensis*." *Immunology Letters* 68 (1999): 391–95.

Snow, J. M. "*Hydrastis canadensis* L. (Ranunculaceae)." *Protocal Journal of Natural Medicine* 2 (2): 25–28 (1997).

Tyler, V. E. Personal communication to Ginger Webb, American Botanical Council, 7 April 1998.

U.S. Fish and Game Department. "Proposal for the Inclusion of *Hydrastis canadensis*, Appendix II CITES (Convention on Trade in Endangered Species)." 1997.

Vogel, V. J. *American Indian Medicine*. Norman: University of Oklahoma Press, 1970.

GOLDTHREAD
Coptis spp.

NANCY AND MICHAEL PHILLIPS

Goldthread didn't readily reveal herself on our northern New Hampshire farm. The mixed balsam fir and spruce woods here certainly provide the expected habitat. Out on walks we would find ground cedar, partridgeberry, twinflower, and myriad mosses—but not the glossy lobed leaves marking the golden roots sought for medicine. We put the case to our friend Andy, a botanical Sherlock Holmes if ever such a sleuth walked the forest floor.

Ergo, we went back a 120-plus years to the time this mountain farm first heard the ringing ax clearing virgin timber to open up pasture ground. Eastern goldthread, *Coptis groenlandica*, is an old-growth plant in its own right. Rhizomes along established roots sprout forth new leaf clusters, thereby allowing the plant to spread. Andy reckoned that any remnant patches we might find today would be traceable directly to the original twining roots that somehow survived decades of dairy cows and workhorses. We headed for rocky ground. Our woods are going through a first succession of shallow-rooted firs that, having toppled in gusty winds, have left a jumbled maze of soil-restoring logs to snag our

way. Moss-covered rocks abound among the ferns, and sure enough, here and there we found the smallest clusters of goldthread, so precious we simply honored its persistence. The hike back led us along an alder bog, where our feet pressed softly into luminous beds of moist moss. Our sleuth surmised: Ground too wet, cows stay back, native plants endure. Goldthread awaited us on the western edge of the bog, where deciduous shade adds to the cool of the evergreen forest. We sensed that roots might be gathered here should an individual in our family or community have a need for this medicine. A spiritual permission from Goldthread herself will take place should such an occasion ever arise.

BOTANICAL FEATURES

Goldthread is aptly named—this dainty little evergreen plant of the Buttercup family has bright gold, threadlike roots. Its lustrous leaves rise from a rhizome base, each stem divided into three leaflets with scalloped, toothed margins. Each leaflet is usually less than $1^1/_2$ inches wide. *Coptis groenlandica*, which grows here in the East from Québec south to North Carolina, stands 3 to 5 inches high. Western goldthread, *C. occidentalis*, grows slightly taller, perhaps reflecting its preference for more mountainous terrain in undisturbed stands of cedar, yew, and grand fir. The whitish flowers of goldthread extend at the end of leafless stems. The five to seven narrow petals eventually fall off, leaving behind a green sepal that hollows into a star-shaped capsule that bears exceedingly small black seeds.

The thin roots form a creeping network of rhizomes from which the aerial parts of goldthread arise. These rhizomes generally spread in the rich organic matter of the forest floor rather than the mineral soil beneath. Goldthread helps loosen up this otherwise impervious mat of needle debris in the cool shade of evergreen woods. Boggier settings find the rhizomes quite at home in beds of sphagnum, often favoring the drier knolls surrounded by sodden ground.

HISTORICAL BACKGROUND

Native Americans had a ready supply of fresh goldthread available throughout the year for either chewing or making tea. The vibrant gold roots, available even in winter under a blanket of snow, would have been as near as any old-growth forest. Good remedies wee naturally shared with the colonists, and goldthread eventually became so popular that more of it was sold in Boston than almost any other indigenous drug. Such esteem fell by the wayside, however, most likely as our forebears' impact on the land altered the availability of this wee plant. The Eclectics didn't lose sight of goldthread, of course, and soon identified the two alkaloids, berberine and coptine, as its primary agents of unstandardized virtue. Equal parts of goldthread and goldenseal, made into a decoction with elixir vitriol added in the proper quantity, was said to permanently destroy the appetite for alcoholic beverages; apparently the prohibitionists ultimately decided on an allopathic approach, though.

MEDICINAL USES

Goldthread has traditionally been used for mouth sores and thrush, which explains its other common names—canker root and mouth root. This strong bitter has also been used for a variety of digestive disorders, worms, jaundice, and as a so-called blood purifier. It is sometimes used in combination with or substituted for goldenseal, another at-risk plant. Both contain berberine, a bitter alkaloid with strong antibacterial qualities. Goldenseal has been considered rare for more than seventy-five years due to unceasing demand, and some herbalists concerned about its survival have suggested using goldthread in its place. This will never be a reasonable alternative on a broad scale, because the fine roots of goldthread can't begin to meet our current (and sometimes erroneous) zeal for goldenseal. Transferring such high demand to goldthread would soon bring about its extinction, so the better solution lies in using cultivated organic goldenseal with sustainable discretion. Recent laboratory studies of a gold-thread indigenous to China, *Coptis chinensis*, show promise against HIV, infectious hepatitis, and certain flu strains.

PREPARATION AND DOSAGE

The simplest way to use goldthread is to chew the fresh root. This is effective for canker sores and mouth ulcerations. Goldthread is more commonly used in tea or in tincture form. Both preparations can be made with fresh or dried plant material. One tablespoon of fresh finely chopped root (or 1 teaspoon of dried root) per cup of boiling water simmered for twenty minutes makes an effective decoction. This tea can then be gargled for mouth sores or applied frequently for thrush. It can also be taken internally as a bitter tonic, 1 tablespoon three to six times a day for an average adult, for chronic stomach inflammation or digestive problems.

There are several ways to make tinctures, and in reviewing the literature concerning goldthread we found different suggested ratios of root, water, and alcohol. Surprise, surprise! When in doubt, the "folkloric method" will always serve: Finely chop the whole plant and put it in a jar. Pour hundred-proof vodka into the jar to completely cover the plant material, with a little extra vodka in the jar so everything can slosh around well (about 1 or 2 inches over the plant material). Close the jar tightly and let it sit for about six weeks, and then strain. Singing healing songs and praying when shaking tinctures each day adds positive intentions to the medicine.

PROPAGATION AND CULTIVATION

Goldthread is a plant of the boreal and transition forests that grows where humans tread lightly, if at all. Spaded clumps—taken only from a vibrant *Coptis* patch—can be carefully transplanted into suitable locations that offer shade and plenty of abundant organic matter. Use trial "hither and thither plantings" to see if your vision is in accord with both the plant and the land. You need to move these delicate rhizomes and their trailing root systems with earth intact to have any chance of success. The seeds are small and easily missed, because the goldthread flower matures quickly. Replenishing native species is an offering of restoration that transcends commercial intent. Nor does the extreme fineness of goldthread roots exactly encourage a medicinal livelihood. Greg Tilford puts this best in his book *From Earth to Herbalist:* "This is a plant to worry about and protect, not to exploit. Goldthread offers us a chance to redefine what 'value' really means and to take the gift of healing to heart instead of to the bank." The Asian species, *C. chinensis*, could offer innovative woodland growers better prospects; its larger roots offer an equivalent medicine. According to Robert Newman, former curator of the Nanjing Medicinal Botanical Garden, this species is cultivated successfully in China but awaits a North American appraisal.

HARVESTING

We first harvested goldthread with Kate Gilday and Don Babineau at their forest home just south of the Adirondacks. The trees here have only recently reclaimed the land first taken from the Iroquois following the Revolution. Goldthread flourishes in a hemlock vale along an open wetland. Prayers are offered to the plant spirits. Hands reach into the soft soil beneath the hemlock duff. Golden roots are revealed trailing from one leaf cluster to the next. Each of us gathers within a small circle of intimacy, fingering the root threads into piles while our thoughts roam deeply into the earth. Our small baskets fill slowly individually, but together we quickly have enough of the very fine roots, rhizomes, and accompanying leaves for Kate to make the pint of fresh tincture she and another community practitioner use every two years. We tuck any neighboring roots back beneath the soil to replenish the tiny radius of our harvest. Goldthread here gains new ground each year, nurtured by reverence and the rich forest compost of undisturbed ground.

UpS RECOMMENDATIONS

- Use cultivated resources only. This plant is slow to grow and very tiny.
- Use barberry as a possible substitute.

REFERENCES

Felter, Harvey Wickes, M.D. *The Eclectic Materia Medica, Pharmacology and Therapeutics.* 1922. Reprint, Portland, Oreg.: Eclectic Medical Publications, 1983.

Felter, Harvey Wickes, M.D., and John Uri Lloyd. *King's American Dispensatory.* 1898. Reprint, Portland, Oreg.: Eclectic Medical Publications, 1983.

Foster, Steven, and James A. Duke. *Peterson's Field Guide: Eastern/Central Medicinal Plants.* Boston: Houghton Mifflin, 1990.

Grieve, Mrs. Maude. *A Modern Herbal.* Vol. 1. 1931. Reprint, New York: Dover, 1971.

Hutchins, Alma. *Indian Herbology of North America.* Windsor, Ont.: Merco Publishers, 1973.

Sutton, Ann, and Myron Sutton. *Eastern Forests, An Audubon Society Nature Guide.* New York: Alfred A. Knopf, 1985.

Tilford, Gregory. *From Earth to Herbalist.* Missoula, Mont.: Mountain Press Publishing, 1998.

HELONIAS ROOT
Chamaelirium luteum

DEB SOULE

I first came upon helionas root, or false uni-corn, when walking in the woods in North Carolina with my botanist friend Doug Elliott in the late 1980s. I was excited to meet this plant and immediately got onto my hands and knees to have a closer look at the white, starry flowers growing on 1- to 2-foot-tall spikes. I thought about how different these small spikes are from the 5- to 7-foot-tall white flowering racemes of the black cohoshes that live in the same neighborhood as helonias root yet flower at different times. I was able to purchase a few dozen plants from Garden in the Woods in Framingham, Massachusetts, four years ago to plant in a woodland garden near my house. Six plants have survived some tough Maine winters under layers of leaf and straw mulch. Every spring when I begin to uncover the area where the helonias root grows, I say a prayer in the hope that my plants have survived in this zone, which is farther north than their normal range. One of the common names for this plant is fairy wand and in late June, when the female plants are flowering, I can't help but smile, imagining a fairy using this flower as a wand.

BOTANICAL FEATURES

Helonias root belongs to the *Liliaceae* or Lily family and grows in moist meadows, bogs, thickets, and woods from western Massachusetts to Michigan and south to Florida. The female and male flowers are small and white and grow on separate stalks. The female flower spike is shorter and straighter than the male flower and blunt at the tip. Each individual female flower consists of six tiny white petals, and a small globular ovary about the size of a grain of hemp seed. The seeds form in an oblong-shaped capsule in the fall. The male flowers are 4 to 6 inches in length and grow on a drooping, plumelike spike—hence another common name, drooping starwort.

The female and male flower stalks arise from a rosette of smooth leaves; veins run lengthwise along each leaf, which is oblong shaped and approximately 8 inches long. The female plant is leafier than the male. The rhizome is the part of the plant herbalists use and its color is a light tan when fresh. The slight upward curve at the tip resembles a stubby horn, which is how the plant received the names false unicorn and unicorn's horn.

HISTORICAL BACKGROUND

Doug Elliott writes about one of the common names for this plant, devil's bit, in his book *Wild Roots: A Forager's Guide to the Edible and Medicinal Roots, Tubers, Corms, and Rhizomes of North America.*

> The name Devil's Bit derives from the bitten-off, knub-like appearance of the rhizome. The name, along with a legend, came from Europe where it referred to a European plant with a similar rootstock. The long, trailing roots of this plant, so the legend goes, possessed not only extremely beneficial healing properties, but extraordinary magic. So beneficial was it for the people who used it that the Devil himself became angered and tried to change the qualities of the root from good to bad. The power and goodness of this plant was so strong, however, that his attempts were always thwarted. Finally, the Devil flew into a rage and personally bit off every one of the roots. His rage was so searing that to this day the roots have not been able to grow back. But the remaining stub is still imbued with good medicine, and every spring it is able to put forth the tall spike of beautiful, blazing-star blossoms as a reminder that the power of goodness can always avert the forces of evil.

In *King's American Dispensatory*, Volume 1, rewritten and enlarged in 1898, pharmacist John Uri Lloyd and Dr. Harvey Felter wrote of helonias root's uses for women:

> In diseases of the reproductive organs of females, and especially of the uterus, it is one of our most valuable agents, acting as a uterine tonic, and gradually removing abnormal conditions, while at the same time it imparts tone and vigor to the reproductive organs. Hence, it is much used in leucorrhaea, amenorrhaea, dysmenorrhaea, and to remove the tendency to repeated and successive miscarriages. A particular phase removed by it is the irritability and despondency that often attends uterine trouble. In painful menstruation it has been found especially adapted to those cases in which there is pelvic fullness, a sensation as if the womb and rectum were distended with blood, and the aching, bearing-down organs feel as if they would fall out of the body.

As so often is the case throughout history, indigenous peoples and women's contributions are often unrecognized and unrecorded. Helonias root is a plant used by Native American women, who passed their knowledge of this plant on to others, apparently through word of mouth. In the 1800s the Eclectics and physiomedicalists wrote about the valuable uses of helonias root. Today's British herbalists recognize the value of this plant as well, for it is included in the 1992 edition of the *British Herbal Compendium.*

MEDICINAL USES

Helonias root contains hormonelike saponins and steroidal compounds, including the hormone precursor diosgenin, which may partly account for its long tradition as a uterine tonic. In my own practice with women, I have recommended that this herb be taken in small doses for several weeks to help restore strength and tone to the uterus after pregnancy, an abortion, miscarriage, or surgery, and for promoting fertility. Women with ovarian cysts or endometriosis may take helonias root with other herbs over several weeks to increase circulation to the pelvic area. Women healing from sexual abuse experiences may find the root, when taken a few times a week, helpful in restoring feelings of strength and vitality in their womb area.

Helonias root is a good remedy for a woman with a prolapsed uterus, because it improves muscle tone. It also acts as a tonic for the genitourinary tract. Helonias root eases nausea and vomiting during pregnancy, too, and in combination with other herbs helps prevent miscarriages. It strengthens the spleen and raises overall energy in the body.

Still, as much as I appreciate the medicine this plant offers to women, I seldom use it anymore. Shrinking habitat coupled with increased demand is causing serious depletion of this already sensitive woodland plant. We need cultivated resources. Unfortunately, no cultivation studies are under way and, even should acres be successfully planted today, it will be years before the *Chamaelirium* root is ready for harvesting. I hope more people will become interested in cultivating this plant so that it will flourish again in protected woodlands and meadows and be accessible to women who need helonias root's medicine.

PROPAGATION AND CULTIVATION

It is possible to propagate helonias root, though at this point I know of no one who is actively engaged in doing so. The only person I know who has successfully started this plant from seed is Heather McCargo, who worked for Garden in the Woods for five years, propagating native woodland plants. The seeds are collected in the fall from the female flower stalks and stored in a dry, dark, and cool place. The seeds are very tiny and need to be gently tamped into moist soil in late winter and kept in a semidark place; they germinate and develop in an indoor setting. The cultivated roots can be harvested in the fall of their fourth year. Until cultivation of helonias root can be assured, no wildcrafting of this plant is recommended.

UpS RECOMMENDATIONS

- Use only cultivated sources.
- Motherwort is a good alternative.

KAVA
Piper methysticum

TANE DATTA

Kava was placed on the United Plant Savers target list in 1997 because wild populations of the plant in Hawaii were being rapidly depleted. The popularity of the root had increased dramatically, and the overall availability of the plant material was diminishing. This was seen by rapidly increasing prices, empty holes in the rain forest where there had once been large thirty- to fifty-year-old *awa* (kava) stands, the development of a black market for stolen awa roots, and the visible destruction of kava's rain forest habitat to make way for large papaya plantations and other development.

The kava plant intrigues me because it grows well in undisturbed rain forests. I am an organic farmer who believes that a healthy society can be based on caring for and nurturing the soil. One way of manifesting this care is finding the highest sustainable value for land; in turn, part of finding the highest sustainable value is understanding the environment well enough to find crops that grow naturally in it. The closer the plant fits naturally in the environment, the less need for farmer intervention such as the addition of fertilizers, pesticides, and herbicides.

This approach led me to look closely at the wide variety of plants already growing naturally in the Hawaiian rain forest and to recognize the value in the plants already existing there. I have since gained a local reputation for selling weeds such as gotu kola, passion vine, mullein, and beach almond. These are plants that some people spend a great deal of effort trying to eliminate.

The early 1990s saw an increasing threat to the rain forest in the form of geothermal exploitation in the heart of the preserves. The popular "Save the Rain Forest" movement organized some festive demonstrations within the lush rain forest. Some of the literature distributed at these gatherings mentioned that if geothermal development was allowed, twenty-six species of rain forest plants would become extinct. I pursued the organizers and asked them *which* twenty-six plants were endangered. After six months of tracking down leads, I finally got the list. Kava was among them.

I thought about my own partial clearing of the rain forest where I live to make room for organic gardens, orchards, and dwellings. I have left quite a bit of original forest, and much of what I cleared was Christmasberry, a recently introduced, strongly aggressive tree in Hawaii. Still, it has always been my desire to compare the value of integrating economic plantings into the jungle with that of clearing land for highly intensive organic beds or orchards. Kava, being a shade-loving understory plant, has given me a chance to try just that.

Kava plays a significant and esteemed role in all Polynesia, of which Hawaii is part. The plant is used medicinally to set the spiritual framework for other healing practices. The ancient kava ceremony recognizes and honors both visitors and the culture they are visiting. Kava's use by the *kahunas* (traditional healers) is valuable in helping individuals and in revitalizing Hawaiian culture, which is indeed resurging: hula dancing, language, traditional foods and practices, and political organizing are all permitted now after long bans.

All of the issues above have combined to bring me into an increasingly complex relationship with kava. Personally, I would like to see:

- The kava I've been planting for the past few years become as valuable as the cultivated areas of my farm;
- kava's use increase on the Islands—possibly decreasing alcoholism and aggressiveness;
- kava cultivation become part of the base for sustainable economic and community development of Hawaii.

I am working toward developing our kava in a way that reverses more than 150 years of colonialism imposed by sugar and pineapple plantations and their domination of the political systems. All these dreams are slowly coming true.

BOTANICAL FEATURES

Kava, an elegant shrub that grows 3 to 15 feet tall, is a member of the Pepper family. It has elongated, jointed stems that are swollen at the joints in a manner similar to bamboo. These swollen joints are called knuckles, and are used in the propagation of the plant. Kava has alternate dark green heart-shaped leaves about 5 to 8 inches long. Left on its own, the plant forms small groves and dominates its area of the rain forest understory.

The plant is sterile, and therefore any patch of kava, no matter how remote, was at one time placed there by humans. There are wide variations in chromosome numbers in the *Piper* genus. *P. methysticum* has a high ploidy[1] level, which could explain its sterility. The original plant was likely *P. wichmanni*, which is the only other plant from which kavalactones have been isolated. Kavalactones, a secondary metabolite in kava, are produced in unusually high quantities, reflecting its close association and dependency on humans for its survival. Dr. Lebot believes kava should be considered, botanically, a sterile cultivar of *P. wichmanni*, which is sometimes used to "stretch" the kava herb.

Kava developed its characteristics by human selection. When the plant was harvested, its stems were left lying out. After the beverage was drunk, if its flavor found approval, the kava was replanted. In this way, characteristics favored by different human groups were selected. These characteristics can be seen biochemically by looking at the various kavalactones and their ratios in the various cultivars.

Each kava variety has its own unique physiological effects. Some are strong, some are weak, some induce deep sleep, and others cause nausea. Some have effects that last only overnight while others can be felt for three days. The different ratios of kavalactones within varieties are responsible for these different effects. Many Hawaiian cultivars are being analyzed according to age and growing location. This will become the basis for a classification system.

The six major kavalactones are:

1. DMY = demethoxyyangonin
2. DHK = dihydrokavain
3. Y = yangonin
4. K = kavain
5. DHM = dihydromethysticin
6. M = methysticum

The composition of different cultivars of kava are being coded based on the sequence of the above numbers. Thus a cultivar such as maha kea, a black kava from Hawaii, may be characterized by the code 426351 based on kavalactone analysis. This indicates that the cultivar contains the highest K, kavain (4); followed by DHK, dihydrokavain (2); followed by M, methysticum (6); and so forth. This system maps out the relative proportions of these six kavalactones. Often the first three kavalactones represent more than 70 percent of the overall total. In some cases, the relative percentage of the first three is relatively close (25, 23, and 22 percent respectively, for example). This places importance on whether a kavalactone occupies one of the first three digits rather than its exact rank. The effects gotten from a 426 would be likely similar to those derived from a 624 or 246.

Ethnobotanical data show that drinkers do not prefer a high percentage of DHM (5) and DHK (2), because the physiological effects are too severe and nausea is often felt. The most appreciated chemotypes have a high percentage of K (4) and low percentage of DHM (5).

Piper wichmanni, which is considered the origin species of kava, contains a high concentration of DHK (2) and DHM (5). The kavalactone content of a kava plant is related more strongly to the cultivar (variety) than to environmental or cultivation factors. In practical terms, this means that the clones gotten from a plant will produce the same effect as the mother plant. *P. methysticum* appears to have developed by farmers selecting for the effects they sought. When they migrated to different regions of Polynesia, they brought their preferred clones with them and continued to develop them.

The many different effects attributed to kava along with the many different names in several subcultures are results of centuries of this process. Ethnobotanists have used the varying characteristics of kava to trace the dispersal of the Polynesian people. The morphological features of the plants have been mapped out in a similar manner as the chemotype. The morphological features used are stem color, internode configuration, leaf color, lamina edges (shape of leaf), leaf pubescence, and internode shape. By correlating the chemical and physical characteristics, a less confusing nomenclature is being developed. This will enable kava users to reliably obtain the effects they are seeking.

HISTORICAL BACKGROUND

Kava usage was first observed by Captain Cook, the European discoverer and recorder of Hawaii. Kava usage was well established and integrated into Polynesian society by this time. Looking at its effects on his crew, he assumed it to be an opiate. Samples taken back to England showed there were no opiates in kava, however, and Western medical interest in it waned.

Kava is used ritually throughout Polynesia as a means of bringing people together or honoring dignitaries. The pope, Hillary Rodham Clinton, and the queen of England have all participated in such kava ceremonies.

For a long while kava was overlooked by Western herbalists and promoted mainly as a legal intoxicant or love drug. The demand for kava in these markets remained low but, along with the native taboos already existing, contributed to a mysterious but tarnished and fearful image of the plant.

Kava's ability to reduce stress and anxiety is rapidly gaining recognition in Western society. *The Wall Street Journal*[2] recently noted the vast amount of sales potential it may have. Kava and St.-John's-wort are being successfully promoted as herbal alternatives to barbiturates and Prozac. This newfound respectability is responsible for the harvesting pressure leading to its endangerment in Hawaii.

MEDICINAL USES

Historically kava has been used in Polynesian culture for a wide and sometimes conflicting range of ailments: to treat headaches; provoke abortions; ease childbirth; treat intestinal problems, urinogenital system infections, cough, skin disease, and gonorrhea; and, of course, to induce relaxation. It is a spinal rather than a cerebral depressant. It has been shown to be an anticonvulsant, local anesthetic, and, in some cases, antifungal. There is a large variance in the constituents of the plant. Synthesized kavalactones do not create the same physiological effects as the natural extract. The constituents work synergistically with each other to such an extent that extracts used without the slightest alteration give much better results than any single isolated constituent.

All parts of the plant can be used, but the root is the most common. The concentrations of kavalactones vary among the stem, leaf, and root. The difference between cultivars overshadows, however, the differences in the plant parts.

Kava is not classified as a drug, because its consumption never leads to addiction or dependency. It has psychoactive properties but is neither hallucinogenic nor stupefacient. It has been classified as a narcotic and a hypnotic. This may help explain the atmosphere of sociability felt when drinking it. In Polynesian society, it is often said that "you cannot hate while drinking kava."

Kava drinking in a cultural context similar to beer drinking is the plant's most common use. Kava drinkers experience a state of well-being and contentment free from physical and psychological excitement. Conversation flows freely, and hearing and vision are improved. Drinkers remain masters of their conscience and reason, and their temperaments are soothed. Kava helps the thought process by relieving nervous tension and allows drinkers to talk through and solve problems of everyday life. The next day, drinkers awaken in excellent shape with no hangover effects.

Excessive consumption of kava can cause temporary oculomotor paralysis; the muscles may no longer respond to control of the mind, walking becomes unsteady, and drinkers look inebriated. The drinkers feel a need to sleep and are often found prostrate at the place where they have drunk. These effects will vary with the cultivar consumed.

Long-term excessive consumption has been found to cause skin lesions, drying up the epidermis and causing areas of severe itching. This is rare and is due in part to allergens that attach themselves to skin proteins. Poor diet (especially a diet lacking in B vitamins), susceptibility to allergies, and the use of undesirable cultivars are also significant factors in this effect. These symptoms disappear as soon as kava consumption is reduced.

Recently European pharmaceutical companies have developed from kava prescription medicines marketed as antianxiety drugs with fewer side effects and higher safety than synthetic drugs in the same classification. Pharmacologically, some studies have shown that kava is active in the hippocampus and amygdala, depressing activity in the area of the brain that governs anger.

Beverage companies are including kava in many enjoyable tea blends. Natural supplement manufacturers are cranking out new formulas;

I have even seen kava incorporated into corn chips. Of course, some of these products do not contain enough kava to have an effect.

Solving the problem in variability and composition of kava's active constituents has greatly increased the potential uses for this herb. Selection of particular cultivars for particular markets is now realistic. An herbalist seeking a specific effect from Hawaiian kava may soon be able to order by chemotype and reliably get the same effect on the next order.

PREPARATION AND DOSAGE

Traditional preparations use fresh root or dried root. In either case the root is broken down by grinding, pounding, or chewing, and then boiled as a tea. The root needs to be kept at a slow boil for at least twenty minutes. The kavalactones stay stable in the heat. About 1 tablespoon of dried powdered kava makes 1 cup of kava tea. The fresh root is stronger. The initial flavor is bitter with a slightly peppery aftertaste. A few minutes after drinking the tea, the tongue becomes numb and the bitter flavor is no longer noticeable. One to 3 cups of kava drunk slowly during an afternoon or evening is usually sufficient for a social gathering.

There are many ritual and ceremonial variations. In many cases, the kava is made in a large communal bowl and served from a single coconut bowl one person at a time according to rank or honor.

Modern preparations by herbal companies include tincturing at various ratios, continuous hot alcohol extraction, drying, freeze-drying, and powdering. Each method favors different plant constituents. It usually takes about 7 pounds of fresh root to make 1 gallon of alcohol tincture.

My favorite natural preparation is to take a young rootlet from an old root and chew it. I like the juicy, sweet, slightly peppery flavor and the quick numbing effect in my mouth. That alone generally enhances my mood.

Pharmaceutical companies extract specific kavalactones and reduce the kava to the familiar pill form of Western modern medicine.

PROPAGATION AND CULTIVATION

Kava propagation is in essence simple. It can only be started from the stem or parts of the stem as a clone. If harvesting is done in the moist jungle and the stems are put back into the ground where the root was, a new clump will grow. In commercial production, just the joints (or "knuckles") on the stem are used. These can be placed in trays filled with cinder and compost and kept in the shade under high humidity conditions. When a bud (small sprout) appears on the knuckle, it is transplanted to a small pot with a similar mixture. Often a single knuckle will have several buds. These are all allowed to grow. The key elements are good drainage, high humidity, and shade. The stem itself holds enough nutrient to support the budding. In the initial propagation stage, before budding, the stem is highly susceptible to bacterial and fungal damage. This seems to stem from stagnant water or air conditions.

Propagation from tissue culture has not proved viable. Some growers make use of fungicides and growth hormones. Others just throw coconut leaves on top of a pile of discarded stems and come back in a month to harvest knuckles with rootlets already growing. Sometimes stems stay dormant in their trays for months and during a full moon, sprout. The success of initial propagation is highly dependent on local conditions.

Once propagated, planting is relatively simple. Plants are placed approximately 10 feet away from each other in holes filled with cinder, compost, and composted manure. The size of the hole varies according to the conditions of the land and the intentions of the grower. In land with good soil a larger hole may be made; much of the plant growth will take place underground. In rocky soils a small hole may be dug, and most of the growth will be expected to take place aboveground. The best growing conditions seem to be in cinder soil in lowland areas with high rainfall and good drainage. Plants in these conditions will grow quickly to large sizes with little disease.

One important factor to keep in mind when growing kava is the large number of cultivars. Each one was developed for specific microclimates and to have specific effects. When planning a kava farm, it is best to grow several varieties known to have the desired effects. After a few years it will be clear which ones grow best under your conditions; these can be propagated further. You can also carry on the traditions of centuries by replanting the plants you like best, and thus developing new cultivars.

HARVESTING

Cultivated kava is harvested after it is at least two to three years old. The whole plant is dug out of the ground. The stems and leaves are cut off and the root is washed. In Hawaii, if the fresh root is to be sent to the mainland, it must be scrubbed meticulously. No particle of dirt is allowed through agricultural inspection, or the entire shipment may be quarantined. Cleaning the root takes as much time as the actual harvesting of the plant.

In good growing conditions, plant roots can reach 20 to 25 pounds in two years. If left in the ground for another five years, a single plant's root can weigh 100 to 150 pounds. Some plants in the wild reach several-hundred-pound sizes. Older plants spread out, with the center sometimes dying. The plant is subject to attack from pigs and rats. They rarely kill the whole plant but can leave it hollowed out. The rats partially chew the bamboolike stems, which fall to the ground and grow again. Some small rootlets grow out from the base of the stem in a manner similar to mangrove roots. In rocky soils, the root builds itself upward in a large mound. If the stem becomes buried by jungle debris, it may put out rootlets and become part of the root corm itself.

The preferred time to harvest the plant is when the roots approach 100 pounds. Larger plants often have rock and debris intermingled with the roots or sections of root that are hard to clean.

Opinion varies as to what influence age has on plants. Chemical analysis indicates that kavalactone percentage stabilizes within two years, and its levels remain the same as the plant grows larger. Yet a thirty-year-old root chunk larger than a man's thigh is impressive to see and daunting to consume. It becomes the focal point of any type of gathering, contributing to the uniqueness and spirit of the kava event.

If the plant is to be dried, it is broken into smaller pieces with a hammer mill or grinder and air-dried. The wet-to-dry ratio is approximately 3:1. Once dried, it may be left in small chunks or powdered. When it's in small chunk form, adding adulterants becomes more difficult.

UpS RECOMMENDATIONS

- Use only cultivated resources.
- Possible alternatives include chamomile, catnip, wood betony, cultivated valerian root, cultivated passionflower, and cultivated California poppy. (It is illegal in California to harvest California poppy in the wild.)

In earlier times the scarcity of kava in Hawaii may have had to do with the fierceness of the taboos set by the ruling elite. Later, taboos set by missionaries along with the colonials' attempt to destroy all facets of Hawaiian culture kept kava supplies low. Between these times, the use of kava spread to common people, who planted and tended their patches deep in the jungles and along hunting and gathering trails. In this way the kava plant became well established in the Hawaiian rain forest. Once planted, kava has a strong ability to survive on its own and slowly spread through the forests.

The current onslaught endangering kava

comes from two directions. On one side large-scale commercial developments that destroy rain forests in Hawaii are limiting its natural habitat. On another side poor, often local, people intoxicated by the prospects of finding plants of 100 pounds or more (worth more than $1,000 each) have been stripping the jungles and often their neighbors' lands. It is hard work to drag 100-pound roots through miles of rough, slippery trails, and it is simple work to replant an area that has been harvested or leave enough plants to regrow in an area. The intentions of the harvesters have changed from a deep cultural reverence for the plant to exploitation of it for quick hard cash. This is the core reason for the endangerment of wild kava in Hawaii.

Balancing these destructive forces has been a slow but steady resurgence of the Hawaiian culture in language, dance, politics, *kahuna* teachings, unity, and spirit. The Hawaiian culture teaches its members to do what is right in your heart and to conserve and replenish what is taken from the forests and the oceans. The state motto translated from the Hawaiian is, "The life of the land is perpetuated in righteousness." Also balancing these destructive forces has been the commercial development of kava as an alternative crop to defunct sugar. Some of the new kava plantations are using certified organic production systems. There also has been organization among kava growers to share markets, stop theft, and create standards that will make Hawaiian kava consistently the highest quality available in the world.

Few plants in the world have such great dependence on humans and such a great effect on humans. It is easy to replant any plant harvested if the harvester cares at all about kava and its environment: It is a matter of simply putting the stems back in the hole left by the removed root and covering them back up. The reasons kava has not been replanted in the wild and the steps now being taken to reestablish and develop kava as a crop in Hawaii may provide understanding that can help some of the other plants on the UpS threatened list. Some of the keys to the protection of kava are:

- The establishment of cultural and ethical values in the harvesters.
- The development of organic kava farms.
- The study and understanding of the plant's chemistry, mode or action, and the resulting refinement of cultivars.
- The development of a growers' association to share production and market information, protect each other from thieves, and protect themselves from the corporate exploitation commonly seen throughout the Pacific islands.
- The willingness of consumers to support organically certified production.
- The development of kava nurseries.
- The convening of gatherings such as the First International Botanical Symposium on kava sponsored by the American Herbal Products Association and Rural Economic Transition for Agriculture-Hawaii or the UpS workshop. These meetings bring local people together to discuss the forces affecting their crops.
- The increase in market value of kava.

The increase in kava's market value is ironic, because the increase in demand for this plant was the driving force in the destruction of wild kava plantings to begin with. Yet the kava market also gives an economic base for the preservation of the plant. Kava's ability to live well as an understory plant in undisturbed rain forest increases the value of undisturbed rain forest, possibly to the point of protecting this ecosystem.

The increase in market demand for kava, properly handled, may increase its abundance and protect its natural environment. This may also be true for other medicinal plants facing similar pressures. Kava production in Hawaii may become a model for sustainable development in which a combination of local growers, government, consumers, pharmaceutical companies, the natural environment, and herbal companies increase the abundance of a plant along with the economic and cultural stability of the residents.

NOTES

1. Kava has a somatic complement of $2n = 130$. In an unpublished study from 1988, Vincent Lebot notes that this is the first time a decaploid has been recorded in this genus. Tane Datta speculates that the high chromosome number allows the mutations necessary for the development of varieties from clonal propagation.

2. Petersen, "The making of an herbal superstar."

REFERENCES

Blumenthal, Mark, and Yadhu Singh. "Kava: An overview." *HerbalGram* 39 (1997): 33–55.

Petersen, Andrea. "The making of an herbal superstar." *The Wall Street Journal*, 26 Feb. 1998 p. 1 Sec. B1.

Lebot, Vincent. "Kava: The Polynesian dispersal of an oceanian plant." Chapter 9 in *Islands, Plants, Polynesians: Introduction to Polynesian Ethnobotany*, edited by Paul Alan Cox and Sandra Anne Banack. Proceedings of a symposium sponsored by the Institute of Polynesian Studies, Brigham Young University, Hawaii Campus. Laie, Hawaii: Dioscorides Press, 1991.

LADY'S SLIPPER ORCHID
Cypripedium spp.

ROSEMARY GLADSTAR

I moved to Sage Mountain in central Vermont in the late 1980s. A farm child of the fertile northern California countryside, complete with apple orchards and oceans, old redwood forests, and weather that the great plant wizard Luther Burbank felt was as perfect as anywhere on earth, I took planting in February for granted and harvesting in November as a fact of life. Having landed quite suddenly, almost by accident it seemed, midway through life, on a large granite outcrop in the northeastern forest (Zone 3), my life as an herbalist took a radical shift. Aside from having to relearn the rules of gardening and adapt to "arctic" land, there was the matter of learning an entirely new ecosystem and the plants and animals it supported. I was full of delight, a child again, as I came to know my new plant neighbors, many of them favorite medicinal herbs I had used all my life but had never seen growing in their native habitat. The mountain ranges here are ancient, ground down through time, and the forests, though resilient and hardy yet, are worn by the continuous cuttings of many generations of wood users. The plant communities reflect this harsh reality; still, they thrive. I felt wonder in getting to know my new surroundings and, throughout the short but riotous growing season, made new plant discoveries every day.

But by far the greatest event was my discovery of the bog, a calcareous pool of shallow, slow-running water that steeped from the cedar grove. We had moved to this rugged terrain in late fall, only a breath or two away from winter. The colorful lushness of the foliage's seasonal spiral dance to earth had past. Shortly after we had settled into our two-room log cabin with an old woodstove and a pile of books, we were hit by the worst—or best, depending on your outlook—snowstorm ever known in these parts then or since. When spring rolled around several long months later, like every other Vermonter I was hungry for the green. It was on one of those early-spring forays that I first discovered the bog. The water filtered between layers of ancient peat moss and supported a rich array of bog and purple-stemmed aster *(Aster nemoralis, A. puniceua)*, spotted joe-pye weed *(Eupatorium maculatum)*, and a variety of sedges, cotton grasses, and rushes. This was my first encounter with sundew *(Drosera rotundifolia)*, bugleweed *(Lycopus uniflorus)*, and a host of other bog-loving plants. Yes, I was in bog heaven. But one plant definitely piqued my curiosity. Still unfurling its large, soft, downy leaves—which looked, except for the down, much like false hellebore—it was scattered throughout the several-acre bog in significant clusters.

I watched for the flower. By the second week in June, still early spring in these parts, the first blossoms began to open. I knew in a moment the treasure that was here and only then began to fully understand the relationship and responsibility I would have with this land. Here, unbeknownst to me when we purchased those 500 acres of wilderness, was one of New England's treasures, the showy pink lady's slipper *(Cypripedium reginae)*. Rare, endangered, protected in every state within its native range, the showy pink lady's slipper was hunted to near extinction by the mid-1900s by herbalists and Eclectics for its gentle, soothing root. Little was known at the time of its amazingly slow reproductive process or the fact that the population stands that were being harvested would never recover their original grandness no matter how careful the harvesting or ethical the wildcrafter.

When I first opened my herb shop in northern California in 1972, the lady's slipper, though officially classified as an endangered wildflower, was still employed in herbal medicine and sold commonly in herb stores. There was no mention of its protected status, and we herbalists certainly weren't aware of such issues at that time. Because it was included in many formulas of the early Eclectics, physiomedicalists, and herb doctors, it was readily adopted into our formulas; you'll occasionally still see a nervine formula containing lady's slipper on the herb store shelf. Upon inquiring, you'll be assured that these products contain lady's slippers from cultivated sources. Part of the problem, of course, is that lady's slippers belong to a large family, so some confusion could arise over the variety. However, all lady's slippers are at best challenging, and at worst impossible to cultivate. Those used primarily in herbal medicine *(Cypripedium reginae, C. acaule, C. calceolus)* are among the more difficult to cultivate. Though possible to cultivate with great care and manipulation, it raises the question: Why would we want to introduce something so rare in the wild and so challenging to grow into our American materia medica? Especially when there are equally effective common weeds and cultivated plants that easily do what lady's slipper is purported to do?

In the ensuing years of discovery of this great and wild land I call my home, I have made many discoveries here that serve to further connect me to the land. I have found stands of bloodroot, blue cohosh, an occasional (though rare) colony of black cohosh, more lobelia than I've ever seen elsewhere, and mossy areas interwoven with the tiny stitches of goldthread. And to my great delight, I have found the other two lady's slippers *(Cypripedium acaule, C. calceulis)* that were commonly employed in early American medicine. When I look out my back door, our woods are filled with trillium, wild leeks, and spikenard, all fairly common plants in these parts. Yet I'm tempted less to pick them than I might have been a quarter of a century ago. Each time I take down my collecting basket, I think about how much of this wild plant must be harvested to make a small mound on the bottom, about how many plants must come with me to make a quart of good medicine. I think of all of my friends, their friends, our students, and their students, all with their collecting baskets and their quarts of medicine. And I think of the large industry that feeds off these "common" wild natives and how many tons of plant material it takes to fill the bottoms of their baskets. Often my thoughts inadvertently turn to the buffalo and passenger pigeon and marsh hen. And more often than not on those collecting days when I might have once headed into the woodlands, I generally head, basket in hand, to the garden instead.

BOTANICAL FEATURES

In 1856 Thoreau wrote, "Everywhere now in dry pitch pine woods stand the red lady's slipper over the red pine leaves on the forest floor, rejoicing in June. Behold their rich striped red, their drooping sack."

This is a plant that elicits poetry and stories from all who have the good fortune to come across it. Even modern technical descriptions of lady's slippers often lapse into the poetic vernacular: "No one expects the queen's slipper to be common, but all should respect the corners of the castle where it lives."[1] And Mrs. W. S. Dana reminisces in *How to Know the Wild Flowers*, "This is a blossom whose charm never wanes. It seems to be touched with the spirit of the deep woods. I recall a mountain lake where the steep cliffs rise from the water's edge; here

and there, on a tiny shelf strewn with pine-needles, can be seen a pair of large veined leaves above which, in early June, the pink balloon-like blossoms floats from its slender scape."

There are many species of orchids—more than twenty thousand, in fact—and they can be found around the world in habitats varying from desert to rain forest, in trees, on the ground, and even underground! The following describes three of our native orchids most commonly used in traditional herbal medicine; they are the species herbalists are currently most concerned about due to habitat destruction and inappropriate harvesting for medicinal purposes.

Lady's slippers are among the most spectacular of all wildflowers, almost shocking in their beauty. All species of lady's slippers, whether growing in bogs or woodlands, are shy, quiet-loving plants that seek out homesites in undisturbed natural habitats. Pink lady's slipper or moccasin flower, *Cypripedium acaule*, is found growing in dry, acidic forests under pines, hemlocks, and other conifers. It is the only *Cypripedium* with basal leaves only; the stalks are leafless. The flower stalk rises to a height of 8 to 20 inches, with the two large leaves at ground level reaching 4 to 8 inches long. These two distinctive basal leaves are downy, large, and deeply plaited; even when not in flower they are quite noticeable in the woodlands. As with all orchids, the flowers are striking, emitting a slight but fragrant scent, attractive to its pollinator, the native bumblebee. The large dark pink sac, or pouch—quite sensual even to those with tame imaginations—makes it a striking candidate for a botanical erotica poster. It is found growing in decreasing frequency in sandy or rocky woods, Newfoundland to Manitoba, south to North Carolina and Tennessee, and west to Minnesota. "All who have found it in secluded haunts will sympathize that each specimen is a rarity, even though he should find a hundred to an acre," Mrs. W. S. Dana wrote nearly a hundred years ago in *How to Know the Wildflowers*.

Showy lady's slipper, *Cypripedium reginae* (queen or royal), considered by many to be the most stunning of all our native orchids—and perhaps the most temperamental—is found growing in calcareous swamps, peat bogs, and open wet woodlands from Newfoundland to Ontario and as far south as Georgia. The luscious pink slipper is formed of white, ovate sepals, the lateral ones united their entire length to form the large pouch or sac. This sac has been likened to a "funhouse tunnel for bees."[2] The sepals are round or oval and waxy white. Variegated crimson and pink stripes cascade over the large white inflated lip. The flowers are supported by a stout stem from 1 to 3 feet high with large elliptic-shaped downy leaves, 3 to 8 inches long. Both the leaves and stems are covered with soft white down, and the flowers, borne as many as three to a stem, are $1^1/_2$ to 2 inches across. A colony of these showy pink ladies growing in a bog emits a sense of deep peace far more effective than any amount of nervine tincture sold in a bottle.

As the name implies, yellow lady's slipper, *Cypripedium calceolus* and *C. pubscens*, has a bright yellow "slipper," or sac, and is found growing in rich woods and thickets from Nova Scotia to Ontario and Minnesota, Nebraska, and south

to Alabama. The large, showy flowers grow on a strong tall stem, $1^1/_2$ to $2^1/_2$ feet high, occasionally reaching a height of 3 feet. The flower stalks generally bear one to three blossoms each. The leaves are oval or elliptic, 3 to 6 inches long, grow up most of the stem, and end in a pointed tip. The sepals are ovate-lanceolate and are usually longer than the lip. The narrow, twisted petals are purple striped, which contrasts beautifully with the yellow flowers. Purple and yellow are traditional colors of royalty and this flower, simple though its lifestyle may be in the heart of the forest, is nothing less than an elegant member of a royal family.

HISTORICAL AND MEDICINAL USES

Author's Note: All references are historical, because no lady's slippers are recommended for use in any form at this time due to the difficulties of cultivation and habitat loss. There are other plants that serve as excellent analogues or substitutes and work as well, if not better, than the *Cypripediums*.

The name *orchid* derives from the Greek *orchis* or "testicle," and in early days orchids and the sac were prized as aphrodisiacs. Timothy Coffey in his wonderful reference *The History and Folklore of North American Wildflowers* cites two early references to the use of orchids as aphrodisiacs, though truly, I'm certain the suggestive appearance of the flower has more to do with its amorous reputation than any of its chemical constituents. In 1500 the German herbalist Braunschweig wrote: "In the mornynge and at nyght dronke of the same water at eche tyme an ounce and a half causeth great hete, therefore it giveth lust unto the works of generacyon and multiplicacyon of sperm." And in 1672 Josselyn commented, "I once took notice of a wanton woman's compounding of the solid roots of this plant with wine, for an amorous cup; which wrought the desired effect."

Lady's slippers were highly valued as an herbal medicine by the Native people, who used the plant as a calming agent; its use was adopted by the early settlers. Its most common name during early American colonization, American valerian, points to its nervine qualities. It was primarily used to treat all manners of nerve disorders, from headaches to nerve stress and epilepsy. Principal constituents that have been identified are volatile oil, tannin, gallic acid, resins, glucose, starch, and inorganic salts. Lady's slipper acquired an undisputed reputation as a safe, nontoxic herb, with no side effects, and thus was considered an excellent medicine for nerve stress and chronic nerve debility. It was frequently used for young children with nerve disorders and specifically for teething.

Joseph Meyer in *The Herbalist* (1918) classified its actions as tonic, antispasmodic, and diaphoretic and considered it a mild, effective tonic for nervous stress. Dr. Christopher, a well-known herb doctor who had great influence on American herbalism through the 1960s and 1970s commonly called the plant nerve root and considered it in his book *The School of Natural Healing* "almost a pure nervine and relaxant. Its action is slow, yet it influences the entire nervous system." It was a favorite remedy of Dr. Christopher's for hysteria, convulsions, nervous exhaustion, and "female weakness," and he included it in several of his well-known formulas. Dr. Felter also felt that lady's slipper was an "excellent tonic for weak women and nervous children" and found it effective for dispelling gloom (behold the beauty!) and inducing "a calm and cheerful state of mind."[3] It seemed to be a favorite remedy of early doctors and herbalists, and frequent references of its affinity for "women's hysteria" and "disorders of weak women" can be found in the old medical textbooks, providing insight into not only the importance of this plant but also the pervading viewpoint of women at the time. My favorite such reference is Dr. Felter's statement concerning menopausal women: "We have been able to accomplish more with it than any drug except pulsatilla in worry, with fear of disaster or insanity, in women passing through this phase of life."[4]

PREPARATION AND DOSAGE

A perfectly safe remedy, lady's slipper could be taken in large dosages, if necessary, with no ill side effects. "They have a peculiar, slightly bitter, and rather nauseous taste, and a somewhat unpleasant odor. Alcohol or boiling water take up their virtues, which, however, are impaired by boiling"[5] The root was generally infused as tea, because the volatile oils were thought to be easily destroyed by decocting (boiling). One teaspoon of the dried root was steeped for anywhere from twenty minutes to an hour in hot water. One wineglassful, three or four times a day was the dose recommended by most of the early herb doctors.

Dr. Christopher felt, too, that the root was best infused. However, he did recommend a decoction (4 ounces of lady's slipper to 1 quart of water simmered for an hour or longer on low heat) with a suggested dose of 1 tablespoon diluted in a wineglassful of water three or four times daily. John K. Scudder frequently recommended a soothing syrup for irritated children made from the yellow lady's slipper, lavender, and lobelia, and felt it was especially useful during teething. He did comment that if nausea occurred, lobelia should be lessened or omitted.

A favorite method of preparation of lady's slipper was a liquid extract and/or tincture, which was officially titled Specific Medicine Cypripedium[6] and administered in doses of from 5 to 60 drops. *Specific medicine* was the term applied to standardized preparations made from alcohol by the Eclectic doctors of the early 1900s. They were "designed for kindly therapeutic effect rather than for intense physiological activity."[7]

Lady's slipper was also powdered and combined with other herbal powders in various formulas. A favorite formula of Dr. Christopher's for seizure disorders was a combination of lady's slipper powder combined with powders of goldenseal root, lobelia seeds, and cayenne. These herbs, two of which are also considered at risk to date, were mixed in equal proportions and encapsulated in #2 capsules. The recommended dose was one capsule every three hours if seizures were imminent. Otherwise, one capsule twice daily, morning and evening, was his recommended dosage.

But perhaps the most effective medicine of all "made" from lady's slippers is found simply in its company and distilled at the place of its origin—the fields, bogs, and thickets that it once populated so abundantly. Here, in the quiet of its home, there emanates a deep and warming peace, likened to that found in the finest of nature's cathedrals, the old-growth forests. Lady's slipper speaks its medicine most clearly, inviting the weary to sit, rest, and drink of the beauty of the moment. The very air around these elegant flowers smells of a sweetness that is almost indiscernible. Not a fragrance, but a sweetness and a stillness so profound that many weary travelers on life's path, discovering a stand of lady's slippers, find their nerves soothed simply by drinking in their presence; they travel on refreshed and renewed.

PROPAGATION AND CULTIVATION

"Cross fertilization," says Darwin, "results in offspring which vanquish the offspring of self-fertilization in the struggle for existence." The Orchid family demonstrates this more clearly than any other group of plants, for no other plant family has taken more elaborate precautions against self-pollination nor developed a more specialized mechanism to attract pollinating insects. And its ingenious techniques have certainly proved successful; an estimated twenty to twenty-five thousand species grow worldwide, each with its own highly developed and specialized mechanism that induces insects to enter into its pure lusciousness. Were it not for human ignorance, sometimes born simply out of love for beauty (picking wild orchid blossoms for the table, or transplanting to the garden, for instance), the Orchid family would continue to thrive in great abundance.

Though many species are still abundant, of the several species used for medicinal purposes through the early 1900s, all are in danger of disappearing due to habitat destruction and unscrupulous collecting of roots for propagation (it seldom survives transplanting) and/or medicinal purposes. Listen to this poetry written in 1900 by Neltje Blanchan:

> The fissure down the front of the pink lady's slipper is not so wide that a bee must use some force to push against its elastic sloping sides and enter the large banquet chamber where he finds generous entertainment secreted among the fine white hairs in the upper part. Presently he has feasted enough. Now one can hear him buzzing about inside trying to find a way out. Toward two little gleams of light seen at the end of the passageway beyond the nectary hairs, he at length finds his way. Narrower and narrower grows the passage until it would seem as if he could never struggle through; nor can he until his back has rubbed along the sticky, overhanging stigma, which is directed forward and placed there for the express purpose of combing out the pollen he has brought from another flower on his back. The imported pollen having been safely removed, he still must struggle on toward freedom through one of the narrow openings, where an anther almost blocks his way. As he works outward, this anther plasters his back with yellow granular pollen as a parting gift and away he flies to another lady's slipper.[8]

This phenomenon is described much more succinctly in the Stokes's *Guide to Enjoying Wildflowers:* "The lady slipper flower is like a funhouse tunnel for the bees, with a one-way entrance, a big chamber with a bright exit sign, and some sticky sweet hairs on the way."

This ingenious method of pollination has one major flaw. There is no sweet nectar to reward the bee for its hard work. So after a few tumbles down the tunnel of love, the bee gives up on the lady's slippers and finds its way to albeit less attractive, but more substantial finds. To ensure good pollination rates, a healthy population of bumblebees in the vicinity is a must. Smaller-sized insects slip too easily through the tunnel and escape the pollen trap set by the ingenious orchids. Once pollinated, the journey of survival has only just begun.

A single lady's slipper seedpod will contain between ten and twenty thousand minute seeds that have been likened to a "mote of dust on the wind." Adapted for wind dispersal, they are remarkably light, and unlike most other seeds, they do not contain their own endosperm, or food reserve. Thus, in order to survive, the seedling must find a dependable source of nourishment during this fragile stage of development. This is where magic and science merge. An odd symbiotic relationship between the lady's slipper and potentially lethal (to plants, anyway) pathogenic fungi has developed over eons of time. In order for the seed to survive, it forms a small corm that waits in dormancy until "invaded" by certain symbiotic soil fungi. The lady's slipper seed may lie in waiting for several years before the right mycorrhiza comes along. Once penetrated, the seedlings feed on this soil fungus called *orchid mycorrhizae* (*myco* means "fungus," and *rhiza*, "root"), digesting it to obtain the nourishment needed for growth. More than six species of *Rhizoctonia*, or soil fungus, necessary to the growth of lady's slippers have been identified thus far.

Bill Cullina of the New England Wildflower Society speculates on the fact that these soil fungi are pathogenic, or disease causing, when they infect nonorchid species, yet have developed a beneficial relationship to the orchids. "It may be that in the distant past these fungi were parasites on orchid seeds, but eventually the seeds developed ways to resist and control this parasitism to their own benefit. In effect, the seeds have reversed roles, now becoming parasites of the fungus." However, the relationship between fungus and plant remains a tenuous one, indeed. The *Rhizoctonia*, though beneficial to lady's slippers at this juncture in evolution, is still a pathogen and, given the opportunity, would happily destroy the tiny seedling. To protect itself, at seed's emergence, the tiny plantlet immediately begins to produce a fungicide to keep the mycorrhizae in check. The relationship between fungus and orchid is a slow underground waltz witnessed only by the creepy-crawlies of the soil world. Over a two-year period the plantlet develops slowly underground,

nourished by its tenuous relationship to the potentially deadly mycorrhizae. As leafs and rootlets develop, one spring day in its third year of growth, the tiny orchid breaks ground, reaches toward the light, and begins photosynthesizing on its own.

Thousands upon thousands of these gorgeous and sensitive native wildflowers have been dug from their ancient home grounds, transplanted to habitats they couldn't possibly survive in, and have slowly—or quickly—died out. This practice still continues, undercover, because they are protected from harvesters in most of their native range. Luckily headway has been made in the past few years in the propagation of the lady's slipper species. And with the right conditions, a bit of luck, and some obliging mycorrhizae, you too can cultivate a garden of exotic slippers. One of my favorite stories, which appeared a few years ago in *Garden Design*, tells of a New Hampshire high school girl who, unaware of the difficulty of propagating lady's slippers, decided to take it on as a high school science project. Discovering that the showy pink lady's slipper was on the endangered list and could only be found in one spot in the entire state of New Hampshire, April Donovuolu, under the guidance of her high school science teacher, decided to tissue-culture it for her science project.

How did she do it? Last spring, with fellow students Tyler King and Katie Sokolski, April won second prize at the prestigious 1996 International Science and Engineering Fair, for successfully cloning a ladies slipper—astonishing the orchid world in the process. By applying rigorous scientific techniques, under the guidance of their teacher, the students succeeded with unheard of two-week seed germination. Now they have 8,000 babies in flasks that will be eventually planted in the New Hampshire woods.

To fully appreciate this phenomenon, you must recognize that for the past century professors, scientists, biologists, and botanists have dedicated a great deal of their lives' work to the process of lady's slipper propagation with little success. That a child should succeed speaks, perhaps, of some mysterious force in the plant kingdom that as yet goes widely unrecognized.

Following are cultivation guidelines for three of the lady's slippers that were commonly used in herbal medicine. Lucky enough to have a wonderful abundance of all three species growing naturally in the woodlands and bogs where I live, I've not attempted cultivation myself. So these guidelines are gleaned from others' experiences. The number one priority, if attempting to grow your own, is to be absolutely certain that your growing stock does not come from wild sources. Plants started from nursery-grown stock have a much better chance of survival, and it is illegal to harvest lady's slippers in the wild.

There are also a number of resources available these days to help you successfully grow a garden of lady's slippers. The New England Wildflower Society is perhaps one of the best and provides cultivation guides as well as plant-

ing stock. A Web site that features extensive growing techniques as well as cultivated planting stock is included in the references (at the end of this chapter), and the UpS nursery directory (at the end of this book) supplies the names of several nurseries that specialize in cultivated lady's slippers.

How To Grow

All *Cypripediums* require shade and a moist, acidic soil, and the northeastern and western coniferous woodlands or a deciduous woodland environment provide conditions as ideal as are found on the North American continent. The degree of moisture and acidity needed by each species may differ, and each species requires its own specialized microenvironment to thrive—complete with its "nurse" mycorrhizae—so mimic the natural conditions as closely as possible for the greatest success.

Cypripedium acaule does best in a very acidic soil (pH 4.0 to 5.0), augmented if necessary with such acidic materials as pine needles or leaf mold. Even if you meet its every requirement, however, it is very challenging to domesticate.

Cypripedium calceolus and *C. pubescens* require a mildly acidic (pH 6.0 to 7.0) soil ranging from slightly moist to boggy, and do best in partial shade and deciduous woods. Some species of yellow lady's slippers thrive in drier soil as well, so again, mimic the natural environment as closely as possible. These are the most successful lady's slipper in cultivation and are best grown from nursery divisions. Kathy Keville states in *The Illustrated Herb Encyclopedia*, "They can be grown in pots if adequate drainage and peat moss are provided. Indoor temperatures should average about 60 to 70 degrees."

Cypripedium reginae needs an acidic (pH 6.0 to 7.0) and very moist soil ranging from boggy to swampy. Its favored habitat includes light shade and calcareous bogs. Though difficult and challenging, it can be cultivated by division and is best grown on raised hummocks over a limy, wet soil. Plant *Cypripedium* in the fall, setting the rhizomes of *C. acaule* and *C. calceolus* 1 to $1\frac{1}{2}$ inches deep and the shallow-growing roots of *C. reginae* only $\frac{1}{2}$ inch deep. Space the plants 1 to 2 feet apart and water them thoroughly, then mulch them lightly with dead leaves or pine needles to retain moisture. Water the plants abundantly while in active growth; reduce moisture after shoots have flowered and begun to wither. Plants must not be moved, because movement disturbs the fragile roots, making them susceptible to root rot. Plants increase by forming new rhizomes; flowers will develop as the clump ages.

HARVESTING

The rhizomes, or fibrous roots, were unfortunately the coveted part of this slow-growing peaceful plant historically. These plants, as only recently discovered, are known to live much longer than originally expected, with mature lady's slippers being up twenty to thirty years old. The numerous cup-shaped leaf scars found on many plants are indicators of great age (see Wise Old Plants by Robyn Klein on page 24). Fleshy rhizomes and roots range in color from orange-brown to brownish. Though variations

exist in different species, most roots of the medicinal species are thick, fibrous, and thickly matted. The roots were traditionally dug in the late summer to fall, allowing the plant to complete its flowering cycle and attempt one final opportunity to fruit. Roots cleaned easily and were sliced and allowed to dry in the shade. Gathering baskets or porous bags were used for this purpose. When roots were thoroughly dried they were stored in closed storage containers, which helped to keep their properties for several seasons.

UpS RECOMMENDATIONS

- No wild harvest is permissible. Use only cultivated resources.

- Cultivated valerian, cultivated California poppy, and cultivated passionflower are good substitutes. Another alternative is lemon balm for its antispasmodic and nervine properties, as well as skullcap, which has antipasmodic, nervine, sedative, and anodyne actions.

Beauty is not "its own excuse for being," nor was fragrance ever "wasted on the desert air." The seer has at last heard and interpreted the voice in the wilderness. The flower is no longer a simple passive victim in the busy bee's sweet pillage, but rather a conscious being, with hopes, aspirations, and companionships. The insect is its counterpart. Its fragrance is but a perfumed whisper of welcome, its color is as the wooing blush and rosy lip, its portals are decked for his coming, and its sweet hospitalities humored to his tarrying; and as it speeds its parting affinity, rests content that its life consummation has been fulfilled.

William Hamilton Gibson,
discoursing on the relationship
of insects and flowers

NOTES

1. Wallner and DiGregorio, *New England Mountain Flowers.*

2. Dana, *How to Know the Wildflowers.*

3. Felter, *Eclectic Materia Medica, Pharmacology and Therapeutics.*

4. Ibid.

5. Felter and Lloyd, *King's American Dispensatory.*

6. Felter, *Eclectic Materia Medica, Pharmacology and Therapeutics.*

7. Ibid.

8. Blanchan, *Nature's Garden.*

REFERENCES

Blanchan, Neltje. *Nature's Garden*. New York: Grosset and Dunlap, 1900.

Christopher, John R., M.D. *School of Natural Healing*. Provo, Utah: BiWorld Publishers, 1979.

Coffey, Timothy. *The History and Folklore of North American Wildflowers*. New York: Houghton Mifflin, 1993.

Dana, Mrs. William Starr. *How to Know the Wildflowers*. New York: Charles Scribner's Sons, 1900.

Felter, Harvey Wickes, M.D. *Eclectic Materia Medica, Pharmacology and Therapeutics*. 1922. Reprint, Portland, Oreg.: Eclectic Medical Publications, 1983.

Felter, Harvey Wickes, M.D., and John Uri Lloyd. *King's American Dispensatory*. Vol. 1. 1898. Reprint, Portland, Oreg.: Eclectic Medical Publications, 1983.

House, Homer D. *Wild Flowers of New York*. Albany: University of the State of New York, 1918.

Keville, Kathi. *The Illustrated Herb Encyclopedia*. Nye, N.Y.: Mallard Press, 1991.

New England Wildflower Society. *From the Garden Newsletter*. Garden in the Woods, Framingham, Mass. 01701.

Wallner, Jeff, and Mario J. DiGregorio. *New England Mountain Flowers*. Missoula, Mont.: Mountain Press Publishing, 1997.

The Cypripedium Garden: Cultural Information on Cypripedium Seedlings (www.infonet.ca/cypr/CULTRINF.HTM" ~).

LOBELIA
Lobelia inflata

CASCADE ANDERSON GELLER

I'm one of those herbalists who actually admire lobelia. I was trained to use and admire it, but the fact is, I had over time departed from using it much. Occasionally I would potentize a cough remedy with a few drops per dose, but the stock bottle of extract grew dusty upon my herb room shelf. Then about a month or so ago, while I was working on this chapter, I awoke with a muscle spasm. I tried to ignore it but it got worse and finally I had to lie still and think of the best remedy. I asked my husband to rub me with *Lobelia inflata* fresh tops extract. I took a few drops orally, too. After five minutes the pain was entirely gone. It could've been my husband's healing hands, but I suspect the lobelia was also doing the work of soothing my spasms.

Recently, on the first morning of a camping trip to the Oregon coast, I awoke with the beginnings of a headache due to tight shoulder and neck muscles after days of computer work. This time lobelia tincture was the first remedy to come to my mind. After my earlier experience with it, I had put the extract back in the first-aid kit. My daughter's young friend was willing to massage my back and neck with the extract, and again I took a few drops by mouth. Within fifteen minutes I was feeling much better, and the headache never materialized.

Though I always stock tincture made from fresh or freshly dried tops, before these experiences I had not been an avid user of lobelia for a number of years. I had forgotten how well it works applied topically after a long day at the computer or after hours of gardening when back muscles become tired. This is the way I love lobelia most: as a topical muscle rub, with perhaps a few drops taken orally. It is a wonderful antispasmodic, but it has many other indications and uses as well, and a rich historical past in the Americas and abroad. Writing this chapter has helped me remember the powerful and feared lobelia once again.

Mention lobelia and for most modern herbalists it tends to conjure up words like *toxic, puking, alkaloids,* and *Samuel Thomson.* It is a good example of the American tradition of demonizing plants that are powerful in action. Far from being a demon, in the right hands and the right dose lobelia is a superb, quick-acting remedy that every practicing herbalist should be trained to know and use.

Fortunately for the plant itself, lobelia's use has been limited, so perhaps the demonizing has benefited its conservation. It is my hope that this chapter will not have the opposite effect by firing up the rapidly expanding herbal consumer market to demand more and more lobelia. At this time United Plant Savers lists lobelia as a to-watch medicinal plant.

BOTANICAL FEATURES

Lobelia is a beautiful name for a beautiful plant with a notorius reputation and a rich historical past. Currently, most texts list the genus in the Campanulaceae or Bluebell family, much noted for their lovely, stand-up-and-be-noticed floral sprays. Lobelias are sometimes relegated to a subfamily, Lobelioideae, within the Campanulaceae, although other works delegate it to the Lobeliaceae family. There are more than 360 species of lobelia found worldwide.

Though the flowers of many lobelias are not large, their flower spikes, which range from the bright, cobalt blues of *L. siphilitica* to the intense red of *L. cardinalis*, are striking. The flowers are noted for their two-lobed upper lip and three-lobed lower lip. The leaves are alternating, and often there is a milky juice in the pinched stems. North American species range from 4 inches *(L. kalmii)* to 4 feet *(L. cardinalis)* in height.

Anyone walking down a flower-bedecked village or city street has seen the bright blue blossoms of lobelia. Because of their long-blooming, lovely flowers, lobelias are popularly planted as ornamentals, especially the trailing hybrids and compacts such as *L. erinus* and *L. fulgens*, which are available in spring and summer in most garden centers in the United States, Canada, and Europe. Other species make lovely garden plants but require a special habitat to thrive.

This August, along Michigan's Muskegon River in the upper region of the Lower Peninsula, I was able to visit both *Lobelia cardinalis* and *L. siphilitica*. *L. cardinalis*, which is seen less frequently, stood out like a beacon with its surprising crimson flowers bathed in the early-morning light along the riverbank. *L. siphilitica* was growing in its standard neighborhood of lowland, moist soil in the shady ditch along the trail. I remembered my "own" childhood patch of *L. siphilitica* at the old Michigan artesian well that was in my "fort." Nibbling on those leaves with their intense acrid bite was a sure way of causing a stir. Playmates would spit and moan. I could understand later how a showman like Samuel Thomson could have gotten so attracted to them.

HISTORICAL BACKGROUND

Lobelia seems to have been added to European and American medicinal repertoire by contact with Native Americans. According to the sketchy information from early European medical botanists and physicians from the 1700s and 1800s, numerous tribes used a variety of species. There is some indication that *L. cardinalis* was one of the few medicinal and ritual plants cultivated by certain tribes, and perhaps even imported to western areas outside its natural range. Writers who denigrate Native American medicine have commented that roots of *L. inflata* were used by the Natives as an emetic. There are reports of different tribes using lobelias as love charms, purgatives, anthelmintics, diuretics, and pulmonary remedies. The Swimmer Manuscript discusses the Cherokee use of lobelia for a shaking condition: A cold-water infusion of the root of *L. spicata* is blown on the scratched skin of the patient. But it was the Natives' use of lobelia as a curative for syphilis that got white medicine fired up about the plant and sent it scurrying across the "Big Water" back to England's Royal Infirmary.

Accounts in 1758 from Dr. Colden testified that less than an ounce of the root of *Lobelia siphilitica* had cured soldiers of syphilis in less than a week. The importance of such news in 1758 would be similar to an announcement today of a quick, successful cure for AIDS. English doctors began to doubt its efficacy and its use was eventually abandoned, but it is of interest to note the words of Charles F. Millspaugh: "The cause of failure may be the fact that the aborigines did not trust to the plant alone, but always used it in combination with may-apple roots (Podophyllum peltatum), the bark of the wild cherry (Prunus Virginica) and dusted the ulcers with the powdered bark of New Jersey tea (Ceanothus Americanus). Another chance of failure lay in the volatility of its active principle, as the dried herb was used."

As a medicine to colonial civilization in the United States, lobelia was an early contender. *L. inflata* was listed in two preparations in the first *United States Pharmacopoeia* of 1820 and maintained two to four listings for one hundred years through the 1920 edition. It was dropped in the eleventh edition of the *Pharmacopoeia* but maintained a listing in the International Protocol Standards published in the *Pharmacopoeia* from the Brussels Conference of 1925. *L. inflata* was maintained in the *National Formulary* until 1960. References to its use as a hypodermically administered preparation in a variety of conditions from threatened abortion to tetanus as directed by Finley Ellingwood, M.D., are cited in the *Digest of Comments on the Pharmacopoeia of the United States of America* and on the *National Formulary* published in 1914.

SAMUEL THOMSON AND THE LOBELIA CONTROVERSY

Instrumental in popularizing and later stigmatizing lobelia was Samuel Thomson (1769–1843), the rabble-rouser and thorn in the side of mid-nineteenth-century college-trained physicians. Thomson credited himself with discovering the emetic qualities of lobelia, though Native peoples had long used it for this purpose. There is little doubt, however, that Samuel Thomson, with his flair for drama and success in treating a wide range of conditions for all manner of people, spurred the use of lobelia as a medicine in both lay and professional medical circles.

Called Thomsonianism, his method of curing used a variety of plants, but most notably the warming powers of capsicum (cayenne) and the puking powers of lobelia. Some have compared Thomson's herbal healing methods to the Heroic System of the 1800s, which involved blood letting and use of calomel, a mercury-based cathartic. Bleeding and purging by the medical profession, along with numerous infectious disease epidemics, helped foster deep discontent with American medicine in those earlier years and helped popularize Thomson's curing. In fact, by the 1830s numerous states had repealed licensing regulations for the practice of medicine, allowing irregular schools and practitioners to flourish. Regular medicine did not really gain strong momentum until the advent of aspirin (1899). Its all-powerful grip was solidified more securely in the early 1900s with the manufacture of sulpha drugs and, more than thirty years later, penicillin.

"Thomson's Improved System of Botanic Practice of Medicine" was patented in 1813. For about $20, a person could purchase the course and have "Family Rights" to use the doctoring system. By 1839, in the heyday of disgruntled medical consumers, Thomson's patented system claimed three million followers. It was perhaps one of the first network marketing schemes in the United States, with agents making a percentage of the profits and texts being dispensed from Thomson's own warehouse. The lineage of herbal correspondence courses had begun and continues to this day as one of the chief ways herbalists in the U.S. and Canada are trained.

Thomson was proud of his down-home roots and neighborhood herb-doctoring ways; he was an evangelist for what he saw as a more sane method of healing. A scrapper who seemed to relish attacking the modern, overly educated form of allopathic medicine, which he saw as detrimental to the real healing of people, Thomson was often embroiled in controversy and battles with authorities.

The most notorious case in 1809 involved a very ill young man, Ezra Lovett, whom Thomson allegedly murdered with the overzealous administration of lobelia. Though Thomson was acquitted, this case has forever left lobelia with a reputation as a poisonous plant and darkened Samuel Thomson's legacy. (For an excellent review of this case with excerpts from the trial records, see Paul Bergner's article in *Medical Herbalism*, Volume 10, Numbers 1 and 2, spring and summer 1998.)

In the mid-1800s the controversy surrounding lobelia also got rolling on the European side of the Atlantic with a prominent Thomson-like practitioner, Albert Coffin, who arrived in England from the United States and set up his own patent herbal system popular with the working class of northern England. So popular, in fact, that it wasn't too long before the toes of the established doctors felt bruised and cases involving lobelia and other herbs gained notoriety. The cholera epidemic of this time gave the medical profession the deaths they needed under Henry VIII's "Herbalists Charter," an edict of the 1540s, to begin prosecuting botanic practitioners. Lobelia was cited as a poison and blamed for more than a dozen deaths.

MEDICINAL USES

Many species of lobelia, named for the Flemish botanist Matthias de L'Obel (who died in 1616), have been used in herbal medicine. The roots of the perennial, *L. nicotianaefolia*, a mid- to high-elevation species from India, are used for scorpion stings, as were the American species.

In Africa the resinous root of the small shrub, *L. pinifolia*, is used for skin diseases. Traditional Chinese medicine offers *L. chinensis*, the root of which is not considered toxic and is used for a range of conditions, from detoxifying poisons to treating end-stage schistosomiasis. *L. decurrens*, a Peruvian species, is noted for its nauseous odor and toxicity. *L. dortmanna*, or water lobelia, now found rarely in the United States and northern Europe, and *L. urens*, heath lobelia, another rare species of northern European damp woods and acidic heaths, are specimens with little medicinal literature to note.

Lobelia inflata was once known as Indian tobacco and though it is not related to *Nicotiana tabacum* or the other tobacco species in the Solanaceae family, it does contain alkaloids with a similar taste and action. Even a tiny taste of a marginal-quality lobelia preparation or, better yet, the fresh or dried plant will wake up the taste buds with a hot, acrid flavor. According to early accounts by botanists, lobelia leaves were smoked either instead of tobacco or as an additive to tobacco and as an antispasmodic and expectorant for respiratory symptoms. Because of its effects on the respiratory tract and similar properties and taste to those of tobacco, lobelia and its alkaloid, lobeline, have been used in a variety of smoking-cessation compounds. The alkaloid has also been used in products to revive drug overdose victims and as a resuscitation aid in newborns.

In naturopathic and herbal practice, lobelia has myriad uses, but chief among most practitioners is its effect as an antispasmodic for smooth or striated muscles. Muscle strains and sprains, menstrual cramps, and even angina pectoris have been treated with lobelia, both orally and topically as a poultice or fomentation. For the youngest infant, lobelia was recommended as a superb remedy for colic. In dry or wet coughs from colds to whooping cough, pneumonia, and asthma, lobelia has been effectively used orally and topically to help calm the spasms without impeding expectoration.

Birth attendants today still use lobelia as a medicinal plant. I know a number of children who were aided in their birth process when their mothers were given a modest oral dose of lobelia extract, which helped relax the uterus. Harvey Wickes Felter, M.D., in his 1922 textbook for the Eclectic Medical College of Cincinnati, writes about the specific relaxing effect of lobelia on a rigid cervical os that is thick, doughy, and unyielding: "This specific effect of lobelia has won many converts to specific medication." In the earlier years of this century, doctors were using hypodermic lobelia for threatened abortion.

PREPARATION AND DOSAGE

Most herbalists find it difficult to give precise directions for dosage of a plant medicine, because there are so many variables—which is why older and more modern texts most often give a range of dosage and frequency. An herb such as lobelia with its already suspect reputation and variable quality adds to the mystery.

My personal suggestion is to start with a very modest dose and see what happens. Some people are very sensitive to the potentially nauseating effects of lobelia, and as little as 3 to 5 drops of potent tincture can cause discomfort. Others can tolerate a sizable dose of $^1/_2$ dropperful (perhaps 30 or more drops) several times a day. For some conditions, a dose that causes nausea may be necessary to achieve the effect of relaxation; the nausea is quickly dispelled. Others may feel nauseated for hours after a dose, making the remedy worse than the condition.

Topical application has never yet caused a complaint of nausea in my experience. Personally, I like to rub it on the affected part and also take 5 to 10 drops of tincture orally when I'm feeling stress build in an area. The following is a topical formula for muscle cramping.

ANTI-CRAMP TOPICAL COMPOUND

20 ml *Lobelia inflata* tincture, cut herb with tops and some seeds

10 ml pure essential oil of peppermint

Shake, blending the mixture in a 1-ounce bottle. Shake well before each application. Apply to any area of spasm with gentle massage. If possible, apply a warm, damp cloth covered with a dry cloth for fifteen minutes. This works well on some sprains, strains, menstrual cramps, and headaches.

The Thomsonian system often used the powerfully relaxing lobelia paired with the stimulating properties of cayenne (*Capsicum* spp.) as a corrective. Dr. Butler, in 1800, said, "The effects of lobelia may be compared to a fire made of shavings, which will soon go out unless other fuel is added; cayenne therefore may be said to keep alive the blaze which the lobelia has kindled." Numerous compounds include these two North American native plants for a variety of conditions and ages. Here is an example of a formula based on the principle of combining dried cayenne and lobelia.

ACID TINCTURE OF LOBELIA WITH CAYENNE

2 ounces lobelia seeds (crushed)

$^1/_2$ ounce lobelia herb

1 teaspoon cayenne

Macerate (soak) the mixture for ten days in 1 pint of malt vinegar, shaking well daily. Strain and bottle for use.

Older texts make reference to the effect heat has on diminishing the medicinal properties of lobelias, though modern texts report that lobeline is readily soluble in hot alcohol. Some of the more than fourteen isolated alkaloids in lobelia seem to be heat sensitive, and some need heat for extraction. Most sources agree that alcohol, water, and some added acid make the best, most stable tincture source of the dried or fresh plant.

The ranges of dosage and modes of administration of lobelia have varied throughout its two hundred or so years of use in the United States. In his excellent article, "Is Lobelia Toxic?" Paul Bergner illustrated the inconsistency of dosage from writers over the years.

PROPAGATION AND CULTIVATION

My grower contacts have primarily cultivated *Lobelia inflata* in the Pacific Northwest, where summers are typically warm and dry. Lobelia fares well in a variety of soil conditions and can thrive even in part shade in a loamy, rich soil. Seeds may be sown in late fall, the way the plant does it, or in spring. Because the seeds are so tiny, finely sifted soil will work best for germination and early growth. Top-sow the seeds and keep them moist. Irrigate twice weekly if summers are dry. Keep patches well weeded. Pest problems have not been noted by western growers. One acre could produce from 1,000 to 1,700 pounds of the dried herb.

Lobelia inflata is adaptable by nature and thus able to grow in the "waste" places created by humans and natural occurences such as flooding. This species normally acts as an annual and self-sows from its multitude of minuscule seeds, so it should fare well in our culture if common-sense wildcrafting procedures are followed. If harvested before the lower seedpods have been able to mature and drop their seeds, populations may be at risk. Wildcrafters should leave some healthy individuals to resow; if seeds have matured, scattering some in the area should ensure new plants for the next season.

HARVESTING

Twenty years ago the average batch of lobelia bought in an herb store was of marginal quality—typically older, dry, bleached-out stems and leaves with few pods, seeds, or flowers. Currently, a much improved quality of lobelia is available thanks to more demand and education of manufacturers, consumers, wildcrafters, and growers.

Dried tops of *Lobelia inflata*, cut when lower seedpods are inflating with seeds in the late summer, cost between $15 and $20 per pound wholesale. Fresh-cut tops in seed are also available from one company by special order and run about $10 per pound wholesale. At this point there is both wildcrafted and organically grown lobelia on the market, but the bulk of what is used in the American market is wildcrafted—a fact that must change if we wish to ensure the continued viability of our wild populations.

Though the roots were commonly used in early colonial days and by the Native Americans, leafy tops in partial seed are fortunately preferred in today's market. *Lobelia inflata* is a midsummer bloomer and the tall, linear flower stalks may produce flowers until autumn. Harvesting should be done in dry conditions, clipping the stalk when the plant is vibrantly producing flowers and the lower seedpods are swollen with seeds. A mower is used to cut the tops in the bud and flower stage in larger operations. Smaller growers use manual tools. Growers who want to collect seeds should do their cutting over a piece of fabric or bucket in order to catch the seeds.

Lobelia dries easily on sheets with a fan blowing, taking five to seven days to dry. Dry the plants indoors in the shade with a temperature not exceeding 90 degrees. Drying times that are extended due to damp conditions will cause the plant to bleach out and lead to an inferior product. Good-quality dried lobelia is green in color. Most knowledgeable herbalists avoid using overly mature, woody stems or bleached-out leaves and stems in their medicines.

UpS RECOMMENDATIONS

- Very limited wild harvest is permissible when no other alternative will do.

- Thyme, cultivated violet, and hyssop are possible alternatives.

As a beautiful native plant, lobelia has work to do outside the realm of human herbal medicine. Its teachings are many and varied, and we have probably only just begun to understand its role in healing. Like so many of the plants demonized by colonizing cultures, lobelia embodies a harmony of light and dark. With proper attention to the details of ethical wildcrafting, lobelia will be able to thrive in the margins of our developed lands and in the few remaining wild spaces we leave. We of United Plant Savers heartfully hope that wild lobelia will continue to flourish and fascinate the generations to come.

REFERENCES

Bensky, d., A. Gamble, and Kaptchuk. *Chinese Herbal Medicine: Materia Medica*. Seattle, Wash.: Eastland Press 1986.

Bergner, Paul. "The London lobelia trials." *Medical Herbalism* 10 (1, 2): 32 (1998).

———. "Lobelia toxicity: A literature review." *Medical Herbalism* 10 (1, 2): 25 (1998).

Birzneck, Ella (president, Dominion Herbal College). *Home Study, Professional*. Burnaby, B.C.: author, 1969. Correspondence course.

Bolyard, Judith L. *Medicinal Plants and Home Remedies of Appalachia*. Springfield, Ill.: Charles C. Thomas, 1981.

Boyle, Wade. *Herb Doctors: Pioneers in Nineteenth-Century American Botanical Medicine and History of the Eclectic Medical Institute of Cincinnati*. East Palestine, Ohio: Buckeye Naturopathic Press, 1988.

———. *Official Herbs: Botanical Substances in the United States Pharmacopoeias 1820–1990*. East Palestine, Ohio: Buckeye Naturopathic Press, 1991.

Cook and LaWall. *Remington's Practice of Pharmacy*. 8th ed. Philadelphia: J. B. Lippincott, 1936.

Evans, W. C. *Trease and Evans' Pharmacognosy*. 12th ed. London: Baillière Tindall, 1983.

Felter, Harvey Wickes, M.D. *Eclectic Materia Medica, Parmacology and Therapeutics*. Portland, Oreg.: Eclectic Medical Publications., 1983.

Felter, Harvey Wickes, M.D., and John Uri Lloyd. *King's American Dispensatory*. 1898. Reprint, Portland, Oreg.: Eclectic Medical Publications, 1983.

Fitter, R., A. Fitter, and M. Blamey. *The Wild Flowers of Britain and Northern Europe*. New York: Charles Scribner's Sons, 1974.

Foster, Steven. *Herbal Bounty! The Gentle Art of Herb Culture*. Salt Lake City: Gibbs M. Smith, Peregrine Smith Books, 1984.

Gilmore, Melvin R. *Uses of Plants by Indians of the Missouri River Region*. 1914. Reprint, Lincoln, Nebr.: University of Nebraska Press, 1977.

Griggs, Barbara. *Green Pharmacy*. Rochester, Vt.: Healing Arts Press, 1997.

Kloss, Jethro. *Back to Eden*. 1939. Reprint, Santa Barbara, Calif.: Woodbridge Press, 1972.

Millspaugh, Charles F. *American Medicinal Plants, an Illustrated and Descriptive Guide to the American Plants Used as Homeopathic Remedies*. 1884–1885. Reprint, New York: Dover, 1974.

Mooney, James. *The Swimmer Manuscript: Cherokee Sacred Formulas and Medicinal Prescriptions*. Washington, D.C.: U.S. Government Printing Office, 1932.

Motter, M., and M. Wilbert. *Digest of Comments on the Pharmacopoeia of the United States of America and on the National Formulary for the Calendar Year Ending Dec. 31, 1912*. Washington, D.C., 1914.

Schauenberg and Paris. *Guide to Medicinal Plants.* New Canaan, Conn.: Keats Publishing, 1977.

Smith, Ed. Personal conversations with author, Herb Pharm, Williams, Oreg.: May, Sept., 1998.

Sturdivant, L., and T. Blakley. *The Bootstrap Guide to Medicinal Herbs in the Garden, Field, and Marketplace.* Friday Harbor, Wash.: San Juan Naturals, 1999.

Tyler, V., Brady, and J. Robbers. *Pharmacognosy.* 8th ed. Philadelphia: Lea and Febiger, 1981.

Uphoff, J. C. *The Dictionary of Economic Plants.* New York: Verlag Von J. Cramer, 1968.

Vogel, Virgil J. *American Indian Medicine.* Norman: University of Oklahoma Press, 1970.

Von Reis, Siri, and Frank J. Lipp, Jr. *New Plant Sources for Drugs and Foods from the New York Botanical Garden Herbarium.* Cambridge, Mass.: Harvard University Press, 1982.

Von Reis Alltschul, Siri. *Drugs and Foods from Little-Known Plants: Notes in Harvard University Herbaria.* Cambridge, Mass.: Harvard University Press, 1973.

Wheeler, Mark. Personal conversations with author, Pacific Botanicals, Grants Pass, Oreg. May 1998.

Windholz, Martha, ed. *The Merck Index: An Encyclopedia of Chemicals and Drugs.* 9th ed. Rahway, N.J.: Merck, 1976.

Youngken. *A Textbook of Pharmacognosy.* Philadelphia: Blakiston, 1943.

The Pharmacopoeia of the United States of America. 11th ed. Easton, Penn.: Mack Printing Co., 1936.

LOMATIUM
Lomatium dissectum

KRISTA THIE

Springtime east of the Cascade Mountains stirs my core, building my fascination with the beauty of the plant world. The desert grays, greens, and dusty browns quicken with new growth and are interspersed with the vibrant color of the three-nerved violet, pink phlox, purple grass widow, and delicate pink prairie star waving in the fresh spring winds. In addition, the rocky scablands bloom with pink, yellow, white, or purple *Lomatium* species flowers.

In my quest to learn about medicinal plants, I was a research assistant for a European-heritage ethnobotanist working with the Native Americans of the Columbia River plateau and began to learn about the importance of the *Lomatium* genus as source of food and medicine. The medical lore of any traditional culture contains the empirical scientific data of local plant medicine noted through centuries of use. That knowledge makes the difference between life and death. Of the nearly seventy species of *Lomatium*, nine grow just outside of my house in the Columbia River Gorge, on the border between the states of Washington and Oregon.

At one point a local wildflower expert with the Native Plant Society of Oregon showed me the yellow-flowered variety of *Lomatium dissectum* var. *multifidum* growing in the road cutbank in The Dalles, Oregon. He also mistakenly taught me that *L. grayi* was another variation of the plant, inadvertently demonstrating to me the importance of checking with several experts and botanical keys to ensure proper identification.

At that time a large herb company asked me to identify *Lomatium dissectum* for it and I mistakenly showed them *L. grayi*. However, through botanical keys and with other help we were able find the tall purple-flowered variety. Then, in a rush to make money, the company collectors ripped the plants from the ground without replanting the crowns or replacing the dirt from the holes, desecrating my treasured meadow and woodland sanctuaries. At least one of the partakers of its new product had to go to a hospital suffering from a severe rash in reaction to its preparation. Was it karma?

Another time I relented to dig *Lomatium* commercially, but only because it was for a "research" project. My terms included that the researchers were to share the data collected from their project with me. However, all I got out of the deal was a bad case of poison oak and phone calls from supposed researchers fighting over money and status.

It was past time for another approach, so I published a book with a title that states my philosophy: *A Plant Lover's Guide to Wildcrafting: How to Preserve Wild Places and Harvest Medicinal Plants*. Now I collect, share seeds, and teach others to grow their own medicine or to buy and make products from organically cultivated plants, stressing that that herbs are to be collected in an ethical way that does not endanger habitat.

BOTANICAL FEATURES

Lomatium dissectum, with its reddish purple umbel flowers and deep green, glossy, fernlike leaves, grows as tall as 5 feet in the western white oak woodlands of Oregon and Washington and lives at about 300 to 1,500 feet in elevation. The yellow-flowered varieties are up to 3 feet tall with yellow-green foliage. There are at least three different growth forms found in rocky soils from Alberta and British Columbia south to Arizona and southern California, including western Montana, Washington, Oregon, Idaho, Wyoming, Colorado, Utah, and Nevada.

The main plant in herbal commerce now, *Lomatium dissectum*, is commonly called *Lomatium* in herb circles, and I'll follow that practice in this chapter. The older scientific names are various combinations of *Leptotaenia foliosa* var. *dissecta*, *Leptotaenia multifidum*, *Lomatium eatonii*, and *Ferula multifida*. Common names include fern-leaf *Lomatium* or desert parsley, chocolate tips (for the reddish brown nubbins of the flower heads), Indian balsam, toza, and cha luksch.

Lomatium dissectum is one of about seventy-five species of the largest genus in the Parsley family (Apiaceae or Umbelliferae). A genus is a group of plant species based on flower, foliage, chemical, and genetic characteristics assembled by botanists to identify plant relationships. The *Lomatium* genus, also called biscuit root or desert parsley, is found throughout and only in western North America, making it regionally endemic. Some species are quite rare and are on threatened or endangered lists. Be sure to learn the rare ones, and do not harvest any of them. *Lomatium* hybridizes and looks different in different habitats, which adds to the difficulty of correctly identifying it. Some of the herb in commerce may not be *L. dissectum* but rather other species of *Lomatium* or *Cymopterus*.

All Parsley family species have an umbel form of inflorescence, like dill. It looks like an umbrella turned inside out by the wind with the cloth blown away. Other species in the family include important food and herb plants such as carrots, cilantro, celery, dill, parsley, fennel, chervil, lovage, Queen Anne's lace, and osha (*Ligusticum porteri*). It also contains several of the most deadly toxic higher plants in the world, including poison hemlock (*Conium maculatum*) and water hemlock (*Cicuta douglasii*). (See Greg Tilford's book *Edible and Medicinal Plants of the West* for a description of the differences.) Check with several experts and botanical keys to make sure you have positive identification before ingesting any of these related Parsley family species.

Parsley family plants generally contain strong-smelling aromatic chemicals, many of which are pleasant or pungent, though poison hemlock smells "mousy" and unpleasant. Each of the eleven species of *Lomatium* growing in my area has a unique scent. Use your eyes to learn these plants, but your nose may be the most important tool to identify the different species. *L. dissectum* has a pungent, resinous smell. Your local native plant society, school instructor, herbarium, or wild-plant expert may help you learn to identify *L. dissectum*. Get outside with the plants and engage in "social botany"—my favorite way to learn about plants, meet great folks, and learn quickly and safely.

HISTORICAL BACKGROUND

As medicine and food, this genus plays an important role in the lives of western Native North Americans. The spring greens or the roots are prepared for food in many ways and are commonly called biscuit root (including *L. canbyi*, *L. cous*, *L. nudicaule*, and *L. piperii*). Northwest anthropological records indicate at least six species were used for medicine: *L. dissectum, L. grayi* (root for colds), *L. macrocarpum* (root as poultice or taken internally for pneumonia; eaten for infertility and magical powers), *L. nudicaule* (seeds for aches, cough, sore throat; whole plant for colds; important Salish medicine and food; fumigant for house against bad spirits), *L. triternatum* or *L. geyeri* or *L. ambiguum* (food and plant tea for colds and sore throats; root as emetic), and *L. utriculatum* (roots chewed for stomach problems and headaches). In addition, the Oregon Trail settlers learned from the Native Americans to rub the leaf and root resin on irritated or chapped skin.

Many people died during the influenza epidemic of 1920–1922. More people survived who used *Lomatium dissectum* than those who did not have access to it. Mr. and Mrs. Percy Train searched for drug sources at the time of World War II and collected extensive information about the use of plants as medicine by the Native Americans in Nevada. Their team demonstrated that *L. dissectum* can inhibit bacterial growth and has a high vitamin C content.

As a horse medicine, charred *Lomatium* root chunks were placed in a nosebag so that the horse would breathe in the fumes. This helped cure lung infections and break up coughing. Externally, the ground-up root was put on saddle sores.

Native Americans would use various plants to stun fish to make them easier to catch. *Lomatium dissectum* roots were mashed in burlap bags; the bags were then put into quiet pools, causing fish to rise to the surface.

MEDICINAL USES

Michael Moore suggests taking *Lomatium* internally for pneumonia, respiratory infections, chronic fatigue syndrome, HIV, and as a douche for *Candida* and other vaginal infections. It kills gram-positive bacteria and shortens the duration of viral infections such as colds or influenza. "Its main value is for respiratory virus infections. Its aromatic resins act as an expectorant, some of the fractions . . . are exhaled as gases by the lungs, and some of the resins are excreted in the bronchial mucus, all aiding lung cleansing and reducing bronchial microbes."

Richo Cech of Horizon Herbs has the following to say about the use of *Lomatium*:

> I've used the tincture of the fresh root as an antiviral for children and for adults. The herb contains furano-coumarins and saponins. It tastes a bit oily, but pleasantly celery-like. Small dosages quickly ameliorate symptoms of colds, influenza, tonsillitis and bronchitis, assist in rapid recovery and prevent progression of these symptoms into more serious disease states (for example, pneumonia). Because of this, I consider it to be an immune enhancing herb as well as an antiviral. Individuals suffering from Epstein-Barr and systemic *Candida albicans* have also reported to me good success in using this herb.

Overuse of *Lomatium* seems to bring on a rash. Richo Cech notes:

> *Lomatium* has accrued a dedicated following, but it is strong medicine, and as with many other very active substances a little bit does a lot of good, and a lot of it can be too much. I refer here to the "*Lomatium* rash" side effect, which is worrisome to the sufferer at best. The rash starts as a reddish bumpiness to the skin, often around the sensitive thighs, midriff, or neck. Even if dosage is discontinued immediately (and with few exceptions we find that the person was taking a very substantial dosage of tincture, in excess of the maximum recommendation of thirty drops three times per day), the rash inevitably increases for several days. Apparently, the half-life of *Lomatium* phytochemicals in the blood system is comparatively long, which makes sense from a doctrine-of-signatures point of view. Cut the root, and the oleoresins slowly ooze out, and the pervasive but not unpleasant odor clings to everything and everyone in the area. In any case, a rash discovered on Monday may still be in full swing on Friday. Generally, it does not itch. In all cases, in the end analysis, the rash is benign, and the skin returns to normal within two weeks. But it can be a long two weeks.

Paul Bergner has further indicated that corticosteroids have "NO EFFECT on the rash, demonstrating that it is not an allergic rash."

Do not use *Lomatium* like a drug; rather, take it in combination with other herbs that support the liver and kidneys, such as dandelion. Also take an expectorant like grindelia and a diaphoretic such as elder to open the pores and lungs and to increase sweating. Regarding rashes, Michael Moore says, "The rashes seem to be a short-term nitrogenous waste-product overload from immunologic stimulation, cytokine excess, or the waste products of viral die-off. If you use other herbs to stimulate waste-product metabolism and excretion, you get no rashes." It is best to take *Lomatium* with help from an experienced practitioner.

PREPARATION AND DOSAGE

Because of my earlier experiences harvesting *Lomatium*, I usually take other, more common herbs for my own healing. The following preparation and dosage notes are from friends and references.

Fara Currim advises making a tea (decoction) with 1 tablespoon of root to about 8 ounces of water, and taking it once a day for three days at the first signs of a cold. It is "foul and oily," so drink with lots of water. Or take the tincture, no more than 30 drops, two to three times per day for five to seven days. Combine it with lots of rest, garlic, and Oregon grape.

Michael Moore suggests, "Fresh Root Tincture, 1:2, Dry Root Tincture, 1:5, 70 percent alcohol, both 10–30 drops, up to five times a day. Cold Infusion, 2–3 fluid ounces, up to five times a day."

PROPAGATION AND CULTIVATION

Plant *Lomatium dissectum* seeds in the fall for spring germination. This can be as late as January, since one to two months of a cold, wet stratification may be enough for *L. dissectum*. Some *Lomatium* species may have immature embryos and may need a warm wet period in which to develop the embryo, followed by a cold wet time (fall through winter) before germinating in the spring (Julie Kierstead, Berry Botanic Garden, Rare and Endangered Seed Bank, Portland, Oregon). Richo Cech has "had it come up after a pretreatment schedule of 70:40:70 with germination in the spring." I've had seeds germinate after one month of warm, wet treatment, one month in the refrigerator, one month out, one month in, and one month out.

Save all the crowns and plant them in your harvest area; or if that is well stocked, put them into your garden for your next harvest. The crown is the top 1 to 2 inches of the root, where the leaves emerge.

Though *L. dissectum* grows in rocky soils, often intertwined with poison oak and western white oaks, it also spreads easily into road cuts. It likes open, disturbed ground. Howie Brounstein told me of one location in central Oregon's Cascade Mountains that was very thick. Some years later a landslide followed exactly the path of the *L. dissectum* population. Now, once again, the plants are sprouting up along the landslide route.

HARVESTING

Harvesting only cultivated roots is recommended. Before wild-harvesting any plant, learn the general distribution of the numbers of plants in your potential harvest area. Where do they live? How many are there? What is the possibility of their destruction by development or other disturbance, such as grazing? If there are large numbers of plants in your area, happily situated, that you can monitor over a long period of time, go ahead and take a few for medicinal use (less than one in twenty). If not, work toward their preservation in the wild and propagate some in your garden first. Meanwhile, use other medicines while the plants are growing. If there are plenty of plants, you may decide to proceed with wild harvesting. After you are done, leave the site looking as if no one has been there by replanting the crowns, filling in holes, and scattering leaves. Say your grateful thanks for the incredible bounty with which we are blessed.

With this slow-growing plant, wild harvesting is viable only for personal and small community use. Any commercial operation should be supplied by cultivated plants. *Lomatiums* are the old growth of the meadows. I've watched plants in my neighborhood for more than twenty years and they never seem to change much from year to year—not in either in distribution or size. Ten years ago I planted crowns in my garden; only in the past two years have they set seeds. The seeds I wild-planted at the same time are about the size of a pencil with two leaves. It will be many more years before they flower, much less have a resinous root the size of my arm, like some of the wildcrafted roots I have seen. Some wildcrafters guess that plants with roots of that size are ten to twenty years old, while others believe them to be thirty to fifty. I would guess that in rocky and marginal soils, they are more likely 75 to 125 years old, and they may live for several hundred years. In moist and rich soil, however, they do grow much faster. One wildcrafter, Michael Pilarski, is harvesting from a large population in an old orchard where the soil was disturbed and the *Lomatium* population has moved in on its own.

As when harvesting any part of a plant for making medicine, harvest when the energy of the plant is present. If you want the bark, harvest in the fall or spring when the plant juices are traveling through the bark to the roots for storage or in the spring when the plant is preparing to open buds. If you want leaves, harvest them shortly after they have opened and look fresh and alive, before the plant starts putting energy into making flowers. Harvest flowers just after they are open, when the bees are still visiting them for sweet nectar and pollen, and before the plant shifts into making seeds.

Cut the root into thin rounds. Dry these by threading them on a string, or let the roots wilt for several days before slicing them into $1/2$-inch thick slices, then dry in a warm place. Store the roots in glass jars with lids and keep in a cool, dark cabinet.

UpS RECOMMENDATIONS

- Use cultivated resources only. This is not a plant that should be "mainstreamed"—its range is too limited.

- Alternatives include cultivated echinacea, arborvitae (*Thuja occidentalis*), St.-John's-wort, lovage, angelica, and rosemary for respiratory concerns and for *Lomatium*'s antiseptic, diaphoretic, and antibacterial properties.

For the present *Lomatium* has a small but dedicated user group. The dangers for its long-term survival lie in the fad-making ability of the popular press and in people using plants harvested from the wild. For example, a northern California rancher has reported seeing decimation of the accessible *Lomatium* species populations in her area because of renewed interest in traditional foods. If we are to harvest plants from the wild, we need to monitor these plant populations to ensure that they maintain or increase their numbers. In other words, harvest only from places where you can also "wild-garden" by reseeding and replanting crowns. Never harvest from any location that sustains less than one hundred *Lomatium* plants, and even then, take no more than five to twenty. Better still, grow your own or buy organic commercial herbs.

A little *Lomatium dissectum* goes a long way. If antibiotics continue to become less effective, the search for virus- and bacteria-killing chemicals will intensify, and *Lomatium* use might expand. It is important that we grow this plant and teach others to do the same. By having a large repertoire of plants with similar actions, we need use only a little and plant abundance will continue to nourish us.

An alternative to *Lomatium dissectum* root is *L. nudicaule* seeds for sore throats and colds. This was a big medicine among the Salish peoples in the Puget Sound area. The widespread plants are plentiful and survive grazing and other minor habitat disturbances. When you harvest only the seeds, the perennial root crowns will produce more seeds next year. In my area, seeds are generally ready to harvest in June and July. Scatter some where you collect. Generally there is enough for both the survival of the plant population and any gatherer.

One of the benefits of botanical medicine is having control over our own health. We can grow and craft our own herbal medicines to strengthen our bodies along with practicing other healing habits such as good rest, nutrition, play, work, and exercise. Growing your own or making your medicine with plants grown via organic farming practices shifts the larger economic picture to one of greater community health. By striving to keep our bodies in balance, we are better able to help balance the planet.

REFERENCES

Cox, Rachel. *Chemical Investigations into the Ichtyotoxic Effect of "Lomatium dissectum,"* Senior thesis. Reed College, Portland, Oreg., c. 1982.

Hitchcock, C. L., and A. Cronquist. *Flora of the Pacific Northwest.* Seattle: University of Washington Press, 1973.

———. *Vascular Plants of the Pacific Northwest, Part 3: Saxifragaceae to Ericaceae.* Seattle: University of Washington Press, 1984.

Hunn, Eugene, and D. French. "*Lomatium*: a key resource for Columbia Plateau native subsistence." *Northwest Science* 55 (2): 87–94.

Hunn, Eugene. *Nch'I-Wana "The Big River" Mid Columbia Indians and Their Land.* Seattle and London: University of Washington Press, 1990.

Lee, T. T., et al. "Suksdorfin: An anti-HIV principle from *Lomatium* suksdorfee, its structure-activity correlation with related coumarins, and synergistic effects with anti-AIDS nucleosides." *Biorg. Med. Chem.* 2 (10): 1051–56 (Oct. 1994).

Lloyd, W. R., and Glenn L. Jenkins. "A phytochemical study of *Leptotaenia multifida Nuttall.*" *Pharm. Arch.,* 13 (1942): 33–38.

McCutcheon, A. R., et al. "Antiviral screening of British Columbian medicinal plants." *Journal of Ethnopharmacology* 49 (2): 101–110 (1 Dec. 1995).

Meilleur, Brian, and Eugene Hunn. "The all purpose genus: *Lomatium* as protein procurer." Working paper, Department of Anthropology, University of Washington, Seattle, Washington, 1983.

Moore, Michael. *Medicinal Plants of the Pacific West.* Santa Fe: Red Crane Books, 1993.

Thie, Krista. *A Plant Lover's Guide to Wildcrafting: How to Preserve Wild Places and Harvest Medicinal Plants,* 6th ed. White Salmon, Wash.: Longevity Herb Press, 1997.

————. *Medicinal Plants of the Pacific Northwest: A Digest of Anthropological Writing about Native American Uses.* White Salmon, Wash.: Longevity Herb Press, 1999.

Tilford, Gregory. *Edible and Medicinal Plants of the West.* Missoula, Mont.: Mountain Press Publishing, 1997.

Train, Heinrichs, and Archer. *Medicinal Uses of Plants by Indian Tribes of Nevada.* Lawrence, Mass.: Quarterman Publications, 1957.

VanWagenen, B. C., et al. "Native American food and medicinal plants, 8. Water-soluble constituents of *Lomatium dissectum.*" *J. Nat. Prod.* (Jan–Feb 1998) 51 (1): 136–41.

Willard, Terry. *Edible and Medicinal Plants of the Rocky Mountains and Neighbouring Territories.* Calgary, Alb.: Mountain Rose Books, 1992.

OREGON GRAPE
Mahonia spp.

RYAN W. DRUM, Ph.D.

In the old days and in some current texts, Oregon grape species are classified in the genus *Berberis*, the same genus as the dreaded alien invader, *Berberis vulgaris*, or barberry. Both barberry and Oregon grape species are in the botanical family Berberidaceae, and all contain various amounts of the important medicinal alkaloid berberine, as well as many other medicinally active alkaloids.

Much can be in a name. Fifteen years ago, after traveling by bus from Vancouver Island, British Columbia, back to my home in the United States, I passed across the U.S.–Canadian border. I was carrying 10 pounds of cut and dried Oregon grape roots harvested by one of my students in a 4-gallon plastic bucket. When a customs officer asked if I had any plant material, I answered in the affirmative, and when asked what kind, I blithely replied "*Berberis nervosa.*" The ever vigilant officer looked it up in his book of forbidden plants and found *B. vulgaris*, barberry—a totally forbidden plant—whereupon he promptly seized my bucket of root pieces and told me I could not bring it into the country; that it would be destroyed immediately as a threat to *American agriculture*. I was

dumbfounded and decided to argue botanically, saying it was a totally different species, used for medicine, totally dry, no seeds, and harmless; he remained unmoved, triumphant. Exasperated, I looked out the window and saw that all of the building borders were heavily planted with a robust horticultural variety of *Mahonia aquifolium*. I quickly pointed this out to the customs officer, then opened my bucket and showed him the total similarity between the plant stems outside and some of the pieces in my bucket. In an unexpected fit of wisdom and clarity, the man agreed that it seemed unreasonable to ban material already growing at the customs station, and let me import it and return to the waiting bus. I was thus quite pleased when the genus name for the various Oregon grape species was changed back to *Mahonia* from *Berberis*.

BOTANICAL FEATURES

The various North American species of Oregon grape tend to be modest, long-lived, woody-stemmed perennials. Handsome, well-behaved evergreen horticultural varieties abound as ornamentals and erosion-control plantings. Most species transplant readily from wild to domestic and semidomestic sites. The northern species, *Mahonia aquifolium* and *M. nervosa*, usually do not favor full-sun locations. Medicinally active *Mahonia* species are abundant from southwestern British Columbia to central California and east to the eastern edges of the Rocky Mountains; except for horticultural and ornamental plantings, I believe they are truly a western genus, not occurring as native plants east of the Rockies. They can be found in both rain forests and arid lands. There are differences among the individual species in regard to both constituent content and medicinal efficacy.

Two long-lived, solitary-stemmed *Mahonia* species live in my bioregion, Cascadia: one taller, at 4 to 10 feet, *M. aquifolium*, and a much shorter species favoring slightly drier mixed coniferous woodlands, *M. nervosa*. Both are abundant and tend to be dominant understory plants in both old-growth and regrowth mixed coniferous woodlands on the lowlands and slopes of the Cascade Mountains. They were used extensively in local folk medicine by both indigenous and recent settlers.

Mahonia nervosa is my favorite species of Oregon grape. I have lived closely and intimately with this wonderful plant for more than thirty years. Like most *Mahonia* species, it has spiny-tipped leaflets arranged in lovely pinnately compound leaves; each leaflet resembles a solitary simple holly leaf. Young spring-emergent *M. nervosa* leaflets are very tender when they first emerge from the apical bud, yellowish to light green, sweet and sour tasting. Children

favor them; rumor claims they have a high ascorbic acid content; goats, deer, and elk devour them. As the leaflets reach full size they become tough, spiny at the margins, and covered on both upper and lower surfaces with a water-repellent, varnishlike coating. This hydrophobic layer sheds water, preventing the puddling of rain, dew, and snow on the leaves, and also protects against topical microbial decay and casual herbivory. It also reduces water loss during dry weather and drought. Mature leaves of both *M. aquifolium* and *M. nervosa* are perennial and persist for many years. They do not turn red each autumn as some authors claim. They do, however, turn a bit reddish when a single leaflet dies, or when a small isolated insect or mechanical trauma has damaged and killed some leaf parenchyma. The wounded area will heal with a dense concentration of red anthocyanins.

Living close to the same *M. nervosa* plants for thirty years has allowed me to observe their varied responses to changes in upper-story canopy density, herbivory from my goats and children, and rare severe cold. Most of the leaves on solitary *M. nervosa* stems will persist for at least ten years, some for as long as twenty years in closed-canopy, nutrient-poor locations. This means they are true evergreens and very efficient in their investment in structure. At least seven leaflet alkaloids further retard microbial consumption of live leaves. Each persistent leaf has a strong wiry petiole that flares at its basal attachment to its respective solitary unbranched woody stem, an arrangement that tends to promote water puddling at each petiole-stem axil. A leaf can be smartly plucked from the stem with a downward snap to reveal the bright yellow fan of the attachment flare. The bright yellow is from the alkaloid berberine, the most abundant alkaloid in *M. nervosa*'s woody stems and rhizomes. The berberine and other alkaloids can be presumed to be a chemical antimicrobial ploy to compensate for the obvious axillary junction water puddling. (Plant material and water together usually equal decay as microorganisms, mostly fungi and bacteria, digest wet plant tissue with extracellular enzymes.)

The bright yellow blossom cluster spikes are edible, tasty, and pleasantly scented. The $^3/_8$- to $^1/_2$-inch diameter berries tend to mature in Virgo with an intensely blue-gray color and dark purple-red skins. Three to nine hard, woody seeds occupy most of each berry. Even when completely ripe (the powder blue color on the outside of the berries tends to develop long before the berries are actually even remotely ripe), the berries start out tasting sweet and then progress to tart, then astringent and even bitter. The resemblance to grapes (*Vitus* spp.) is superficial at best. The intense berry color and flavor can yield tasty, pretty jellies and wines with appropriate processing and added sweetener. Indigenous *Mahonia* berry use seems to have been situational; the berries were eaten fresh and dried as available, but they were seldom sufficiently abundant to be a major, reliable food source.

MEDICINAL USES

Before proceeding to the topics of therapeutics and harvesting, I'd like to discuss the powerful constituent reality of *Mahonia nervosa:* The combined nine or more alkaloids in the soft bark's inner tissues and occasionally the inner wood (and seldom in the inner pith of the emergent stems) of *M. nervosa* are extractable in aqueous and water-alcohol solutions. The resulting extracts have demonstrated strong, broad-spectrum antimicrobial activity against viruses (herpes, hepatitis), bacteria (both gram negative and gram positive, as well as *Chlamydia*), fungi *(Candida)*, and protozoa (amoebas, *Giardia*, malaria).

Francis Brinker has published an excellent, thorough, and well-referenced discussion of *Mahonia* alkaloids and their respective therapeutic applications and potentials, particularly berberine. Berberine is the most abundant and therapeutically dominant Oregon grape alkaloid; it is soluble in cold water, and less soluble in ethanol than in water. Hypercautious, nonpracticing authors warn of a potential toxic hazard from the use and consumption of *Mahonia* teas or extracts due to this berberine presence. These authors offer no references to primary sources or referenced case studies that might provide authentic empirical data demonstrating genuine human health hazards from the use of *Mahonia*. The potential hazards are extrapolated apparently from caged-animal experiments using isolated, purified berberine, not simple extracts of *Mahonia* species. The berberine in animal experiments was often administered either subcutaneously or intravenously—procedures that both tend to be outside the usual scope of practice for most herbalists. There are no known reports of adverse reactions to *Mahonia* teas or extracts from herbal practitioners or users that

I can locate. The most probable hazard is the miscarriage potential, although no cases have been reported. The relatively poor body uptake of berberine reduces its potential hazards.

Mahonia is most commonly used in medicine in the form of teas and extracts of stem and rhizome pieces both externally and internally. Some folk traditions do use *Mahonia* leaf teas, powders, and extracts. I do not, yet. One of the best summaries of the real therapeutic uses of *Mahonia* is in Dr. Christopher's book *The School of Natural Healing*. Dried leaf has reportedly been used as an antimicrobial styptic for skin abrasions and to topically calm herpes and psoriasis skin lesions. I usually recommend strong *M. nervosa* decocted tea for herpes and psoriasis patients; the functional dosage is roughly 1 to 2 8-ounce cups of a two- to twelve-hour-steeped decoction two to four times a week. This usually results in a noticeable lessening of symptom severity. Less-defined eczema and rashes often resolve with two to ten weeks of *M. nervosa* tea use. The action here may be due to a combination of improved liver and kidney excretory function, antifungal or antibacterial activity, and possibly mild thyroid stimulation.

Simple aqueous and ethanol-water extracts of *Mahonia* exert a gradual positive effect on all body symptoms and tissues. The primary actions are improved biliary flow and excretion, enhanced kidney function, antimicrobial action, and spasmolytic toning of smooth-muscle tissue. The improved bile flow in particular results in better digestion, better appetite, and better elimination of stool, and, in women, a lessening of PMS symptoms.

Recently a forty-year-old woman came to see me about some chronic health problems. She complained of episodic poor circulation and cold hands. I examined her hands, looking for Raynaud's signs and spotting nothing much, although her hands were a little cool. One middle finger was warm, reddish to purple, and a bit puffy and inflamed looking, especially around what appeared to be a recent deep puncture wound. I asked her about the finger. She said that she had decided not to mention it to me, since it was so much better than it had been a day or two previous. The puncture wound had occurred several days earlier and was approximately 3 millimeters wide and 8 deep. It had bled a bit but remained open, although it was not enough of a bother to cover. A day or two later she cleaned a lot of fish and crabs, and twenty-four hours after that the punctured finger was very swollen, red to purple in color, hot, and painful. I was seeing her finger about thirty-six hours after the maximum swelling and discomfort. The wound and finger looked to be in recovery, but the heat seemed to indicate some residual infection. I asked her to come by or send word if the finger worsened. Three days later, a neighbor contacted me and said that the woman's entire hand had become hot, swollen, and throbbing with great pain; it was reddish purple in color with a prominent red line forming on her inner wrist. I immediately went into the nearby forest and harvested several pounds of mature *M. nervosa* stems and underground rhizomes. I bundled them carefully for transport and wrote out directions for preparing and using strong *M. nervosa* decoctions, both internally as a decoction and externally as a hot soak for her hand. Most of her friends and family were not supportive of her choice to use herbs instead of flying off to the mainland to receive emergency medical attention and a probable strong, intravenous antibiotic treatment. Certainly the ghastly appearance of her hand was alarming. She resisted and persisted with the Oregon grape regime I had suggested. She was very much against using prescription antibiotics. If her symptoms had seriously worsened, I would have either tried stronger herbs or conceded to intravenous antibiotic(s) in an obviously life-threatening situation. Previous success in using Oregon grape to treat apparent localized gram-positive infections allowed me a certain confidence. Her symptoms did not noticeably improve until twenty-four hours had passed, but they then improved rapidly until most had subsided within five or six days after starting the Oregon grape treatment. Soreness, discoloration, some cavitation, and shedding continued for eighteen to twenty days; complete resolution and superficial healing had occurred by week five with no recurrence. The woman continued to drink at least 12 ounces of strong decoction daily through week six.

Decoctions of Oregon grape's woody parts become progressively stronger medicinally from prolonged steeping (twenty-four to seventy-two hours) and repeated short daily reboiling (one to two minutes). I have also redecocted the same batch of stem and root material three times, with strong tea still produced from the third decoction. A good strong *Mahonia* decoction is a dark orange-brown color with a mildly bittersweet flavor. It can act as both a mild diuretic and a laxative.

IMPETIGO

When children (or, rarely, adults) present with obvious impetigo sores, I treat them with an equal mixture of strong tinctures of Oregon grape and grindelia applied topically four to six times daily until resolved. Sanitary rigor improves the likelihood of positive outcome.

A thirty-year-old woman came to see me. Her arms and her modestly exposed chest, neck, and face presented numerous angry raised sores and eruptions, along with attendant scars from previous sores. The sores had first appeared abruptly nearly a year previously. No one consulted medically seemed to know how to treat them successfully. Since she was finishing acupuncture school at the time, I was surprised. For her. I felt that a suggestion of teas and prolonged external soaks might result in poor compliance, so I recommended tinctures. Unsure of the exact nature of her presentation but suspecting one or more infectious gram-positive bacteria, probably *Staphylococcus aureus* (a bacterium I had worked with in graduate school), I had her use an equal-parts mixture of usnea and grindelia tinctures topically on all sores and inflamed surfaces. Internally she took a 5 cc dose of strong *Mahonia* tincture three times a day. In a week she was 80 percent better; in two weeks, 90 percent better; within a month all symptoms had resolved, and she was amazed. Everything had cleared up and there was no recurrence in the four years until I saw her again. She had continued to take the *Mahonia* tincture for six months. Today she bears no signs of a once-terrible disfigurement.

GIARDIA

Giardia is an octoflagellated protozoan spread usually by infested water and occasionally by food. It is parasitic in humans and attaches to the cells of the mucosa of the small intestine. The presenting symptoms of great abdominal discomfort—loose stools, belching, intense borborygmus, and bouts of constipation—can range from debilitating to barely noticeable, or a *Giardia* carrier may be apparently asymptomatic. For known, tested *Giardia* cases I use strong-steeped Oregon grape decoction taken once or twice a day in 12- to 16-ounce doses for four weeks and then suggest a retest for *Giardia*, continuing to take the tea until the test results are known. If the test comes back negative, consider having a retest in a week or two to help rule out a false negative. If the test comes back positive, continue the *Mahonia* teas until a negative test is obtained, testing once every four to six weeks. The most persistent case in my experience took four months of daily decocted tea to resolve. I have not obtained *Giardia* clearance with tinctures of *Mahonia*. The decocted Oregon grape teas apparently do not kill the *Giardia* cells, but rather render the intestinal environment *Giardia* unfriendly; the little rascals detach and leave in the stool. In my experience all compliant cases of known *Giardia* infestation have cleared when treated with strong *M. nervosa* decoction as determined by stool examination.

GUM DISEASE

Some periodontal gum disease can be suppressed or even cleared by persistent treatment with strong *Mahonia* decoctions. The procedure is simple: Hold an ounce or more of the decoction in the mouth for fifteen to twenty minutes at least once daily, although twice daily is better, morning and evening.

PROPAGATION AND CULTIVATION

Transplanting is done by burying 4- to 6-inch-long stem tips with buds. The pieces are buried vertically with an inch or less of the growing tip emergent above the soil; the soil should be well tamped around the stem. Underground rhizome sections 4 to 6 inches long can be planted 2 to 4 inches deep, laid out horizontally. The pieces to be planted should be cut and planted in due haste to prevent desiccation; keep them moist and cool between cutting and planting. Water the new plantings and keep the soil moist until new growth appears. Richo Cech of Horizon Seeds says, "To grow Oregon grape from seeds, the seeds must first be removed from the fruit and washed. Then the seeds are planted in the fall, midwinter, or early spring in an outdoor nursery bed. Germination is in the early spring in cold soils. We timed the germination period once at seventy days."

HARVESTING

More than twenty years ago I began commercial harvesting of Oregon grape—stems and rhizomes of *Mahonia nervosa*. At first I used a full-strapped, serious spading fork (Bulldog Tools, England) for about a year with great effort and frustration. Then I harvested only the underground rhizomes under the mistaken assumption that the emergent stems had little or no medicinal value; I did notice that the inner bark of the older stems was bright yellow-orange, indicating substantial amounts of berberine if not other alkaloids. I checked with other herbalists and phytochemists, who assured me that all of the woody material below the terminal-leaf bud scales was suitable for harvest and extraction. That immediately meant a lot less waste and much greater time and effort efficiency in harvesting.

By the second year of harvest, I had also made a lot of observations about how *M. nervosa* likes to grow. This particular species of *Mahonia* with solitary woody stems is a relatively long-lived perennial, with individual stems persisting for up to 150 years. The plant spreads deliberately by shallow sharp-tipped rhizomes, which may grow 10 to 20 feet underground radiating outward and back from their centers of origin to form a multilayered, loose mesh of many interconnecting woody rhizomes. These tend to persist in several distinct sizes, some barely enlarging in diameter for decades after they first grow out from a center of origin. An individual rhizome may emerge as an apparent new plant 20 or more feet from a growth center. A single propagation center can spread out over many acres as one continuous or visually intermittent stand of what to the casual observer presents as individual plants. In the Pacific Northwest, in areas where this plant is extemely healthy and abundant, a respectful harvest of mature stems and roots may be accomplished without noticeably diminishing the stand. I can go back to areas that I harvested five or more years ago and upon casual observation find that it looks like none had been harvested. The many small bits and pieces of rhizomes left in the soil sprouted new stems. However, in marginal habitat—mesic to zeric forests with full canopy, or especially arid areas with complete forest canopy—it may take twenty years after harvest for the plants to attain harvestable regrowth.

On older rhizomes, you'll find dense woody spherical masses, 1 to 2 inches in diameter with very dark orange wood and inner bark. From one of these masses a dozen or more individual colonial propagative rhizomes may grow. I save these masses for the strongest medicine and for replanting.

Stems and underground rhizomes of *Mahonia nervosa* are quickly harvested by simply tugging on mature stems in the hope and expectation that the stem will lift easily from the ground with a long, thick underground rhizome attached at right angles to the vertical axis of the stem. This is not always the case, so it is best to leave the resistant stems and to move on. Trim the harvested stems of scaly apical growth, and cut the remaining wood carefully into 18- to 24-inch linear pieces. The individual cut pieces are laid flat across the longitudinal axis of a polyester plastic mesh feed bag laid out flat on the ground. Do not stuff the pieces into the bag; this would result in a lot of unacceptable bruising and scuffing off of the thin bark layers containing the alkaloids. I prefer to harvest on cloudy, cool days to prevent drying of the harvested sticks. The sticks are wrapped up in the plastic bag as a protective cover, tied with a piece of baling twine, and placed carefully in the shade. The plastic feed bag wrap also retards drying. As soon after harvest as permissible, very carefully wash the harvested material by repeatedly dipping, agitating, and turning the roots and rhizomes in tubs of cold water; usually you can simply lift entire bundles off the unwrapped plastic bag and place them whole in the washing tub. No brushes are used, since this might scuff off the delicate bark. After washing, hand-cut the sticks into 4- to 8-inch pieces and quickly place them in brown paper bags for shipping fresh, or cut the sticks into 2- to 4-inch pieces for drying on cloth-sheet-covered wire-screen drying racks. I try to keep the drying temperature between 70 and 90 degrees. With circulating air, drying takes eight to twelve days. After drying, store the pieces in airtight containers kept in a dark and cool (50 to 60 degrees) spot. The fresh material loses about 50 to 60 percent of its weight with drying.

Although one species (*Mahonia aquifolium*) grows in full sun, the majority of the species are found associated with old-growth and second-growth coniferous forests and are dependent on the forest habitat for their survival. These plants are extremely sensitive to harvest and should be taken only very sparingly from abundant stands. After harvesting the root, the leaves can be trimmed back and the crowns replanted.

UpS RECOMMENDATIONS

- Limited wild harvest is permissible.

- As a direct substitute for Oregon grape, the non-native plant barberry (*Berberis vulgaris*), which is common in the eastern United States, can be used. Barberry contains a similar concentration of the antimicrobial alkaloid berberine, and like Oregon grape, it promotes the secretion of bile thereby improving digestion of fats.

- Dandelion (*Taraxacum officinale*) and yellow dock (*Rumex crispus*) are common weeds that have a similar liver-stimulating and digestive effect.

Few of us realize that the greatest hazard to *Mahonia* species, at least in the Pacific Northwest, does not come from medicinal harvest or simple loss of habitat from logging and developmental human settlement sprawl. It comes from the nearly twenty-thousand non-timber-forest-products (NTFP) industry workers who pick mushrooms and "brush." The lovely long-lasting *Mahonia* leaves are prized for floral displays; hundreds of huge shipping containers full of only the best *Mahonia* leaves are exported each year from West Coast rain forests. More than 90 percent of brush pickers are recent immigrants or migrant workers; English is often a distant second language. These people cannot be expected to protect the resource. Their relative poverty also mitigates against the niceties of protecting the plants; they are more concerned with picking more pieces to protect their families. There are several well-intentioned efforts to organize these people to not only raise their wages and improve their working conditions, but also to raise the pickers' awareness of sustainable harvesting. I have great hopes for these efforts.

REFERENCES

Brinker, Francis. *Native Healing Gifts*. Sandy, Oreg.: Eclectic Medical Publications, 1993.

Christopher, John R, M.D. *School of Natural Healing*. Provo, Utah: BiWorld Publishers, 1979.

Drum, R. *Three Herbs* (audiotape) West Hurley, N.Y.: Creative Seminars, (914- 679-6885), 1995.

Duke, J. *Handbook of Medicinal Herbs*. New York: CRC Press, 1985.

McGuffin, M., C. Hobbs, R. Upton, and A. Goldberg. *Botanical Safety Handbook*. New York: CRC, 1997.

Moore, Michael. *Medicinal Plants of the Mountain West*. Santa Fe: Museum of New Mexico Press, 1979.

Tilford, G. *Edible and Medicinal Plants of the West*. Missoula, Mont.: Mountain Press Publishing, 1997.

Turner, N. *Food Plants of British Columbia*. Victoria, B.C.: British Columbia Provincial Museum, 1997.

OSHA

Ligusticum canbyi

GREGORY L. TILFORD

It's a magical place where nature awakens imagination with a deluge of sensory input. Whenever I am there, I find myself in silent contemplation. With my head tilted toward the sun, I close my eyes to feel the dampness of the earth rise around me, combining with clear mountain air and the icy warmth of alpine sunshine. The fragrance of sweet meadow grasses fills my lungs with each deliberate breath, and every cell of my body is slowly filled with a magical feeling of completeness. In my mind's eye a great bear steps away from a nearby stand of lodgepole pine, and when I listen intently enough, I can hear the whispering songs of a thousand happy spirits—all singing in harmony with the bees, the mountain bluebirds, and the earth itself. This is the home of osha, *Ligusticum canbyi*, the great bear medicine of the Salish, Blackfeet, and Cheyenne. It is a place where healing occurs spontaneously—where respect, admiration, and humility are rewarded with the lessons of great elders. I visit osha as often as I can—sometimes to harvest a root or two for my personal apothecary, but usually just to heal by being in the sacred place where it lives. Indeed, the plant itself is a powerful herbal medicine, but I have

come to know this plant as much more than a physical healing device.

Osha (*Ligusticum canbyi* or *L. porteri*) grows in one of nature's grand classrooms—in high, moist mountain meadows and bogs, where the effects of human encroachment are compounded by a continuous struggle to survive. In the Rocky Mountains, at elevations between 6,000 and 10,000 feet, life succeeds only if allowed by nature's intent and design. Winter is very harsh, the spring and summer are very short, and the plants and creatures that live here are specially adapted and critically dependent upon one another. It is a place where humans are outsiders—where our intellect is overshadowed by the raw powers of nature. It is a place where the deepest level of healing does not come from the exploitation of the plants themselves, but from our efforts to understand the ways of their source.

For years I have been trying to learn how everything interrelates in osha's fragile environment, but such lessons come slowly, even if I spend a good part of every day in nature's classroom. I have watched the way osha draws pollinating insects toward the earth, to benefit its plant neighbors as well as itself. I have seen how in early summer osha feeds the winter-weary moose, bears, deer, and birds from its foliage and fruits. And I am just beginning to learn how all of these creatures serve one another, and osha in return. Now, after decades of quiet observation, two things stand out as the most valuable lessons I have learned: that I still know very little about the ways of osha's world; and that my lack of knowledge makes me a dangerous visitor in osha's environment.

In osha's world most of what we regard as "resource management" amounts to little more than the kind of speculations a kindergarten student might make. And as a result, we see osha and its habitat disappearing under human pressure. Osha offers herbalists a valuable gift: an opportunity to step beyond the boundaries of the human self so we can help ourselves and others heal as part of the large whole we call the earth.

BOTANICAL FEATURES

Several species of *Ligusticum* inhabit North America, but only two are recognized by herbalists as superior medicines: *L. canbyi* (Canby's lovage or osha) and *L. porteri* (Porter's lovage or osha).

Osha (pronounced *oh-SHAW*) presents us with characteristics typical of the Parsley family—umbrella-shaped inflorescence of tiny white flowers on top of hollow, 1- to 3-foot stems that bear fernlike, pinnately compound leaves. The basal leaves are up to 8 inches long and are finely divided two or three times into

deeply lobed leaflets. Leaves of the upper stem are smaller and with fewer divisions. Many of the other *Ligusticum* species are smaller plants, with leaves that are more finely divided and carrotlike (such as *L. tenuifolium*). Beach lovage (*L. scoticum*), a common circumboreale species that occurs at low elevations in Alaska and the western provinces of Canada, is quite different from other North American species, with leaves that are twice divided into threes to give an appearance that is more like celery. It is used primarily as a food spice and a carminative, similar to the uses of fennel (*Foeniculum vulgare*).

For many years I was hesitant to harvest and use osha, for reasons other than its at-risk status. With the exception of beach lovage, *Ligusticum* species share a frightening resemblance to their extremely poisonous cousins, hemlock parsley (*Conioselinum* spp.), and poison hemlock (*Conium* spp.). Differentiating osha from these deadly impostors depends strongly on personal familiarity and practical experience, and until a level of absolute comfort is reached in identifying osha, the self-reliant herbalist is well advised against making a potentially fatal mistake. To begin the identification process, learn to use a botanical key. Then, you can begin associating "stand-out" characteristics. First, unlike its poisonous cousins, osha has a well-defined, brown taproot (tapered like a carrot), the upper third of which has distinctive growth rings. Second, the root crown is surrounded by hairlike dead leaf material. And third, the root has a spicy, celery-like fragrance that closely resembles that of its cultivated relative, lovage (*Levisticum officinale*).

177

HISTORICAL BACKGROUND

Ligusticum translates to "from Liguria," a province in Italy where *L. scotium* may have originated. Some historians argue that this species of osha was carried throughout Europe and the Mediterranean countries by the Scots, while others believe that it was the Romans who distributed the plant. According to Alaska herbalist Janice Schofield, in her book *Discovering Wild Plants*, Aleut and Athabascan Indians know this species as *petruski*, a Russian name that suggests that the herb was introduced to them by Russian explorers.

The name *osha* is a North American word meaning "bear." The plant was probably given this name by tribes of New Mexico and the southernmost reaches of osha's range, where it has remained a popular medicine to date. It is likely that *Ligusticum porteri*, *L. canbyi*, and other native species earned the name from human observations of bears eating the plants. Many First Nation cultures recognize the bear as a very powerful totem that brings forth strong medicine. Observations of the great animal using osha in a time of need would indeed be very impressive. The Indians used osha as an antiviral medicine, and they eventually shared these attributes with white settlers.

MEDICINAL USES

Given the effectiveness and regional popularity of this herb, it's amazing that more scientific study has not been done on osha. Perhaps this is why it remains a well-known medicine within its bioregional range (from the Rocky Mountains westward), but a relatively obscure one in the eastern half of North America. This may also explain why market pressure has not wiped out osha entirely.

Like many plants that have been found to possess an exceptional capacity to heal, osha has become somewhat of a "designer herb." In addition to being a time-proven antiviral and expectorant remedy, this herb brings an intriguing name and history to the marketplace. Osha-the-Ancient-Indian-Bear-Medicine is very attractive to a growing audience of people who are increasingly concerned about the continuing rise in virus-related illnesses, and who see osha as a rediscovered Indian secret capable of stamping out viral infections. This of course is not true, and like many herbs with a rich history and provocative name, hundreds of pounds of osha root are probably being wasted for purposes that don't justify its harvest.

Osha works its best magic when employed within narrow therapeutic parameters. Specifically, it is an excellent respiratory antiviral for cases of infection that are characterized by a dry, raspy, bronchial cough. The volatile oils it contains (primarily pthalides) are very warming, expectorant, and anesthetic to the upper respiratory passages, providing quick stimulation to the mucous membranes and making coughs wetter and more productive. Osha also has phytosterols that help relieve upper respiratory inflammation. In China *Ligusticum wallichii*, a species very similar to our *L. porteri*, is used to lower blood pressure, induce uterine contractions, and inhibit postpartum bleeding. Most notably, though, osha possesses antiviral and antibacterial constituents that help shorten the duration and moderate the severity of many types of respiratory infections.

Osha also has very good carminative properties, and is an excellent gastric antispasmodic, but its usefulness here is overshadowed by the existence of equally effective and less endangered alternatives such as fennel (*Foeniculum vulgare*), angelica (*Angelica* spp.), or culinary lovage (*Ligusticum* or *Levisticum* spp.). Likewise, nettle (*Urtica* spp.), shepherd's purse (*Capsella bursa-pastoris*), yarrow (*Achillea millifolium*), and raspberry leaf (*Rubus* spp.) are all useful for slowing postpartum bleeding; blue cohosh (*Caulophyllum thalictroides*) serves as a uterine stimulant and is much easier to cultivate.

PREPARATION AND DOSAGE

The active constituents of osha are poorly water soluble, so the root must be chewed or made into a tincture. The latter option is the best choice, because it eliminates the possibility of spoilage and thereby reduces subsequent waste. To make a good, strong tincture from the dried root you will need a menstruum strength of at least 70 percent alcohol. The chopped or ground root is then macerated at a ratio of 1:5—that is, 1 part herb (by dry weight) to 5 parts menstruum (by liquid volume). I like to make my tincture from the fresh roots right in the meadow from which they are dug. This makes optimum medicine, and helps me weigh my harvest impact against my actual needs. I dig a root, chop it up, put it into a jar, and cover it with a 1:2

ratio of 70 percent alcohol. I listen to the birds for a moment, smell a wildflower, then look at the empty space I have created and the footprints I have pressed into the delicate soil. From this I reconsider my need for more; a few ounces of tincture will last us for years. Usually, I end up digging much less than I had intended.

PROPAGATION AND CULTIVATION

Osha is extremely difficult to cultivate. It prefers high elevations, and seed viability is typically very low. In my experience, only about 10 percent of the seeds can be expected to germinate in the wild, out of which only a few seedlings will survive to reach maturity. The complex natural growing medium that wild plants require cannot be replicated by humankind, making cultivation a very iffy proposition. Nevertheless, if you live in the mountain West, or Pacific Northwest, you might give osha a try in the garden (seeds are available from Horizon Seeds; see the end of this chapter). You will need rich, moist, slightly to moderately acidic soil and partial shade, preferably from conifers. Seeds are sown on top of the soil in late fall, cupped-side up. They must be kept moist until they germinate. When they are an inch or so tall, the plants should be spaced 1 foot apart. If and when they are established, they will become drought tolerant.

HARVESTING

Osha lives in a delicately balanced habitat that does not tolerate the effects of human encroachment. Harvest should be limited to the periphery of large, healthy stands, preferably from the edges of a well-established trail (I follow the moose routes). Soil compression is a primary concern here; if your feet leave a lasting impression, chances are you are damaging delicate root systems and interfering with a rich, subterranean microcosm. Be aware of any evidence of animal forage, while keeping in mind that the moose, bears, and other wildlife need osha more than we do. Roots should be conservatively gathered, using a hand trowel. A visible change in the appearance of the stand means that you have harvested too much. Mature plants might be ten to twenty years old, meaning that osha's interdependent roles in its habitat are well established. You should therefore monitor the long-term effects of harvest for several years. Is there regrowth since your last visit? Did the seeds from the plants you harvested germinate and take hold? Is there any new evidence of human impact or increased animal use in the stand? These are questions that wildcrafting herbalists need to ask themselves during each subsequent visit to osha's home. From the answers, we can learn to work in symbiotic harmony with nature and give for all that we receive from her bounty.

If you decide after all considerations to dig osha, it should be done in the late summer or fall, after the plant has bloomed and the seeds have fully ripened (you will be able to shake them from the umbels). After digging a root, lay the umbel-bearing stem of the plant onto the soil in the exact same spot from which it was dug. This will allow the seeds to germinate

and reproduce in a close-to-natural manner. The roots can be cut in half lengthwise, and dried on newspaper in a warm, airy portion of your home. When completely dried, they can be stored in a plastic bag or glass jar for a year or more, but it's best to use them as soon as possible.

UpS RECOMMENDATIONS

- Use the wild plant only when absolutely necessary; otherwise use only cultivated resources.
- Thyme, elecampane, marsh mallow, lovage, angelica, and rosemary are all good alternatives.

In many isolated areas of the mountain West, osha still stands in dense abundance. However, if we view the plant from a perspective that encompasses its entire range, it is becoming increasingly scarce, and we can see that market pressure is forcing the harvest of younger roots.

Osha is being harvested from the high mountains (9,000-plus feet) in New Mexico and Colorado by the tons each year, much of which is being exported to Mexico. To reach and carry out the roots, pack animals (and I suspect ATVs) are used to enter very delicate ecosystems that scientists and herbalists admittedly know little about. In other words, the environmental damage caused when we harvest osha may be more serious than its overharvest.

The future survival of osha and the fate of its special environment rest in the hearts and minds of those who recognize it for what it really is—a precious gift of healing, a teacher, and a representative of environmental health. To save osha from extinction, herbalists must do much more than make concessions relative to its use. We must extend our holistic healing efforts beyond the human self to include the health of green allies and their habitats. The only way of assuring that osha is being harvested with respectful attention to its environment is to harvest it yourself, and only for your needs. And to use osha for anything but its unique indications—dry coughs that are secondary to a respiratory virus—would constitute waste of a valuable and almost endangered medicinal ally.

In most instances cultivated lovage *(Levisticum officinalis)* serves as an excellent alternative, and should be used as such. However, while substituting a cultivated herb for osha may help relieve pressure upon its remaining stands, this barely begins to address the issues of habitat destruction. All herbalists, being delegates of nature's healing provisions, have a responsibility to protect the source of our craft. This starts with getting to know the plants themselves, learning and sharing the ways and needs of their world, and becoming involved as active guardians of the environment we share with them. Most of all, it means living as interconnected components of the living biosphere we call earth.

REFERENCES

Moore, Michael. *Medicinal Plants of the Mountain West.* Santa Fe: Museum of New Mexico Press, 1979.

Schofield, Janice. *Discovering Wild Plants—Alaska, Western Canada, the Northwest.* Seattle: Alaska Northwest Books, 1989.

Tilford, Gregory L. *Edible and Medicinal Plants of the West.* Missoula, Mont.: Mountain Press Publishing, 1997.

———. *From Earth to Herbalist.* Missoula, Mont.: Mountain Press Publishing, 1998.

Willard, Terry. *Edible and Medicinal Plants of the Rocky Mountains and Neighbouring Territories.* Calgary, Alberta: Mountain Rose Books, 1992.

OSHA SEEDS

Horizon Herbs
P.O. Box 69
Williams, OR 97544-0069
(541) 846-6704

PARTRIDGEBERRY
Mitchella repens

SUSUN S. WEED

Take a walk with me through my woods: a third-growth white pine, oak, ash, deciduous forest. We'll have to walk for a while to get to where the partridgeberry grows. It's hard to find her near the house. Let's go on the trail that leads to the swamp, where it is always shady and cool.

BOTANICAL FEATURES

Look here, nestled in the roots of these big oaks, here in the needle duff of these white pines, here in the shelter of this graceful hemlock. See those oval, paired leaves, each on its own little stem, each about the size of my thumbnail, with a lighter stripe down the middle? Look around and you'll see strings (as short as a few inches or as long as a foot) of these small evergreen vines sewing the forest floor together for acres and acres. Her name is *Mitchella*, and she is one of the most common understory plants of regenerating forests throughout the Catskill Mountains. My Peterson's field guide says she is found as far south as Florida, as far west as Texas and Minnesota, and as far north as Nova Scotia. According to Hutchens and Millspaugh, *Mitchella* has been found in Mexico, as far south as Guatemala, and in Japan, too.

If you visit in the summer (mid- to late June here in the Hudson River Valley, late July at higher elevations, April way down south) and get close to the ground, you'll see the fuzzy, firm-textured, white or blushing pink, paired flowers of *Mitchella*. Their lovely starry faces with dainty petals (mostly in fours, but sixes are common, and threes and fives have been seen) arise from half-inch long white tubes and four-toothed calyxes found at the growing tips of the plant. Two sweetly scented flowers, each with four short stamens and four stigmas, share an ovary, and the small tasteless, persistent red berry they coproduce shows two scars and bears four to eight seeds. There's been a lot of buzz about her sexuality. As early as 1868 Mr. Thomas Meehan reported in the *American Journal of Pharmacy* that *Mitchella* has some male flowers and some female flowers. But I don't find anyone nowadays who agrees with his observation.

Yes, the partridges do eat the berries, and yes, her leaves are always small, green, and leathery. And that does make her easy to confuse with other small, waxy, leathery, native plants.

She isn't pipsissewa *(Chimaphila umbellata)*, although many herbalists avow that they can be freely substituted for each other. Here's pipsissewa, under the pines in the old mule trail through the quarry. She stands up while *Mitchella* reclines. Her leaves are alternate, while *Mitchella*'s are opposed. And pipsissewa leaves are bigger, longer, and very strongly toothed, altogether different from *Mitchella*'s jolly little ovals, which sometimes extend a bit into a heart shape.

And she isn't true wintergreen *(Gaultheria procumbens)*, either—although they do both go by many of the same names: partridgeberry, deerberry, checkerberry, teaberry. And both have small oval, waxy, evergreen leaves and red berries that stay all winter. But wintergreen is upright, with alternate, slightly toothed leaves on a little woody stem, while *Mitchella* sprawls, rooting at her nodes as she goes, putting down first whitish, then brownish, threadlike fibrous roots. The perennial rhizomes help every rooted node send out new shoots until the ground is matted over with *Mitchella*. There's wintergreen, those little plants over there by the rotting log. Small as they are, *Mitchella* is smaller yet.

You wouldn't confuse her with this pretty plant over here in the swampy area if you were in the field, even though *Mitchella* can grow in very damp environs. These leaves are large and heart shaped with a scalloped edge and a taste of roses. And the sunny yellow flowers change her leaves to lyrelike. But in the library you could get confused. Because *Senecio aureus*, golden ragwort—or liferoot, as we prefer to call her—is also disrespectfully called "squaw weed."

What a surprise to be told this prolific perennial plant is at risk. What a delight to be asked to introduce her to you. And to share with you a story from my adopted grandmother, Yewenode Two Wolves, She Whose Voice Rides the Wind, also known as Twylah Nitsch.

When the white man first came to the longhouses of the people of the Peaceful Nations, they could not speak intelligently. They made signs to say they were in need. When they pretended to be tying strings under their chins, we brought them feather headdresses; but they did not want those. When they motioned to their chests, we brought them bone chest plates; but they did not want those. Then they made much show of pointing to their genitals—what we call "squaw" when we wish to make fun—and so at last we knew what they wanted. How surprised we were to hear them refer to the women by this crude word: *squaw*. How harshly it falls upon our ears to hear you repeat it.

After hearing this story, I started calling her *Mitchella*, even though my books referred to her as "squaw vine" (a name I now understand is the same as saying "schmuck vine"). I could also call her checkerberry, deerberry, twinberry, two-eyed berry, two-eyed chequerberry, creeping checkerberry, odor berry, stinking berry, foxberry, boxberry, chickenberry, cowberry, partridgeberry, pigeon-berry, snakeberry, teaberry, one-berry, partridge vine, winter clover, running box, or hive vine. *Mitchella* is in the Rubiaceae family, and is the only member of her genus, named in honor of Dr. John Mitchell, an early American botanist.

HISTORICAL BACKGROUND

Mitchella is especially notable for the number of encyclopedic and specific books that do not include her. She is not mentioned in the classic European herbals, of course, but neither is she to be found in modern European herbals, most of which include such indigenous American plants as echinacea and cimicifuga. *Mitchella* is not included in *Edible and Useful Wild Plants of the United States and Canada* by Charles Frances Saunders (1920) nor in Steven Foster's *Forest Pharmacy, Medicinal Plants in American Forests* (1995); she is not even mentioned once in the *Encyclopedia of Natural Medicine* by Murray and Pizzorno. *Herbal Drugs and Phytopharmaceuticals* by Max Wichtl does not include *Mitchella*, and neither does *Major Medicinal Plants* by Julia Morton, nor the new (1998) *Physician's Desk Reference for Herbal Medicines*. And although it is continuously cited as a plant used by American Indians, Frances Densmore (1928) did not find it used for food, medicine, art, dye, or charms by the Chippewa. It arrived late in the *National Formulary of the United States* (1926) and remained listed barely twenty years (1947).

Early references to *Mitchella* include a mention by Cotton Mather in the early eighteenth century, and one by Dr. Barton at the end of that century. Erichsen-Brown cites Rafinesque, 1830, commenting on the use of the leaf tea as a mild diuretic against dropsy and gout, and the berries as a popular remedy against diarrhea. An 1849 "Report on the Indigenous Medical Botany of Massachusetts" by Stephen Williams says much the same. By 1861 *Gunn's New Domestic Physician* listed all the currently accepted uses: diuretic, astringent, tonic, parturient. The *Canadian Pharmacy Journal* included *Mitchella* in a list of medicinal plants of Canada in 1868. Maude Grieve included it in her 1931 *Modern Herbal* (although I doubt that Grieve ever saw the plant, because she claims it has "clover-like leaves.") Mrs. C. F. Leyel (1943) suggested daily use during the last month of pregnancy, following the example of Cherokee women. *Mitchella* is included in Foster and Duke's *Field Guide to Medicinal Plants* (1990). As of the summer of 1999, *Mitchella repens* (folia and radix) is an item of herbal commerce, with a wholesale price of $15 to $20 per pound.

MEDICINAL USES

Internally, the leaves (sometimes the berries) have been used to remedy a variety of urinary and uterine problems, hormonal problems, digestive problems, and nervous system problems. Externally, the berries (occasionally the leaves), mashed with fat, are applied with much success to heal nursing moms' sore nipples, treat sore eyes, and ease rheumatic pain. The *National Formulary* listed *Mitchella* as an astringent, diuretic, and tonic.

Vogel tells us, "Most investigators have found Indians reluctant to give details of such remedies [female medicine], as is indicated by Speck's cryptic note [1905] on the use of this plant *[Mitchella]* by the Penobscots: non-specific—to be steeped." Other reported American Indian uses include the Montagnais (1915) using berries against fever; the Chippewa (1928) smoking leaves; the Iroquois (1916) eating berries; the Ojibwa (1933) using as nonspecific medicine; the Menomini (1923) using leaf tea against insomnia; and the Iroquois (1970) using berries as parturient.

In the *Eclectic Materia Medica*, both *Extractum Mitchellae* and *Syrupus Mitchellae Compositus* (containing *Mitchella*, *Helonias/Chamaelirium*, *Viburnum*, and *Caulophyllum*) are listed. (Compare this formula with the similar one from Clymer, following.)

Mitchella has been cited as useful to aid in childbirth, prepare for childbirth, increase uterine contractions, prevent miscarriage, ease nervousness leading to miscarriage, interfere with habitual miscarriage, promote full-term fetal development, ensure smooth, easy delivery; nourish the uterus, restore the uterus, relieve enfeebled uterine nervous systems, correct uterine derangements including dysmenorrhea, amenorrhea, and menorrhagia; moderate the menses, relieve menstrual pain, stop genital discharges, reduce profuse menstruation, counter fibroids; alleviate diarrhea, hemorrhoids, varicose veins, and phlebitis; alleviate constipation; counter suppression of urine, stimulate the kidneys, ease difficult or scanty urination, relieve excessive water retention, edema, and dropsy; relieve insomnia; increase lactation; and improve energy.

It doesn't take much imagination to connect *Mitchella*'s unusual flowering characteristic—two flowers make one berry—with human fertility. Every reference book I consulted insists that *Mitchella* was called sq—— vine because Native American women used it. Dr. Smith in the *Botanic Physician* of 1860 states the general paternalistic view: "I first obtained knowledge of its use from a tribe of Indians in the west part of New York. The squaws drank it in decoction for two or three weeks previous to and during delivery, and it was the use of it that rendered that generally *dreaded* event so remarkably safe and easy with them." (My italics.)

James Duke and Steven Foster report that *Mitchella* is primarily used in cases of delayed, irregular, or painful menses, and difficult childbirth. R. S. Clymer reports that American Indian women used *Mitchella* as a tea or infusion throughout pregnancy to assure proper development of the child, render parturition both safe and easy, and at the same time develop lactation. He advocates continual use of the tea or tincture during pregnancy and for the entire course of lactation, especially if the woman suffers from "unpleasant nervous reflexes."

I devoted half a page to this "renowned uterine tonic" in my first book, *Wise Woman Herbal for the Childbearing Year*, including a recipe from Jeannine Parvati Baker, who says:

> A woman with an "incompetent" cervix who had lost five babies and delivered all her others early took this formula faithfully, and carried full term. Combine one ounce each: false unicorn root *(Chamaelirium luteum)*, wild yam root *(Dioscorea villosa)*, partridgeberry leaves *(Mitchella repens)*, and one-half ounce

cramp bark *(Viburnun opulus)*. Simmer for 20 minutes in a quart of water. Take one wineglassful every four hours until symptoms of miscarriage cease. They will.

"Mother's Antispasmodic Compound #410," suitable for the last six weeks of pregnancy, contained *Mitchella* and was sold by Indiana Botanic Gardens for most of the twentieth century. Most authors boast that *Mitchella* facilitates labor, while just as many swear that it stops labor and forestalls miscarriage. Many authors say that *Mitchella* is to be used when there is debility, exhaustion, or irritability; yet it is classified as cooling and relieving of congestion.

Mitchella is widely recommended to prevent and stop miscarriage. Jethro Kloss teams it with wild yam and raspberry for this purpose. R. S. Clymer uses *Mitchella* frequently in his classic *Nature's Healing Agents*. Here are some of his formulas.

CLYMER: TO RELIEVE MENSTRUAL HEADACHES

(use every three hours)
Tincture of *Anenome pulsatilla*, 1–3 drops
Tincture of *Mitchella repens*, 8–15 drops
Tincture of *Leonurus cardiaca*, 8–25 drops

CLYMER: TO PREVENT MISCARRIAGE

(use as required, or 3–4 times a day throughout the pregnancy)
Tincture of *Aletris farinosa*, 2–40 drops
Tincture of *Viburnun opulus*, 5–20 drops
Tincture of *Caulophyllum thalictroides*, 5–15 drops
Tincture of *Mitchella repens*, 5–15 drops

CLYMER: AGAINST MENORRHAGIA, DYSMENORRHEA, AND MENSTRUAL PAIN

(use 3–4 times a day)
Tincture of *Aletris farinosa*, 10–40 drops
Tincture of *Mitchella repens*, 5–15 drops
Tincture of *Polygala vulgaris*, 1–15 drops

DR. CHRISTOPHER: AGAINST DYSMENORRHEA

(Simmer herbs in 4 cups water, gradually reducing to 3 cups. Sweeten, cool, bottle. Use 2 fluid ounces, 3–4 times a day.)
$1/2$ ounce *Mitchella repens*
$1/2$ ounce *Rubus ideaus*
$1/2$ ounce *Arctostaphylos uva-ursi*
$1/2$ ounce *Hydrastis canadensis*
$1/2$ ounce *Populus tremuloides*

Alma Hutchens makes a telling remark: "It is best to combine *[Mitchella]* with other herbs." And, as Mildred Fielder says: "Even the whites recognized it as a *minor* drug." (Emphasis mine.) Consider the actual worth of *Mitchella* in formulas such as this one against chills and fevers: goldenseal, Peruvian bark, and *Mitchella*. Or this one for sore nipples: glycerine, tincture of myrrh, and partridgeberries. Or this for sore eyes: witch hazel leaves, raspberry leaves, *Mitchella* leaves. The more I read about *Mitchella*, the more obvious it became that it was not a critical ingredient in any of the formulas in which it is found. Every Dr. Christopher formula including *Mitchella*, save one, also contains *Caulophyllum*, *Chamaelirium*, *Cimicifuga*, or *Trillium*, roots well known to have a powerful effect on the female reproductive system. (Because these indigenous American roots are suffering from severe overharvesting, they ought not to be considered substitutes for *Mitchella*.)

It seems to me that *Mitchella* has few strengths. All of her properties are mild, and better represented by other, much more common, and often far more effective plants. She is a uterine tonic, especially during late pregnancy, but so are common weeds such as raspberry, dandelion, yellow dock, and motherwort. She is astringent, and has been used against skin problems and sore eyes; but oak, witch hazel, even blackberry are better astringents, and more common. She does have a mild diuretic effect, and has been recommended for those dealing with kidney stones, gravel, and other urinary ailments—the mother tincture is used by homeopaths to treat those with irritated bladders,

kidney pain, and dysuria—but yarrow, nettle, and horsetail are not only more easily gathered in quantity, but also more effective in my experience.

CONSTITUENTS

Saponins, resins, bitters, tannins, mucilage, dextrine, minerals, vitamin C.

ENERGETICS

Cooling, drying; also decongesting, astringing, restoring.

PREPARATION AND DOSAGE

Most authors suggest the whole fresh plant tincture: a deep orange-red liquid. American Indian women are reported to have drunk a strong tea, freely. It is rather tasteless, with the slightest hint of wintergreen to it. Grieve, Christopher, and Lloyd prefer the decoction. A few authors, including Lewis, maintain that the berries are preferable to the leaves, and were the primary part used by American Indians. Collecting a lot of berries seems a formidable task because, even in a good year, they are by no means profuse. Most authors assume little toxicity, but the herb is rarely used in quantity or for long periods of time, so toxicity is less likely to develop.

The dosage of *Mitchella* varies according to the strength of the remedy and the inclination of the herbalist. A tea of 1 teaspoonful of dried leaves steeped for fifteen minutes in 1 cup of boiling water must be consumed lavishly, at least 3 cups a day, for effect. Of a strong tea, made by brewing an ounce of the dried leaves in a quart of boiling water for four hours, as little as a cup a day may prove effective. Reduce the strong tea by half (a decoction) and 2 to 4 ounces daily is the dose. If you make a medicinal vinegar from the fresh leaves, 1 to 3 tablespoonfuls per day is all you'll need. The dose of dried leaf tincture is 1 to 3 drops twice a day, while the dose of fresh leaf tincture is only 5 to 15 drops, which may be taken up to three times a day.

Most books, including mine, follow the standard advice: Use *Mitchella* for the last six weeks of pregnancy. But some authors, including Dr. Christopher and Jeannine Parvati Baker, maintain that it is safe, and more effective in many cases, to use *Mitchella* throughout pregnancy. Otherwise, it is used only as needed to relieve symptoms.

FOR SORE NIPPLES

Two ounces of fresh herb is boiled in 2 cups of water until reduced by half. The herb is strained out and as much fresh good cream as there is decoction (about a cup) is added. Then the whole is boiled down to the consistency of soft salve, and used to anoint the breast before and after nursing.

CULTIVATION AND PROPAGATION

Sowing *Mitchella repens* from seeds is quite rewarding. The plant is dioecious, with male and female flowers on different plants. In order to produce berries, both a female and a male plant must be present. The bright red berries contain numerous yellowish seeds. These seeds do not remain viable in dry storage, but must be kept in the fresh or semidried berry or in moist peat moss in the refrigerator to retain their fertility in storage. The seed is an extended multicycle germinator, and must be removed from the berry prior to planting, because the fruit of the berry contains germination-inhibiting compounds. Fresh seeds planted in the fall will show some germination the following spring, but many of these seeds will remain quiescent until the next spring, and even after three years new plants will come up. *Mitchella* has developed this long, sporadic germination cycle as a survival response to environmental disturbances such as drought or fire. The plant relies on birds to remove the seeds from the fruit, and to transport them to likely growing places in the forest shade. In domestic culture the seeds may be planted directly in the shade garden, in outdoor nursery beds, in the forest, or in an unheated greenhouse. The patient gardener may expect germination as the winter-cold ground warms into spring.

To propagate the plants from stem cuttings, simply snip off a rooted stem from a mature plant and transplant this to the desired location. The rooted stem is buried shallowly in the soil, with leaves up toward the sun, and mulched with rotted leaves or rotted bark mulch. Always water the cutting immediately after transplant, and keep it moist until the new plant is well established. Remember that this plant is actually a clone of the parent. In order to maintain more diversity in the cultivated population, it is a good idea to obtain cuttings from numerous individuals and intersperse these plants with others, grown from seeds. This will help assure the presence of male and female plants and preserve genetic diversity.

Mitchella is a delightful plant for the moist shade garden, and prospers in many localities far removed from its native range. It also does well in the partial shade of deciduous forests, and will tolerate the acidic soils of conifer forests. When planted in the garden or agri-forest, it will benefit from a yearly application of organic compost and rotted leaf mulch. Because it ceases to grow when ground moisture is used up, it makes sense to water the plants during drought, to assure ample production of the leaf and stem that make the medicine.

HARVESTING

Because partridgeberry is an evergreen perennial plant, you can harvest its leaves anytime you need them, even during the winter. New growth on the vines occurs during the early summer, concurrent with blooming, and continues until the berries are formed and red, usually late autumn; I generally avoid harvesting during this time. (Unless I am actually using the flower of a plant, I tend to leave it alone while it is "having sex.") David Hoffmann, one of the few authors to address this question, states the opposite: Harvest the plant only while in flower!

Most authors agree that the fresh plant is preferable, especially for making salves and tinctures. To dry the leaves for teas and decoctions, spread in a layer on a screen or shallow basket and air-dry out of the sun, but at room temperature or warmer.

UpS RECOMMENDATIONS

- Use the wild-harvested plant only when necessary; otherwise use only cultivated resources.

- Motherwort and catnip are good alternatives. Also, use instead raspberry leaf for childbirth preparation and peppermint for painful periods and colitis.

REFERENCES

Bethel, May. *The Healing Power of Herbs*. Wilshire Books, 1978.

Christopher, Dr. John R. *School of Natural Healing*. Springvale, Utah: Christopher Publications, 1976.

Coon, Nelson. *Using Plants for Healing*. Emmaus, Penn.: Rodale, 1979.

Clymer, R. S., M.D. *Nature's Healing Agents*. 1905. Reprint, Philadelphia: Dorrance, 1963.

Densmore, Frances. *How Indians Use Wild Plants for Food, Medicine and Crafts*. 1928. Reprint, New York: Dover Publications, 1974.

Duke, James A. *The Green Pharmacy*. Emmaus, Penn.: Rodale, 1997.

Ellingwood, Finley. *American Materia Medica, Therapeutics and Pharmacognosy*. 1898. Reprint, Portland, Oreg.: Eclectic Medical Publications, 1983.

Erichsen-Brown, Charlotte. *Use of Plants for the Past 500 Years*. Aurora, Ont.: Breezy Creek, 1979.

Felter, Harvey Wickes, M.D., and John Uri Lloyd. *King's American Dispensatory*. 1898. Reprint, Portland, Oreg.: Eclectic Medical Pub, 1983.

Fielder, Mildred. *Plant Medicine and Folklore*. Tulsa, Okla.: Winchester, 1975.

Foster, Steven, and James A. Duke. *Peterson's Field Guide: Eastern/Central Medicinal Plants.* Boston: Houghton Mifflin, 1990.

Grieve, Mrs. Maude. *A Modern Herbal.* 1931. Reprint, New York: Dover, 1971.

Hoffmann, David. *The New Holistic Herbal.* Rockport, Mass.: Element Books, 1995.

Holmes, Peter. *Energetics of Western Herbs.* Berkeley: Artemis, 1989.

Hutchens, Alma. *Indian Herbalogy of North America.* Windsor, Ont.: Merco Publishing, 1973.

Krochmal, Arnold, and Connie Krochmal. *Guide to Medicinal Plants of the United States.* New York: Quadrangle, 1973.

Lewis, Memory, and Walter. *Medical Botany.* New York: Wiley and Sons, 1977.

Leyel, C. F. *Elixirs of Life.* London: Faber and Faber, 1943.

Lust, John. *The Herb Book.* New York: Bantam, 1974.

Mabey, Richard. *The New Age Herbalist.* New York: Collier Books, Macmillan, 1988.

Miller, Amy Bess. *Shaker Herbs.* New York: Potter, 1976.

Mills, Simon. *Dictionary of Modern Herbalism.* Rochester, Vt.: Healing Arts Press, 1988.

Millspaugh, Charles F. *American Medicinal Plants, an Illustrated and Descriptive Guide to the American Plants Used as Homeopathic Remedies.* 1884–1885. Reprint, New York: Dover, 1974.

Vogel, Virgil J. *American Indian Medicine.* Norman: University of Oklahoma Press, 1970.

Weed, Susun S. *Wise Woman Herbal for the Childbearing Year.* Woodstock, N.Y.: Ash Tree, 1986.

PIPSISSEWA
Chimaphila spp.

STEPHEN HARROD BUHNER

There is an inescapable feeling to old-growth forest that all who have been touched by it know. We have no words for it, yet it is as real, and as important, as the first kiss of our beloved or the touch of an elder's hand. It comes into the body as the breath into the lungs and is as necessary for life. Even the memory of it is redolent with the scent of ancient soil. When freshly encountered, a part of us remembers in its timeless presence who we are and that we do have purpose in the world.

Such old-growth forests are now only tiny islands surrounded by the roiling waters of our modern world. Each year angry currents nibble away the edges of the wild banks that still front them, and the islands become smaller still.

I was fortunate to live for a decade in one such protected enclave of wildness that had not known the ax. Within it, in that incredible diversity, I first used herbal medicines and discovered that more resided in spiritually inhabited landscapes than I knew; there is also healing there for the ills of humankind.

Eventually I had to leave that wonderful land and move to the Pacific Northwest to land neither so lucky nor so protected. There, that won-derful first home still taught me, but this time by its absence. I had, over the years, come to trust the medicinal bounty that had surrounded me. I knew the plants and their healing well, and human physicians were a rarity in my life. But when I moved to a distant land and eventu-ally became ill, I found myself without the heal-ing allies upon which I had relied for so long—and I became very ill indeed. I knew then what it had been like when the Native Americans, displaced by forced removal, became strangers in a strange land. The part of the self that relies on the medicinal bounty of plants reaches out and finds . . . only strangers. It is a feeling of great vulnerability. Such a knowledge base takes years, if not generations, to rebuild. In a des-peration that I am sure they must have also felt, I began learning the plants of my new home, making a relationship once again with the deep healing of Earth and forest. Eventually I pre-vailed upon two local foresters to take me for a walk in the woods in which they worked each day, woods that they know as well as I know my own hands.

It was here that we came upon a small plant with a beautiful flower and shiny leaves with the taste of wintergreen. The foresters' eyes lit up. They picked a leaf and rubbed it and held it under my nose, urging me to smell. And so I met pyrola, a plant of which I had not heard but which now entered my world. Thus the healing world that I had left began to come to me again in new forms. Slowly I found forests—not so protected as those I had known, but still old and deep. And within them I found that feeling I had missed. Under their shade and the slow dappling of sunlight, within the emerald green that exists in deep, healthy forest, I found new plants and new healing allies. Pyrola is one of them and, after a time, I was lucky enough to meet and begin to know pyrola's close relative pipsissewa.

BOTANICAL FEATURES

Pipsissewa's main recognizable features are its small size, its deep green leathery leaves, and its mild wintergreen smell, released when the leaves are crushed. Its Latin name, *Chimaphila*, is from the Greek *kheima-phileo*, which means "winter loving" and refers to the hardy evergreen leaves that can be found, like uva-ursi, throughout all seasons of the year. In fact, the common name for nearly all the pipsissewas and their close relatives the pyrolas and gaultherias is *wintergreen*, because of their similarity of appearance, their evergreen nature, and the unique smell they all possess that we now commonly call wintergreen. Pipsissewa seeks deep-shaded forests and the loamy, uncompressed soil formed from years of undisturbed leaf and needle composting. It grows from creeping rootstocks that slowly

move through the deep forest soil, putting out sometimes dense clusters of plants. The plant itself is a spokelike whorl of dark green leathery leaves with jagged, sawtoothed edges around a creeping, greenish woody stem. It puts up a brownish flower stalk in May or June, producing beautiful deep pink and white flowers. It is a tiny plant compared to the forests in which it grows, rarely exceeding 12 inches in height. The jagged leaves are 2 to 3 inches long, the flowers $1/4$ to $3/4$ inch across. The plant grows throughout the northern latitudes of the world. The primary species in the United States is *Chimaphila umbellata*, but there are two others. The spotted wintergreen *(C. maculata)*, long known in Europe, has whitish mottling along the leaf veins and grows in Arizona, Utah, Nevada, Mexico, and the eastern United States. Little pipsissewa *(C. menziesii)*, is found only in the Pacific states, from British Columbia to southern California. The leaves of little pipsissewa are slightly spotted and not so whorled in appearance; they are more alternate and less pronouncedly toothed.

HISTORICAL BACKGROUND

Pipsissewa was originally termed *Pyrola maculata* and considered a part of the Ericaceae family. Between the seventeenth and nineteenth centuries its name was changed to *Chimaphila maculata*. As earnest Ph.D. students in the twentieth century sought new topics for dissertations, the entire plant world began undergoing reclassification. As part of this the pipsissewas and pyrolas have been given their own family—the

Pyrolaceae or Wintergreen family. Most herbals and botanic reference books still list it among the Ericaceae. As with so much of this reclassification, there is much foolishness—the Wintergreen family, for instance, doesn't contain the one plant universally considered to be the "real" wintergreen, *Gaultheria procumbens*.

Historically, pipsissewa has been used for medicine throughout its extensive range by all ancient and indigenous peoples. It was well known in Europe and more than thirty indigenous tribes routinely used it as an indispensable part of their materia medica in North America, primarily as an analgesic, for hemorrhages, and as a urinary antiseptic and tonifier.

Along with the other wintergreens and birch sap and twigs—which also have that distinctive wintergreen taste—the pipsissewas were long used in "diet" drinks, that is, beers fermented specifically to aid the gastrointestinal tract. Birch was the first wintergreen flavored plant used in root beer: The tree was tapped like the maples and sassafras root bark boiled in the sugary sap to produce the now recognizable flavor of a "root" beer, then the whole was fermented and bottled and consumed as a spring tonic beer. These beers were quite popular. The flavor and tonic effects of the plants caught on, and any species with that familiar taste was soon incorporated into the making of herbal beers. With the temperance movement and prohibition, these herbal beers and "diet" drinks became sodas, not fermented alcohol beverages. Unfortunately, the slow-growing and hard-to-propagate pipsissewas are still being hunted by companies that dig up 100-ton lots for incorporation into "natural" sodas. The plants

are no longer used for their medicinal effects but solely for the flavoring that comes from only a few of their chemical constituents—a flavoring that could be supplied easily from more sustainable resources.

MEDICINAL USES

The many species of pipsissewa have been used for healing as long as there have been human diseases. In 1633 Gerarde-Johnson commented:

Pyrola [meaning pipsissewa] is a most singular wound hearbe, either given inwardly, or applied outwardly: the leaves whereof stamped and strained, and the juice made into an unguent, or healing salve, with waxe, oile, and turpentine, doth cure wounds, ulcers, and fistulas, that are mundified from the callous and tough matter, which keepeth the same from healing. The decoction hereof, made with wine, is commended to close up and heale wounds of the entrailes, and inward parts: it is also good for ulcers of the kidneys, especially made with water and the roots of comfrey added thereto.

The Eclectics, botanic physicians of the nineteenth century, used pipsissewa (which they called chimaphila) as a diuretic, tonic, alterative, and astringent. Specifically they used it for genitourinary conditions attended with catarrh and foul discharge. They felt it of special benefit in urinary tract infections, prostatic irritation and inflammation, and gonorrhea.

Nowadays, the plant is used almost exclusively for urinary tract infections (UTIs) that have proved intractable to other forms of treatment and are accompanied by pain and inflammation. One of pipsissewa's chemical constituents, arbutin, hydrolyzes in the body to the urinary antiseptic hydroquinone, which is excreted by the kidneys and thus passes through the bladder and urinary tract, where it contacts the inflamed and infected tissues directly. Pipsissewa is quite kind to inflamed urinary tract tissues, being milder than uva-ursi and much less vigorous than juniper berries. For this reason it has found a continuous presence among contemporary herbalists in the treatment of UTIs.

The plant is also strongly astringent, meaning that it dries and contracts moist and bleeding tissues. This makes it of special benefit internally for bleeding from stomach ulceration, birthing, or gum disease. For bleeding external wounds it may be powdered and placed on the wound itself. External application of the fresh plant will irritate the skin—it was traditionally used as a vesicant and rubefacient by both the Eclectics and indigenous healers.

The smell we call wintergreen is produced by plants containing methyl salicylate, the early forerunner to aspirin. All plants containing it were traditionally used for their analgesic properties, and pipsissewa was no exception. This analgesic or pain-relieving action makes it a good herb to use for bleeding or urinary tract infections accompanied by pain. Historically, many indigenous people also used it during the onset of colds and flu to help with the aches and pains of those diseases and to stimulate sweating so as to move the disease more rapidly through the body and bring down fever.

PREPARATION AND DOSAGE

Pipsissewa is used primarily either tinctured or as a tea. For a fresh plant tincture, add the fresh plant to twice its weight of pure grain alcohol; for instance, if you have 4 ounces of plant, add 8 ounces (liquid measure) of alcohol. For a dry plant tincture, add the dried plant to five times its weight of a 70 percent alcohol-water blend. Thus, if you have 4 ounces of dried plant, add 20 ounces of liquid—14 of pure grain alcohol and 6 of water. Use only spring-, well, or bottled water for tinctures. Let steep two weeks and then decant, pressing all the liquid you can out of the plant material. For UTIs use a full dropperful (30 drops) of the tincture per 150 pounds of body weight three times a day. Though some people do not like it, the tincture (and tea) is a unique combination of three flavors: at first bitter, then drying, then a wonderful sweetness only faintly reminiscent of wintergreen.

For tea, chop the dried plant coarsely and use a full teaspoon per cup of water. Do not boil; steep only. For UTIs, colds, and flu, 2 or 3 cups should be consumed throughout the day. If you wish to use fresh plant for tea, add a handful of chopped herb to a quart of water for sun tea.

For postpartum hemorrhages or stomach ulceration, drink as much of the tea as you can comfortably until the bleeding stops. Both the tincture and tea are unusual but not at all unpleasant to the taste.

PROPAGATION AND CULTIVATION

Though the plants produce seeds it is nearly impossible to propagate from them. Pipsissewa (like osha, *Ligusticum porteri*) resents domestication and continually frustrates human insistence that it get with the renewable-growing program. It exists in a nicely symbiotic relationship with the forest, soil, and plants among which it grows; without an exact duplication of that environment, it simply will not cooperate with humans. Mature plants, along with some of the creeping rootstock that produce them, can be dug up and transplanted to an identical forest ecosystem (this may also be tried with the seeds). If the plants like you and the fates smile upon you, they might even agree to grow there. Short of that, they should simply be left to go on their plant way without interference. If you have them growing in abundance where you live, by all means use them for the healing of your family and friends. Commercial harvesting and industrial use are actively discouraged—the declining plant populations, their difficult and shy nature, and their slow growth all point to a necessary protected status. The plant is considered endangered in New Hampshire and rare in Canada; it is protected by law in New York state.

HARVESTING

Because of the endangered nature of pipsissewa, only the top third of the aboveground plant should be harvested, and then only selectively. Harvest the flowering plant and tincture fresh, or dry loosely out of the sun. Try to harvest only from the periphery of healthy plant stands—pipsissewa cannot grow in compacted soils, and the human foot compacts soils quite nicely wherever it treads. Be aware that harvesting of pipsissewa, because of its endangered status, is illegal in some states.

UpS RECOMMENDATIONS

- Use primarily cultivated resources.
- Possible substitutes are uva-ursi, goldenrod, and gravel root.

Pyrola species are abundant and may be used almost identically, with identical results for both UTIs and pain. Uva-ursi, while not as mild in its action, is as effective for urinary tract infections and is an extremely abundant plant. It, too, is extremely astringent—it has been used to tan leather in many places around the globe—but it lacks the analgesic action of pipsissewa because it contains no methyl salicylate. A mix of 2 parts uva-ursi and 1 part black birch twig tincture should duplicate the actions of pipsissewa quite nicely.

If we do not protect plants such as pipsissewa, especially those unwilling to become domesticated, we may all find ourselves as the relocated Native Americans did: strangers in a strange land with no healing allies to help us in our illnesses, in forests empty of birdsong, and devoid of that smiling diversity of life that is the hallmark of the old-growth forest and the habitat of pipsissewa.

REFERENCES

Coffey, Timothy. *The History and Folklore of North American Wildflowers*. New York: Houghton Mifflin, 1993.

Erichsen-Brown, Charlotte. *Medicinal and Other Uses of North American Plants*. New York: Dover, 1979.

Felter, Harvey Wickes, M.D., and John Uri Lloyd. *King's American Dispensatory*. Vol. 1. 1898. Reprint, Portland, Oreg.: Eclectic Medical Publications, 1983.

Foster, Steven, and James A. Duke. *Peterson's Field Guide: Eastern/Central Medicinal Plants*. Boston: Houghton Mifflin, 1990.

Hutchins, Alma. *Indian Herbalogy of North America*. Windsor, Ont.: Merco Publishers, 1973.

Millspaugh, Charles F. *American Medicinal Plants, an Illustrated and Descriptive Guide to the American Plants Used as Homeopathic Remedies*. 1884–1885. Reprint, New York: Dover, 1974.

Moerman, Daniel. *Native American Ethnobotany*. Portland, Oreg.: Timber Press, 1998.

Moore, Michael. *Medicinal Plants of the Mountain West*. Santa Fe: Museum of New Mexico Press, 1979.

Tilford, Gregory. *From Earth to Herbalist*. Missoula, Mont.: Mountain Press Publishing, 1998.

Vogel, Virgil. *American Indian Medicine*. Norman: University of Oklahoma Press, 1970.

PLEURISY ROOT
Asclepias tuberosa

JOANNE MARIE SNOW

It's a cool, cloudy autumn day in New England. I relax here in my apartment and think back on my many experiences with pleurisy root, or butterfly weed (as it's commonly called). Because the plants have long since gone to seed, I sit surrounded by the many photographs that I have taken of pleurisy root throughout the years.

To further connect with the plant, I place some dried root into my mouth. My body enjoys the bitter taste, and yet there's something deeper that I need and desire to commune with—the mystical and magical aspects of the plant, the plant's spirit. To do this, I close my eyes and meditate on the plant. My mind flashes to summer. I'm sitting beside the plant in awe of its vibrant orange flowers. I become lost in its color and form. What a miracle that such beauty exists. I reach deeply to meet with the plant. I ask the plant my question: "What is it that you want me to share?"

My mind goes back further, to the first time that I became acquainted with pleurisy root. I had been studying the medicinal qualities of plants for just a few years, but I'd been "hanging out" with plants my whole life. Still, I didn't have much experience using plants medicinally,

and I was looking forward to experimenting more with them. I had come down with a bad cold while working nights as a nurse's aid and going to college full time during the day. I thought about taking echinacea and a few other herbs, but I really wanted to find out exactly what some of the other herbs I had been studying could do. My major at the time was biology, and I was having a lot of fun learning and doing experiments, so I figured I'd do a little experimentation on myself.

I decided not to treat my symptoms and to allow myself to get sick, which didn't take long given my schedule. I waited until my chest was so sore that it hurt to breathe. It almost felt like I was going to have a heart attack. I don't recommend this type of experimentation, but I was young and going through a Thomsonian phase! I rarely got ill, so here was my chance to find out how well these herbs could work.

I sat bleary eyed at the kitchen table, jars of herbs and herb books spread out around me. Most of the herbs I had wildcrafted; others, such as pleurisy root, I had purchased. I started to put together a formula, wondering perhaps if my experiment had gone too far. Would these herbs work? I had faith that they would, if I picked the right ones. I decided to use a blend of science and intuition to make my selections.

I knew I needed a really good lung herb as a primary component of the formula—something that would break up my congestion and get my fluids moving. I had some coltsfoot that I had wildcrafted myself, but something told me that this wasn't quite what I needed. When I picked up the jar of pleurisy root, though, I felt a big "yes." At first I didn't want to use the plant, because I hadn't harvested it myself. I was trying to be a purist, using only what I wildcrafted or had grown. However, the root tasted nice and strong, and my body seemed to badly need and want it. So I gave it a try.

I made my bitter brew, thinking of all the green witches who had done the same throughout the ages. I thanked the plants for their gift, thinking, "I hope this works." Amazingly, within a few hours my congestion began to loosen, and the pain decreased. By the next day I was feeling much better; the pain was gone and I was breathing easier.

What an incredible herb—not only a gift of beauty for the heart and soul, but a profound healer for the physical body as well! I certainly had found out about the power of pleurisy root and the effectiveness of herbs. My experiment was complete, and I felt no further need to let myself get sick again.

BOTANICAL FEATURES

Pleurisy root is a member of the Milkweed (Asclepiadaceae) family. Leafing through a field guide might give you the impression that this is a small family. However, there are about two thousand species in the Milkweed family. The vast majority of them grow in tropical and subtropical areas.

Pleurisy root is an erect perennial herb that grows from 1 to 2 feet in height. The stems are hairy, simple or branched. One of the key characteristics of this plant is that it has a watery juice—not the milky juice of most milkweeds. The leaves are alternate along the stem and are oblong and narrow in shape; they're 2 to 6 inches long.

The most telling characteristic of this family is its unique flower structure; pleurisy root is no exception. The plant has vibrant orange-red to yellow flowers that attract butterflies, hence the name butterfly weed. The flowers are arranged in flat-topped clusters (umbels) borne at the end of the branches. I'm going to go into some detail describing the flower parts. They are so astounding that they deserve the extra attention. To be honest, they demand it!

The flowers have five petals, which are fused at the base and deeply divided. They curve backward to conceal the calyx (sepals). Above the petals is a crown. Botanically, the crown is known as a gynostegium, which is formed from the fusion of the anthers (male) with the stigmas (female). How profound! I wonder if, in an etheric sense, the plant would help us to unite our inner male and female natures? I'll have to work on that one, and I'd also like to ponder what doctrine of signatures would be represented in this feature. Each gynostegium is surrounded by five nectar horns that consist of an upright hood and a protruding crest. The petals and the gynostegium combine to create a unique flower that you really have to see to believe.

I remember the first time I tried to describe a common milkweed flower, which is similar to this one. I had thought myself a pretty good botanist, but the only parts I could readily identify were the petals and sepals. The intricate beauty and complexity of these flowers astound me. No matter how many times I've examined them, each time fills me with fresh awe.

The fruit is a hairy, narrow, spindle-shaped, 4- to 5-inch-long pod called a follicle. The follicles contain numerous milkweed-type seeds. Each has long silky hairs that carry it majestically through the wind; the seed can give itself up to the currents in the faith that it will fall in a place where it can propagate and grow. I think that there's another doctrine of signatures in there somewhere.

The root is a rhizome with a knotty, branched crown. It has ringlike markings and is grooved lengthwise. The color is grayish brown on the outside and whitish on the inside. The dried root doesn't have much of a smell. It does have a bitter, almost acrid taste when you first put it in your mouth. I find that after chewing it for a while, it loses its bitterness and has a nutty, almost carrotlike flavor.

HISTORICAL BACKGROUND

Members of the Milkweed family have been used as medicinal plants for thousands of years. This is reflected in the generic name *Asclepias*, which is from the Greek name Aesculapius (Askepius), referring to the god of medicine. Aesculapius was an actual person, a physician who became deified in the eighth century B.C.E. In Greek mythology Apollo taught medicine to Chiron the centaur, who taught his healing skills to Aesculapius. The genus was named to honor both Aesculapius and the medicinal properties of the plants that are part of the family.

In North America pleurisy root and other native milkweed species were used extensively by Native Americans for a variety of purposes. The Omaha and Ponca called the plant *makan saka* (raw medicine) and *kiu makan* (wound medicine). As the common name indicates, Native Americans used it to treat pulmonary and bronchial troubles. It was also chewed and used as a poultice on wounds. Other tribes used it as a laxative, heart medicine, and antidiarrheal, as well as for stomach and intestinal pains.

The colonists learned about the plant's uses from Native Americans. It soon became a popular folk remedy for bronchitis, pleurisy, and other lung ailments. The Eclectic physicians of the late 1800s and early 1900s used pleurisy root as a diaphoretic, expectorant, diuretic, laxative, tonic, and carminative.

According to Felter and Lloyd, "It was one of the most common of the indigenous medicines employed by the Eclectic fathers." They used it to treat intercostal neuralgia, rheumatism, pneumonia, bronchitis, stomach problems, diarrhea, and dysentery. Pleurisy root was listed in the *United States Pharmacopoeia* from 1820 through 1905, and in the *National Formulary* from 1916 through 1936.

MEDICINAL USES

As its name implies, pleurisy root is used to treat various lung and bronchial conditions. It's not as widely used today as in the past, which befits its to-watch status. However, it brings great relief (as I found out) to people who have congestion and infections that have settled in the lungs. It is used to treat infections such as bronchitis and pneumonia. According to herbalist Matthew Wood, it's particularly useful to treat the lingering aftereffects of these conditions.

Pleurisy root reduces inflammation, promotes diaphoresis, induces expectoration, and has antispasmodic properties as well. It helps increase fluid circulation in the lungs—which is especially helpful for a dry, nonproductive cough when there's a feeling of tightness in the chest.

There has been little investigation into the pharmacological effects of pleurisy root's constituents. Low dosages of the extracts have been shown to cause uterine contractions in laboratory animals. Historically, it has been used for gynecological conditions; its effect on an animal's uterus may explain why. However, because of its ability to contract the uterus, its use during pregnancy is not recommended.

PREPARATION AND DOSAGE

The rhizome of pleurisy root can be used fresh or dry. According to my copy of the *United States Dispensatory*, printed in 1851, pleurisy root "yields its properties readily to boiling water." Even though roots are generally decocted, pleurisy root is prepared by an infusion. Use $^1/_2$ to 1 teaspoon of the chopped root to 1 cup of hot water and let it steep for at least ten minutes. This can be taken two or three times a day. According to the *British Herbal Pharmacopoeia*, the dose for a tincture (1:10 in 45 percent alcohol) is 1 to 5 ml, three times a day.

However, it's important to remember that dosage varies with each individual. This is especially true with tinctures and extracts. Many commercial products come with recommended doses ranging anywhere from 10 to 60 drops, two to three times a day. I've found that for me, just 5 drops of pleurisy root tincture taken two or three times a day works fine. The important thing is to start slow and listen to your body.

If you want, you can easily make your own tinctures. There are several ways to do this. The easiest is the "folkloric" method, which produces quite effective medicines. Finely chop the cultivated fresh or dried rhizome. Put it in a jar and cover with brandy or vodka. Completely cover your mash, and then add another 2 inches of alcohol to top it off. Cover with a tight-fitting lid and let it sit for four to six weeks. Shake it a few times a day. I "talk" to mine, invoking age-old magic. Sometimes I'll put various crystals and minerals around the jar to enhance certain qualities.

Pleurisy root contains cardiac glycosides and can produce nausea, vomiting, and diarrhea if taken in too high a dosage. I feel it's better to start with a low dose—5 to 10 drops at a time—for all herbs. You never know how the body is going to react. Because of its cardiac glycosides, pleurisy root is not recommended for people who are taking cardiac medications; it may interfere with such treatment.

PROPAGATION AND CULTIVATION

Pleurisy root can be propagated easily by seeds or root division in the spring or fall. Fresh seeds require a period of cool, damp stratification; mix them with peat moss and put them into a refrigerator for ten to twelve weeks. Older seeds don't require this process. You can sow the seeds outside or in.

To sow, put the seeds in a container (if inside) and cover to depth. (The depth of a seed refers to the width of the seed when it's lying on its side; therefore, put just the amount of soil that's equal to the seed's width over it.) Germination usually takes place within two or three weeks. Unlike mature plants, which prefer dry conditions, seedlings need to be kept moist until they are well established.

When the seedling has five to six leaves, it's ready to be moved to its permanent location. (I recommend a permanent location because the plant doesn't like to be transferred. It can be moved, but the roots are thin and break easily, so the plant will take awhile to come back.) Pleurisy root prefers well-drained, sandy soil. According to the New England Wild Flower Society's cultivation guide, it likes a pH of 4.5 to 5.5. Plants should receive half a day of full sunlight at the very least. The soil should contain 25 to 30 percent sand to a depth of approximately 1 to 2 feet. Mature plants like dry conditions. Water once a week only if you've gone a few weeks without rain. Pleurisy root will not flower during its first year of growth; it spends this time developing its root system.

For more specific information concerning growing pleurisy root in your area of the country, check with your local garden club or wildflower society.

HARVESTING

The cultivated rhizome is usually collected in the late fall, after the energy from the aerial parts has gone back into the root. Among herbalists there are always differences of opinion, so while some herbalists feel pleurisy root is best collected in the spring, most collect it in the fall.

The rhizome is long and thin and tends to break easily. Dig around it carefully to pull up the whole root. When harvesting from your cultivated beds, break off the piece of rhizome that holds the bud (which is next year's growth) and replant it. This way you'll ensure the plant's continued survival.

The next step is to thoroughly clean the root, giving special attention to the knotty sections to make sure all the soil is removed. To dry the root, cut it into thin sections. Because it's so long, slicing it longitudinally works quite well.

UpS RECOMMENDATIONS

- Use cultivated sources only.
- Elecampane is a possible substitute.

Pleurisy root is currently on the United Plant Savers To-Watch List. Where I live in New England, it's rare to find it growing in the wild. Thankfully, this plant is fairly easy to cultivate. It's grown throughout the United States as an ornamental and for the butterflies it attracts. Its bright orange flowers fill my heart with joy and wonder and are a blessing to us all.

REFERENCES

Felter, Harvey Wickes, M.D., and John Uri Lloyd. *King's American Dispensatory*. Vol. 1. 1898. Reprint, Portland, Oreg.: Eclectic Medical Publications, 1983.

Gledhill, D. *The Names of Plants*. 2d ed. Cambridge, U.K.: Cambridge University Press, 1989.

Hamel, Paul B., and Mary U. Chiltoskey. *Cherokee Plants and Their Uses*. Sylva, N.C.: Herald Publishing, 1975.

Kindscher, K. *Medicinal Wild Plants of the Prairie: An Ethnobotanical Guide*. Lawrence: University of Kansas Press, 1992.

Newall, C. A., L. A. Anderson, and J. D. Phillipson. *Herbal Medicines: A Guide for Health Care Professionals*. London: Pharmaceutical Press, 1996.

Wheelwright, E. G. *Medicinal Plants and Their History*. New York: Dover, 1974.

Wood, G. B., and F. Bache. *United States Dispensatory*. 9th ed. Philadelphia: Lippincott, 1851.

Wood, Matthew. *The Book of Herbal Wisdom: Using Plants as Medicines*. Berkeley: North Atlantic Books, 1997.

SLIPPERY ELM
Ulmus fulva or *U. rubra*

PAUL STRAUSS

Plants rule! Without them there would be no life as we know it on earth. Plants are the only living things that produce food and medicine and untold numbers of other necessary products by eating dirt, air, sunlight, and water. Plants have no need for verbal communication, shoes, war, taxes, or a short trip to the store. In many ways, I see them as a higher life-form. Self-sustaining, plants are environmentally safe and generate their own energy. Oh what it must feel like as a plant is bathed in the first rays of morning's sunlight. "Plants," as Scooter Cheatham reminds us, "are the only organisms that make protoplasm, the very substance of all living cells from raw elements, the vital umbilical link that sustains all life."

One of my favorite plants, *Ulmus fulva*, commonly known as the slippery elm tree, would certainly demonstrate the sustaining nature of the plant kingdom. This amazing tree is on my "top ten list of useful plants" because I have seen it help so many. But unfortunately, it is in demise in much of its native habitat. Where I live in the fertile foothills of the Appalachian Range, this is sadly evident.

The culprit is a fungus, *Graphium ulmi*, commonly known as Dutch elm tree disease. The carrier, the elm bark beetle, arrived on North American shores in a boatload of logs from Europe around 1930. Dutch elm disease has affected not only the slippery elm but most native elms as well. Urbanization, logging practices, and mining also contribute to the ever decreasing numbers of this giving tree.

BOTANICAL FEATURES

The range of slippery elm, also known as red or Indian elm, extends from Québec in the east to North Dakota in the west and then southward to Florida and Texas. It prefers rich soil and substantial rainfall and can attain a height of 60 feet with a trunk diameter of up to 2 feet. The tree's form resembles the classic vase shape of the American elm, but is smaller in stature.

The bark is thick, brownish gray, and longitudinally fissured into braided ridges. It is the inner bark of the tree that has long been valued for food and medicine—but given the increasingly at-risk nature of the species, its branches may be used instead of the main trunk's inner bark. On my farm I have found that I can use the inner bark of trees that have contracted the disease and will be dead in a year or so. The inner bark is mucilaginous with a sweet, earthy fragrance and flavor.

Slippery elm flowers in that first delicious warmth of late March or April before the leaves appear. Flowers are small, fiery explosions of dark red anthers with reddish purple stigmas. The leaves are dark green, sharply pointed, and rough; the pointed edges of the leaves themselves have points. These doubly serrated leaves are much larger than the American elm, measuring 5 to 7 inches long and 2 to 3 inches wide. The greenish brown seeds, also larger than those of its sister tree the American elm, measure in at around $3/4$ inch and are flat and circular in shape. The seeds can be profuse. Leaf buds, visible through the plant's dormancy, are downy with red hairs.

Both slippery and American elm are dominant succession species, moving quickly into old pastures and hay fields along with sassafras and locust, common trees in this area. Strong and beautifully grained, the wood of slippery elm is hard and reddish in color. I have learned from some of the old-time woodsmen in the area that it is suitable for outdoor use and will last much like white oak. The close-grained wood of the elm weighs approximately 43 pounds per cubic foot—in comparison to white oak, which is weighs about 48 pounds. This spring I will remove some of the recent standing dead elms (victims of Dutch elm disease), mill them, and use them for decking and siding. The tree makes a hot-burning firewood, as well, and I have cut up many of the dead trees for the woodstove.

In the forest surrounding my farm I am fortunate to still have some large older slippery elms that have not succumbed to the Dutch elm tree blight. I fear this may be a short-lived situation and that these trees, too, may go the same route as the American elm and the American chestnut. For many years it seemed that slippery elm was resistant to the blight, and that only the American elm would succumb. However, in the past ten years this has proven false as more and more of the slippery elms are showing signs of the disease. The slippery elm's increased resistance and ability to withstand the disease for so long may be due to the fact that it's a much harder and stronger wood than the American elm. Virtually all of the older American elms have died in my area. Though there are still a few young trees around, they are decreasing rapidly in number. The elms seem to get the disease around ten years of age and die off in a two-year period. But I have seen younger trees affected with the disease as well.

HISTORICAL BACKGROUND

Slippery elm is truly one of the most versatile plants in the herbal kingdom. An important "tree of plenty," it is renowned for its beauty, medicine, and food; it seems to help everything it touches. Its herbal actions are demulcent, expectorant, emollient, diuretic, and nutritive in nature. Slippery elm has a long history of use as an herbal medicine; it is still listed as an official drug in the *United States Pharmacopoeia* and is also sanctioned as an over-the-counter drug. It is one of nature's best demulcents, its effectiveness proven

AN IMPORTANT BEE FOOD

Each spring on the farm there is an excitement like none other, the joyous screams of the land's rebirth. Along with the crocus, cress, trout lily, and hepatica, the elms and maples are some of the first flowers to bloom. I have always heard this awakening before seeing it. Honeybees maul the elm flowers. There is a roaring buzz as the bees work this early food source. At one time, in addition to my domestic bees, there was a plentitude of wild hives in the forest around the farm. Tragically, there are no wild hives left, due to trachial and varroa mites. But that is another sad story.

This pollen from the elms is a vital food for early-spring brood rearing, creating greater hive numbers. A larger colony at the beginning of summer means a stronger and more productive hive.

through eons of use. It contains mucilage cells, starch, tannin, and calcium oxalate. These constituents penetrate and cover exposed and irritated surfaces, aiding in the healing process. Having an emollient action, it tends to soften and relax inflamed tissues and is specific for inflamed conditions of mucous membranes of the bowels, stomach, throat, and kidney.

In 1832 the insatiably curious and observant German traveler and botanist Prince Maximilian (for whom the Maximillion sunflower is named) had this to say about slippery elm:

A kind of bark which is now used is that of the slippery elm. If chewed or softened for a moment in water, it dissolves into a viscous slime and is found useful in dressing wounds. It is cooling and allays inflammation. It is said to have been applied with success in cholera and is now sold as a powder in all apothecary shops. A teaspoon of this bark in boiling water makes a very useful beverage which is sweetened with sugar and has the same effect as linseed.

The soft inner bark of the elm was employed by the Thomsonians (followers of a system of herbal medicine practiced by Dr. Samuel Thomson in the early 1900s) during labor, as a lubricant for the midwife's hands. They also used slippery elm and lobelia (*Lobelia inflata*) mixed with a small amount of soft soap to bring boils and abscesses to a head so they could more easily be lanced and drained.

Slippery elm also formed an important ingredient in an original Ojibwa formula for cancer, now known as the Essiac formula, that is still widely used. It is reported that during the Revolutionary War surgeons used the inner bark as a source of quick energy, and that in 1776 soldiers who had lost their way supported themselves for twelve days on a jelly prepared with the bark of slippery elm and sassafras.

MEDICINAL USES

Slippery elm's inner bark is excellent prepared as a tea and used as an enema and vaginal douche for irritated membranes. It has also been used effectively in suppositories by mixing the powdered bark with warm water and forming pieces about $1/2$ inch thick by 1 inch long. The powder mixed with water makes an excellent poultice for wounds, burns, boils, and ulcers. The tea is also an effective wash for chapped hands and face.

The inner bark ground into a powder and prepared like cereal with either milk or water is recommended for an ulcerated stomach, general weakness, those recovering from illness, bleeding of the lungs, and bronchitis. Because of its mucilaginous nature, slippery elm's properties are readily available during the digestive process. It is easily digested, has as much nutrition as oatmeal, and is an excellent food source for infants and children with digestive disturbances. It is also a mild and harmless laxative for children, causing no griping or pain. Its action is so gentle that it can be retained by the most sensitive stomach when no other food or medicine is tolerated. If desired, it may be flavored with cinnamon, nutmeg, and/or honey.

Slippery elm is a superior medicine for sore throats and coughs. For the greatest effect, chewing on the soft inner bark while swallowing the fluid is recommended. Slippery elm lozenges have been on the market for a hundred years and can still be found in most natural food stores.

In times of starvation and hard winters, many native and pioneer people stayed alive by using the inner bark of this amazing tree as a food source. On spring walks I collect the young seeds and find them to be edible. Though this information is not available in any herbals I've read, I've experienced these tasty seeds to be perfectly palatable and safe.

In a recent herb class we sliced and braided the inner bark and made ropes, necklaces, and bracelets; they proved to be strong but became

slimy when wet. Perhaps a portable skin care product? In conversation with David Winston, a New Jersey herbalist, I confirmed my feelings that slippery elm had indeed been used in nonmedicinal ways. It was commonly used by Native peoples, who removed the mucilage by beating the fibers and then wove it into rope, clothing, or coverings. Clearly, slippery elm is a tree of many uses.

PREPARATION AND DOSAGE

There are many ways to prepare slippery elm bark; a few have already been mentioned. Some of the most common methods are listed here.

TEA

The general formula of 2 ounces of bark steeped in 1 quart of boiling water for an hour or longer, strained and used freely, is a good one for both ingested teas and enemas.

CAPSULES

Finely powdered bark may be encapsulated in gelatin or vegetable capsules. A general recommendation is to take two capsules three times daily.

POULTICE

To make a poultice, add warm water to the powder and make a thick, viscous paste. This may be applied to wounds, burns, and boils to soothe and heal.

NUTRITIVE GRUEL

To make a nourishing gruel, bring 1 cup of milk

to a simmer. Add 1^1/$_2$ teaspoons of powdered slippery elm and 1 teaspoon honey to the milk and stir until it reaches the boiling point. Remove this from the heat. Stir the gruel a few seconds more, adding a pinch of cinnamon powder if desired. This is yummy and very good for young children.

ELM OOZE

Whole pieces of bark may be simmered in a little water until a thick, gelatinous slime is produced. When cooled, this healing "ooze" may be used for raw, chapped skin and wounds.

I always keep pieces of slippery elm in my jacket pockets as a chew, and find this is one of the best ways to use the herb.

PROPAGATION AND CULTIVATION

Given the current status of the elm population in general, along with the incredible usefulness of slippery elm, it is imperative that we begin planting this tree as part of our sustainable farm and garden practices, much as we plant comfrey and Jerusalem artichokes. Though slippery elm is still susceptible to Dutch elm disease, it remains healthy and usable for the first several years of its life. Thick, young stands of trees could be thinned and used as medicine, while older, more disease-susceptible trees could be used for building and firewood. These plantings should not only be considered for aesthetics, and for food and medicine, but also as a source of seed stock to ensure the future survival of this most giving tree.

Slippery elm seeds may be sown as in their normal cycle in the spring of the year, in an 18-inch raised peat moss soil and sand bed. The beds may need a wire top for the protection of the young seeds and seedlings. You can expect some light germination that summer and a greater germination the following spring. Expect a 10 to 25 percent germination rate. Transplant the trees into tree tubes within the first month of germination (this soil should be a well-drained potting soil). They may be field-planted after a year or two, depending on the size of your chosen tree tube. Always keep the tree watered during drought, and routinely check for insect predation and signs of fertilization needs.

At this juncture we don't have enough information regarding how slippery elm is faring in other bioregions. This information is necessary and will be useful in assessing a planting schedule. Please pass any reports on to us at:

United Plant Savers Botanical Sanctuary
Attention: Paul Strauss
35703 Loop Road
Rutland, OH 45775

THE UPS SANCTUARY PLANTINGS

In early November 1998 UpS at its botanical sanctuary in Meigs County, Ohio, planted five hundred one-year-old trees to better understand this plant's possible cultivation. One year after the initial planting we have lost only two trees, yet 1999 has been a very tough year to be on a farm in Appalachia: Besides the Y2K babble and buzz, we have experienced the worst drought in more than one hundred years. Still, the slippery elms went through the year without watering.

But what has set them back and changed their form was the plague of the seventeen-year locusts (cicadas); now most of the trees will have multiple trunks rather than a main one. Certainly this is a strong species able to handle most of nature's traumas but whose one main weakness now is the Dutch elm tree disease. Hopefully, our plantings may help us better understand and defend against this. To top all of these natural calamities, on July 25 we had a twister take out 30 acres of mature timber. Certainly that bears out the truth "what don't kill ya, makes ya stronger." This fall we will replace those trees that look the weakest with our own sanctuary-raised specimens.

HARVESTING

When possible, slippery elm should be harvested in the spring, when it is at its greatest potency. Make sure that you have positively identified the correct species before harvesting. Many trees have a soft inner bark, but only slippery elm is so full of rich mucilage. Always be conscious of the plant's energy, especially when harvesting material for medicine. Thanking the plant or making an offering helps keep this process clear and open, thus recognizing the unseen reality that affects our existence so deeply. We humans must recognize the value and energy of other life-forms as much as our own. The proverb, Do unto others as you would have others do unto you, should include the green world as well, and is most appropriate when harvesting medicine.

Harvest only where there is an abundance of plant material. Never gather from roadsides or polluted areas. Unless harvesting from an area being cleared for a building or pond site, never girdle or strip the tree, as this will cause its sure death. When gathering the inner bark of trees, harvest only from the branches, not from the main trunk. In this way you will minimize damage to the tree. You may strip the trunk bark from a tree that has recently contracted the Dutch elm disesase. The preferred tool for gathering inner bark is a drawknife, but a sharp pocket or kitchen knife will suffice for smaller amounts. The outer bark is scraped away, exposing the medicinal inner bark. This is harvested in 3- to 5-inch strips by angling the blade against the hard inner tissue and stroking downward. This is the same process used for gathering the inner bark of most medicinal trees, such as white oak.

UpS RECOMMENDATIONS

- Limit wild harvest to trees struck by natural disaster such as storms; otherwise use cultivated resources only.
- Possible substitutes include marsh mallow, comfrey, and mullein.

Thirty years ago when I first moved to my farm in the beautiful hills of southeastern Ohio, I shared traits common to many of the back-to-nature people of my generation. I had limited knowledge, but I possessed a thirst that drove me to be as self-sufficient as possible. Some kids went to college; I went to the farm. I'll never get to graduate. As I reflect over these past decades, I realize that I have learned more by doing, by relying on the process of trial and error, than through books or teachers. The land has a way of revealing itself as you interact with it. In essence, I married the land.

I believe it is time again for more people to consider a farm or small piece of land as an option in life. It is wonderful opportunity to help at-risk native plants. Conscious interaction with the earth, rather than unconscious exploitation of its riches, is critical if modern society is to slow its downward spiral toward ecological disaster and mass human devastation.

Though you won't end up with a degree, a life centered on the earth is most rewarding, giving you a unique opportunity to view the interconnection of all things and the dancing circles of life and death—to be endlessly humbled, amazed, and confused as you reap what you sow and watch as the earth teaches you to better attune your physical and nonphysical senses. People must relearn the tunes and rhythms of nature and rekindle their sense of wonder. Let nature nurture you, be your medicine and your guide.

REFERENCES

Culrose Peattie, Donald. *A Natural History of Trees of Eastern and Central North America.* New York: Bonanza Books, 1969.

Cheatham, Scooter. *Useful Wild Plants* 1, 2 (Jan. 1993; newsletter of useful wild plants of Texas).

Hutchins, Alma. *Indian Herbalogy of North America.* Windsor, Ont.: Merco Publishers, 1973.

Grieve, Mrs. Maude. *A Modern Herbal.* 1931. Reprint, New York: Dover, 1971.

Lucas, Richard. *Nature's Medicines.* West Nyack, N.Y.: Parker Publishing, 1973.

Osol, Arthur, and George Farrar. *United States Dispensatory.* 24th ed. Philadelphia: Lippincott, 1947.

SPIKENARD
Aralia racemosa

❧

KATE GILDAY

Years ago, when my children were young, I would drive them to visit their friends on the other side of the small town we lived in. Much of the town was composed of a state forest, with many dirt roads crisscrossing the area. It was on such a road that I first met spikenard. A single plant, tall and graceful, waved to us from the edge of the woods. For weeks I just passed by, at first simply noticing this new roadside plant, too busy or preoccupied to stop. But its gentle waving continued, catching my eye each time I drove by, until one day I pulled over to meet this new friend.

Three ravens croaked a greeting as I approached the sun-dappled area under the tall maple and beech trees shading the roadside. Immediately, I felt an attraction to this beautiful dancer that moved ever so gently in the warm summer breeze. Several of her stems leaned over, heavy with racemes of starlike blossoms in full bloom. Honeybees, wasps, and other flying insects were busy pollinating as they visited the fragrant flowers, hard green fruits already developing at the bottom of the flower stalks.

The long stem held a beautiful purple-red color that blended with the green, especially at the leaf nodes where other stems emerged. This coloring made me wonder if the plant was used to calm or enervate the body—having an action on the nervous system—or perhaps the circulatory system. The large, heart-shaped leaves reminded me of the shape of the pelvic area. Could this medicine plant possibly act on the reproductive system? Perhaps it could be used as an herbal ally for women. What was this new plant friend and why had I never seen this beauty before? I tucked these thoughts and questions away and felt sure that more would be revealed as I came to spend time with and use this new medicinal plant. I felt such a heart and womb connection with this plant, and wanted to learn more. Leaving a seashell at its base, I said thank you to the plant and promised to return.

Soon late summer was upon us, a busy time of harvesting and canning. One early morning I slipped off to check on the spikenard plant, hoping there would be a few ripened berries. Indeed, when I arrived I found the spikenard in full fruit, with several branches heavily laden with bunches of red to dark purple berries bending toward the ground. The berries certainly looked edible. Cautiously, I placed one in my mouth and was pleasantly surprised at its succulent, spicy flavor. I nibbled a few more of these aromatic and tasty treats, then decided to check my reference book once again for edibility. (I later found reference to using the berries to make a wild jam!) Thinking I would try to grow more of these plants, I brought a small bunch home to save for seeds to propagate the following spring.

I had been watching for more spikenard plants since my first meeting, as I wandered backwoods trails and drove down shaded dirt roads. But that summer and fall I did not see another. It was not until the following late spring that I encountered several spikenard plants on my way to a newfound nettle patch. The little-used dirt road had been cut through a hardwood forest, rich with a variety of shade-loving plants including stoneroot (*Collinsonia canadensis*) and spikenard growing along the roadside. The following week I returned with a small group of students to study the plants in the area and dig spikenard root. We chose one plant that had been partially dug up by the snowplow that winter. The roots were deep and strong, but easy to dig because of the location. When we unearthed the large roots, the air filled with an earthy, spicy fragrance, inviting us to taste the richness held there.

We brought the roots home, cleaned and sliced them, and simmered them in honey for an hour. Pouring off the spikenard honey, we were left with candied spikenard root. Yummy! I thought of those candied slices as a little energy tonic and would nibble on them from time to time. Four years later the candied slices still hold the flavor of spikenard and the beauty and fun we had the day we prepared them.

Since then I have kept my eyes open when in spikenard country, often stopping to say hello, photograph, or simply sit and even dance with the plants. Spikenard has become a dear friend that I occasionally use as a medicine, but more often simply enjoy as good company. And she continues to wave as I pass by.

BOTANICAL FEATURES

Spikenard is a perennial plant of the Ginseng family. It is found in the rich woodlands throughout most of the temperate regions of North America, east of the Rocky Mountains, from Québec south to Georgia, west to Kansas, and north to Minnesota. It is a singularly striking plant, with a smooth, arching stem, dark green or reddish in color, 3 to 7 feet tall with spreading branches of large compound leaves made up of many light green, heart-shaped leaflets. There is a prominent sheathed joint at the point each branch meets the main stem, giving it a zigzag look.

The large, elongated clusters of white flowers bear dozens of tiny, white-petaled blossoms in mid- to late summer. The dark purple berries are ripe by summer's end or early autumn. The berries have a spicy and pleasant flavor. The thick, aromatic rootstock or rhizome is light brown and quite fleshy, with numerous long, thick roots.

HISTORICAL BACKGROUND

The root of spikenard was once used to flavor root beer—not the soda we are familiar with, but a healthy beverage country folks would make with different combinations of familiar roots such as burdock, dandelion, sassafras, wild sarsaparilla, and spikenard. A real tonic/alterative that tasted good, too! This spicy root was official in the *National Formulary* from 1916 to 1965, where it was listed as a stimulant and diaphoretic.

Several Native American tribes used spikenard root as a decoction to treat a variety of respiratory conditions such as asthma, coughs, and lung ailments, and also kidney trouble, rheumatism, and syphilis. The decoction was used to aid urinary problems in older males. Perhaps this gave rise to the name old man's root. The roots were also used to flavor other medicines, and the fall-dug root was a food source.

As a dermatological aid, the root would be crushed and poulticed on boils, infections, swellings, and wounds. As a gynecological aid, the root decoction was used as a female reproductive tonic to strengthen the uterus; to treat menstrual irregularities, miscarriage, prolapsed uterus, and uterine pains; and as an abortifacient. It was often used a few months before the time of childbirth to tone and relax the pelvic area, helping ease and shorten the time of labor and delivery.

MEDICINAL USES

The decoction has been used alone, or in combination with other alteratives, to build or purify the bloodstream, and to treat pimples, acne, skin eruptions, and syphilis. The roots can also be made into an excellent cough syrup, again alone or with other cough and sore throat herbs such as wild cherry bark (*Prunus serotina*), coltsfoot (*Tussilago farfara*), thyme (*Thymus vulgaris*), and elecampane (*Inula helenium*). The decoction acts as an expectorant and also helps cut the viscosity of lung secretions.

I have prepared the root as a decoction and fresh tincture, using it occasionally with those whose creative or reproductive energy seems stagnant and who also suffer with a respiratory or sinus congestion. These folks often experience a feeling of being unable to move or shift, stuck in a rut or in rigid thinking. Spikenard promotes a relaxation and flowing that unbinds the tension behind the stagnation. This allows for a healthy release of fluids, whether it be sinus discharge, lung expectoration, proper circulation in the pelvic area, or menstrual flow that had been stopped up. Phlegm stuck at the back of the throat, fears that trigger respiratory problems, and women who are approaching menopause with their "brakes" on are other examples. Energetically, spikenard has a fluid grace and assured strength to share.

PREPARATION AND DOSAGE

A tincture is prepared with the fresh root 1:5 in 50 percent alcohol. Decant after six weeks and store away from heat and light.

Last summer I prepared a flower essence of spikenard, sitting with the plant for a while to learn of the vibrational qualities of the essence of this plant. The experience was both very relaxing and expansive. The description I share here is some of what I learned. Spikenard essence is that of present-moment awareness. It allows the experience of the present to effortlessly guide you to the next moment. It helps you dance gracefully through life's challenges as you let go of resistance, feeling a sense of fluid motion. This is a graceful guardian of the forest.

PROPAGATION AND CULTIVATION

I could find no information on the cultivation of this particular *Aralia* species. According to Richo Cech at Horizon Herbs, cultivation of California spikenard (*A. californica*) needs extra care. "Sow seeds outdoors in fall or very early spring, or subject to six weeks cold, moist conditioning (place seeds in damp sand in a covered plastic container in the refrigerator) before sowing in a warm place. From start of cold conditioning, the seeds usually take about seventy days to emerge. Space seedlings 4 feet apart."

I would also scarify the seeds very lightly with a fine-grained sandpaper to possibly increase germination. This simulates the action of a wild turkey's digestive system on the spikenard seeds; these birds eat the spikenard berries and "plant" them in the wild through elimination.

HARVESTING

The ripened berries can be harvested as a trailside nibble in late summer and early fall. Eat only a few, leaving some for the wildlife and others to hopefully germinate the following year. Bring some berries home to cultivate for your woodland garden.

The thick, aromatic roots of the cultivated species should be dug in early spring when the first shoots emerge, or in autumn once the plant has begun to die back. The roots are quite extensive, so dig deep and wide, being careful not to break the roots with your shovel. One plant can provide enough rootstock for several people. The roots can be split lengthwise, chopped in $1/4$- to $1/2$-inch slices, and dried on screens or in baskets in a warm, dry area. Once dried, the roots should be stored in an airtight glass jar, away from sunlight. If you do harvest this plant, please plant some of the berries at the site of the gathered root.

UpS RECOMMENDATIONS

- Use the wild-harvested plant only when necessary; otherwise, use cultivated resources only.
- Possible alternatives include cultivated ginseng (*Panax ginseng* or *P. quinquefolium*), Siberian ginseng, cleavers for skin concerns and as a diaphoretic and alterative, as well as chickweed.

I would love to see more people cultivating spikenard in the wild and simply taking the time to notice and sit with this beautiful plant. Spending time with the wild plants, especially the native woodland plants, helps us slow down, appreciate the quiet presence of the trees and plants, and hear the whispers of the ancient ones—a place and a way to re-member. In my limited experience and deeper feelings, I believe we do not have to harvest the actual plant to enjoy its gifts. Time with spikenard or using a flower essence can have a subtle or dramatic effect on the body, emotions, awareness, and vital essence. It is in making and taking the time that we truly open to the healing the plants offer us.

Of Spikenard

Graceful dancer
catches my eye
waving from the woods.

Tall and stately
reaching through sun-dappled shade,
beckoning with stars and hearts
She holds me in the moment.

I taste the breeze
she floats upon
And know the richness
of forest soil
holding her here . . .

REFERENCES

Cech, Richo. *Horizon Herbs, Strictly Medicinal Growing Guide and 1998 Growing Catalog.* Williams, Oreg.: author, 1998.

Elliott, Doug. *Wild Roots: A Forager's Guide to the Edible and Medicinal Roots, Tubers, Corms, and Rhizones of North America.* Rochester, Vt.: Healing Arts Press, 1995.

Foster, Steven, and James A. Duke. *Peterson's Field Guide: Eastern/Central Medicinal Plants.* Boston: Houghton Mifflin, 1990.

Hutchens, Alma R. *Indian Herbalogy of North America.* Windsor, Ont.: Merco Publishers, 1973.

Moerman, Daniel. *Medicinal Plants of Native America.* Vols 1 and 2. Technical Reports No. 17. Ann Arbor: University of Michigan Museum of Anthropology, 1986.

STONEROOT

Collinsonia canadensis

MARTIN WALL

I remember my first experience with stoneroot very clearly. I was working at an herb shop in central North Carolina that served a mix of rural and city people, many of whom were elders who had learned about herbs from their parents and grandparents. It was through one of these elders that I was introduced to stoneroot. I suggested it to a couple of people for hemorrhoids, and it worked. As a matter of fact, it worked so well that it became one of our most popular remedies. Sometime after that, a customer who had suffered from seasonal allergies reported that his sinuses were better after taking stoneroot. At first I thought it must have been something else; then I read in an old book written by an Eclectic physician how the herb could tone mucous membranes, which are filled with capillaries. It was becoming clear that stoneroot was useful for far more than just hemorrhoids.

BOTANICAL FEATURES

Stoneroot is an herbaceous perennial growing in the rich deciduous forests of eastern North America, from Wisconsin, Ontario, New York, and Vermont in the North to Louisiana and Florida in the South. In North Carolina it is found mainly in the mountains and the piedmont. It prefers moist areas, often growing in stream corridors. I have found stoneroot growing in pockets of woods along creek banks even in the middle of the city. The largest and presumably oldest plants I have seen were in a protected area of the Blue Ridge Mountains near Asheville, North Carolina. Some of these grandfathers and grandmothers were nearly 5 feet tall measured to their top leaves.

Stoneroot is a member of the Mint family, Lamiaceae, and therefore shares some of the characteristics of that family. It has somewhat square stems, more so between leaf nodes than in the lower part of the stem. The corners can be somewhat rounded, but four flat sides can definitely be observed. The stem rises to a height of from 2 to 5 feet from a very hard, thick rhizome with many attached rootlets. The plant can be multistalked, putting up several aerial stalks. The root is so hard that it takes the sharpest snips to cut it—hence the name stoneroot. The leaves are arranged as opposite pairs, with the pairs tending to alternate at 90 degrees to one another. They are ovate to elliptical in shape, have coarsely serrated edges, and are strikingly large when mature. The largest leaves at flowering can be nearly a foot long and 7 inches wide. Usually there are three or more pairs of leaves at flowering. The numerous yellowish flowers are also striking, having stamens and stigmas that protrude noticeably beyond the fringed lower lip. The flowers are on a terminal panicle, and appear in late summer. The flowers and crushed leaves have a lemony scent.

There are three other members of the genus *Collinsonia*. They are *C. serotina*, *C. tuberosa*, and *C. verticillata*. None are common in the Carolinas except *C. canadensis*. The USDA's PLANTS database lists no synonyms for the Latin name *Collinsonia canadensis*, but common names abound. They include stoneroot, richweed, collinsonia, horseweed, horse balm, knob-root, citronella horse balm, ox-balm, heal-all, hardback, and knot-root.

HISTORICAL BACKGROUND

The Swedish naturalist Carolus Linnaeus, the developer of the binomial system of nomenclature, gave stoneroot its Latin binomial name in honor of amateur botanist Peter Collinson. But stoneroot was known to the Native peoples of North America long before European colonization. Uses ranged from the treatment of colic to swollen breasts. According to one report, the Cherokee boiled the roots and leaves "with the whole plants of *Camptosorus rhizophyllus* and *Asarum canadense*. The infusion is applied to the breast and is also drunk to cause vomiting which is believed to reduce the swelling." After that, we have extensive record of use by the Eclectics for such things as "minister's sore throat" and varicose veins. Stoneroot is currently not a major commercial herb, appearing primarily in formulas for poor venous tone, laryngitis, and other uses similar to the Eclectics'.

MEDICINAL USES

The primary part of stoneroot used is the root (rhizome and roots); the leaves are used to a lesser extent. It is considered much better when prepared fresh and is sometimes prepared as a fresh extract from the entire flowering plant— roots, leaves, and flowers. During the Eclectic era, some practitioners used what was called Aromatic Collinsonia, prepared from the entire fresh flowering plant. According to tests done at Herb Pharm, there is good reason to use the leaf along with the root:

The Herb Pharm Analytical Laboratory performed a chromatographic comparison of Collinsonia fresh root extract in comparison to an extract of the fresh, mature aerial portions of Collinsonia. The constituents tested were terpenoids and saponins. Both in terms of the quantity of these constituents, as well as the specific types of constituents present, the fresh root and the aerial portions were shown to be very similar in their makeup. This provides scientific support for the traditional practice of using the whole plant, and supports the ecologically conscientious practice of making medicine with the renewable portion of the plant.

By using the entire plant, there is less dependence on roots, with a subsequent preservation of plant resources.

Stoneroot's actions are alterative, tonic, stimulant, diuretic, diaphoretic, antispasmodic, and astringent. Some also consider it antilithic, about which there is some debate. Some of its chemical constituents are alkaloids, saponins, tannins, resins, volatile oils, and the polyphenol rosmarinic acid. The primary indications for stoneroot's use are poor venous and mucous membrane tone, and engorgement due to capillary dilation. Stoneroot can be useful in nearly any ailment arising from these conditions.

Hemorrhoids, piles, anal fissures, and varicose veins all respond well to treatment with stoneroot due to its tonic action on the venous system. If the condition is too advanced, only symptomatic relief can be expected. The herb is considered especially useful if these conditions arise during pregnancy. Stoneroot is also considered to have a tonic action upon the heart, with application in rheumatic heart conditions, noninflammatory edema of the pericardium, and mitral valve backflow or regurgitation.

A gargle of stoneroot tincture diluted in water is considered a classic remedy for "minister's sore throat," a condition of inflammation of the vocal cords due to overuse. It also proves of benefit in chronic laryngitis. Stoneroot can be of tremendous benefit to sinusitis due to venous engorgement and catarrh of the capillary-filled mucous membranes.

Stoneroot benefits a wide range of conditions of the female reproductive system. Lloyd and Felter list it as appropriate for "amenorrhea, dysmenorrhea, menorrhagia, vicarious menstruation, prolapsus uteri, leucorrhea, threatened abortion, and pruritis vulvae, dependant on varicosis." In the male, it benefits prostate conditions due to poor pelvic circulation.

Collinsonia has been used as a part of a treatment for urinary calculi. There is debate over whether it actually helps reduce the stones or just eases the irritation they cause. In any event, care must be taken not to cause harm by trying to force stones out by it's diuretic action.

Lloyd and Felter reported *Collinsonia*'s use to treat poor digestion due to low gastric output and poor tone of the digestive organs. There was some belief that stoneroot helped increase innervation of the gastric tissues, resulting in better gastric secretions. The Eclectics believed stoneroot to have a soothing effect upon the vagus nerve (the tenth cranial nerve, with connections to many internal organs) and all tissues to which it traveled.

The bruised fresh leaves have been used as a poultice, resulting in one of stoneroot's common names, horse balm. Stoneroot's leaves can be applied to "burns, bruises, wounds, ulcers, sores, sprains, and contusions."

The *Botanical Safety Handbook* lists *Collinsonia canadensis* root as a class one herb, which is defined as an herb "that can be safely consumed when used appropriately." There are, however, a few references to the fresh plant being emetic in the literature. I was trying to determine how emetic the fresh leaves might be in preparing this monograph, so I did a little *Collinsonia* leaf eating. Reading that small amounts of fresh plant could be emetic, I began rather modestly with a square inch of leaf. It had a strong lemony taste, and I felt a little queasy after eating some. After about twenty minutes without emesis I tried some more. That day I consumed one entire leaf, containing about 12 square inches. I have since eaten as many as two large leaves and have not noticed any queasiness since that first test. Perhaps the thought of throwing up made me uneasy that first day.

PREPARATION AND DOSAGE

The entire fresh plant—roots, leaves, and flowers—should be extracted in grain alcohol, pure water, and glycerine. An herb-weight to solvent volume ratio of 1:2.5 or better is preferred. The solvent, or menstruum, should be around 80 percent alcohol, 10 percent glycerine, and 10 percent water. The glycerine will help prevent precipitation of constituents due to the tannins in stoneroot. The fresh plant material will supply enough water to dilute the final alcohol content to around 40 to 50 percent, depending on the relative amounts of tops to roots.

The dried roots should be decocted by adding from 1 teaspoon to 1 tablespoon of herb to a cup of cold water, heating to a boil, and simmering for fifteen minutes before straining, cooling, and drinking.

A poultice of the fresh leaves is prepared by bruising and applying them to the affected part.

PROPAGATION AND CULTIVATION

There aren't many people who have propagated stoneroot commercially, but there are a few. Tim Blakley of the National Center for the Preservation of Medicinal Herbs has successfully propagated it from seeds, cuttings, and root divisions. Robyn Fletcher of Gardens of the Blue Ridge has also propagated stoneroot, although he says the demand is light for stoneroot as a bedding plant.

Stoneroot can be grown from seeds, but is more difficult than root cuttings. Tim Blakley has seen 60 to 75 percent germination with bottom heat and mist. The plants seem to grow pretty well from seeds in established areas, according to both Blakley and Fletcher. Fletcher says their established beds provide a nursery for young plants, but that it is difficult to intentionally germinate stoneroot seeds. Blakley also reports that stratification with a long cold period is necessary for good germination. A harvestable root can be grown from seeds in about four full years.

Root divisions seem to be the most productive way to go, according to both Blakley and Fletcher. Using very sharp shears to snip the roots between buds, it is possible to get several divisions from each mature root. When roots are dug, divided, and replanted in the fall, harvestable roots are available in three years—allowing three full seasons for growth. Older roots can get quite large, according to Fletcher. He says some of the plants in their seedbeds are eight or nine years old and their roots are as big as his fist!

No matter how stoneroot is propagated, it needs rich, moist soil and shade. It doesn't need as much shade as ginseng, but at least partial shade is required. I have seen it growing along the sides of forest service roads where more sun reaches the forest floor. The few plants I have do just fine in the shade of an oak tree, where they get a little direct sun early in the day, and later, some afternoon shade. The soil is well protected by a layer of leaf mulch.

HARVESTING

The roots should be unearthed in the fall as the aerial portions start to die back, or the entire plant can be harvested as the first flower begins to open for the preparation of whole-plant extract. The roots should be cleaned in cool water immediately to remove soil before it dries in hard-to-reach places. The consensus on stoneroot is that fresh is better, so the plants should be processed immediately. However, if the roots are to be dried, they should be laid out on a screen in a warm, dry, shady place and rotated occasionally to allow for even drying. Cutting the roots while fresh will be easier than trying to do so once they are dry.

UpS RECOMMENDATIONS

- Use primarily cultivated resources; some limited wild harvest is permissible.
- Good alternatives include European horse chestnut (*Aesculus hippocastanum*), red clover, sweet clover, garlic, and parsley root.

Stoneroot currently has in its favor a lack of popularity among the general public. It is an herb that is relatively unknown outside herbal circles, as was black cohosh just a few years ago. As herbs continue to become more popular, the virtues of stoneroot are sure to become more appreciated. This will put an increasing strain on the wild populations that supply the current demand. Two options for harvesting stoneroot are available to us: the use of the whole plant instead of just the root, and dividing and replanting a portion of the roots harvested in the wild until cultivated sources become more available. Relying more on the renewable parts of stoneroot will help reduce consumption. Since the aerial portions offer significant medicinal action, this would seem a logical move. Dividing and replanting a portion of wild-harvested roots will help control depletion as well.

At the same time, the loss of suitable habitat continues at an alarming rate. In much of the East the wild places where many of our medicinal herbs grow are becoming more and more scarce. If the human population continues to encroach upon the last remaining wild places, one day there may be no more. The solutions to human problems are complex, but the earth depends on us finding solutions. As for stoneroot, the dual factors of increasing demand and accelerating habitat loss could bode ill for it. As with most wild-harvested medicinal herbs, I feel the future of stoneroot lies in cultivation. As we move into an era of cultivating plants we once collected in the wild, our knowledge of how to grow them will surely increase. It can be done, but we must not forget the importance of protecting and preserving the environment in which these plants live. It is, after all, the same environment in which we live.

REFERENCES

Amarquaye, Ambrose, and Richard A. Cech. "Study on Stoneroot." Williams, Oreg.: Herb Pharm Analytical Laboratory (Ed Smith, director), 1997.

Felter, Harvey Wickes, M.D. *Eclectic Materia Medica, Pharmacology and Therapeutics.* 1922. Reprint, Portland, Oreg.: Eclectic Medical Publications, 1983.

Felter, Harvey Wickes, M.D., and John Uri Lloyd. *King's American Dispensatory.* 1898. Reprint, Portland, Oreg.: Eclectic Medical Publications, 1983.

Foster, Steven, and James A. Duke. *Peterson's Field Guide: Eastern/Central Medicinal Plants.* Boston: Houghton Mifflin, 1990.

Grieve, Mrs. Maude. *A Modern Herbal.* Vol. 2. 1931. Reprint, New York: Dover, 1971.

Hoffmann, David. *The New Holistic Herbal.* Rockport, Mass.: Element Books, 1995.

Hyam, R., and R. Pankhurst. *Plants and Their Names.* Oxford, U.K.: Oxford University Press, 1995.

McGuffin, Michael, Christopher Hobbs, Roy Upton, and Alicia Goldberry. *Botanical Safety Handbook.* New York: CRC Press, 1997.

Radford, A. E., H. E. Ahles, and C. R. Bell. *Manual of the Vascular Flora of the Carolinas.* Chapel Hill: University of North Carolina Press, 1968.

Taylor, L. A. *Plants Used as Curatives.* Cambridge, Mass.: Botanical Museum of Harvard University, 1940.

USDA, NRCS (1999). The PLANTS database. National Plant Data Center, Baton Rouge, La. 70874-4490.

SUNDEW
Drosera spp.

JANICE J. SCHOFIELD

Appreciating sundews requires humility. You must sink to your hands and knees, shrinking your ego and opening your eyes to the wonders of a miniature plant that thrives in the acidic, nutrient-poor conditions of a sphagnum bog. On a sunny day you will discover *Drosera*'s jewels: Dewy drops with ruby centers extend from each leaf and shimmer like diamonds. Perhaps you'll notice an unfortunate fly that mired its feet in the superglue-strength dew. Sundew patiently waits for the insect's struggle to cease; the presence of protein signals leaves to close and digest the airborne-expressed meal.

I've been fascinated with and appreciative of sundews ever since our first meeting. I feel fortunate to live in the midst of their American stronghold, yet even in the last frontier of Alaska, "progress" marches, bringing new roads, bog drainage, and disruption of native habitat. Sundew's diminutive stature and its intimate relationship with sphagnum bogs place it at severe risk from both zealous foragers and wetland developers. In Germany *Drosera* is threatened with extinction, and harvest is strictly prohibited. In the United States only 3 to 5 percent of carnivorous plant habitat is estimated to remain. My fervent wish is that as appreciation of this fascinating healing herb grows, more efforts will be expended to expand preservation of its native habitat, to practice sustainable foraging, and to promote cultivation.

BOTANICAL FEATURES

Droseraceae, the Sundew family, is comprised of four genera of carnivorous herbs; these plants attract, capture, kill, and digest flies, gnats, and moths. The largest genus, *Drosera*, (from the Greek for "dewy") is of worldwide distribution and includes about eight dozen (mostly perennial) species. American natives include *Drosera rotundifolia*, *D. brevifolia*, *D. capillaris*, *D. filliformis*, *D. intermedia*, and *D. linearis*.

The circumboreal *Drosera rotundifolia*, commonly called round-leaved sundew, is of amazing adaptability, extending in range from northern Florida to Alaska's Arctic Circle. This diminutive herb has a basal rosette of round leaves fringed with dewy, insect-trapping hairs. Botanist Lewis Clark writes:

> Like small green frying pans, the leaves
> contain chlorophyll for sun-chemistry,

but the sparse roots pick up from their watery surroundings very deficient amounts of minerals, and compounds of nitrogen and phosphorous. Hence the plant must make up this deficiency, and this is only possible in its wet habitat by a supplement of insect fare.

Though sundews can live without insect protein, those with access to entomologic feedings produce more robust plants and higher quantities of seeds. Clark further explains how the modified leaf hairs are gland-bearing filaments that secrete, and are enclosed by, chlorophyll derivatives of ruby red fluid:

> The colour is attractive to small crawling and flying insects, which are at once trapped. Then the tentacles bend inward, the leaf-edges curl, and the insect's juices are soon assimilated by digestive enzymes. Finally the leaf flattens, the chitinous husks of the insects blow away, and the glistening beads again appear.

In the late 1800s, Charles Darwin studied sundew in depth (his *Insectivorous Plants* includes more than three hundred pages devoted to *Drosera*). Darwin found that raindrops and inorganic materials had a negligible effect on sundew, but if the leaf was touched by a protein material (like a fly) the tentacles were rapidly stimulated.

Sundew's white to pinkish flowers (petals may vary from four to six, though five is most common) are borne on a stalk 2 to 8 inches high. Flowers, which open singly, may number from five to twenty-five per stalk. *Drosera*'s French name, rosée du soleil, as well as its English name sundew, refers to the flower's fondness for blue-sky days; in cloudy and cool weather the buds remain patiently closed. Other common names range from daily dew and moor grass to red-rot and youth root.

HISTORICAL BACKGROUND

Sundew was regarded as a remedy for "consumption of the lungs" in the sixteenth century. However, Gerarde warned of its "biting nature" and ballyhooed diet as the preferred consumption treatment. Other writers, such as Geoffroi, promoted *Drosera* infusions for asthma and lung ulcerations. The *Medicinal Flora of Rafinesque* recommended sundew juice to remove warts and corns. Schenk and Valentin recognized *Drosera*'s value in coughs, bronchitis, and pulmonary disease.

Kwakiutl men are reported to have made a complex love charm with *Drosera* and other herbs to make women fall in love with them. Interestingly, when flower essence practitioner Jane Bell prepared sundew flower essence[1] (after waiting four years for sundew to flower), she reported feeling oneness with divine love through the process. "I had the concept before of being one with God, but the attunement with sundew gave me an all-encompassing experience of it. There was no separation between me and the Beloved. My experience was of looking at a luminous, Buddha-like figure, and it was looking back at me with the same eyes of wonder and heart of

Divine Love." Sundew flower essence, says Jane, "teaches us how to bring strength and tenacity of the ego into harmony and balance with the wisdom and guidance of the higher self, so that they can function together in unison and bring us ever closer to our reunification with the source of all life." Feeling oneness with love, with life . . . the paths are as diverse as a love charm, a flower essence, or simply sitting and observing sundew in the bog.

MEDICINAL USES

A variety of species of *Drosera* (including *D. rotundifolia, D. anglica, D. peltata*, and *D. ramentacea*) are used medicinally. Constituents include fourteen napthaquinone derivatives, including plumbagin, ramentaceone, and ramentone. (This is similar to Venus's-flytrap, which is used in Germany for cancer.) Sundew's medicinal properties are classified as antispasmodic, antibacterial, and antiviral.

Additional actions listed in the *British Herbal Pharmacopoeia* include demulcent and expectorant (with relaxing effect on bronchial musculature, such as in asthma attacks). Indications include asthma, bronchitis, pertussis, and gastric ulceration. Sundew is generally used in combination with other herbs.

In organoleptic tests (determining properties of an herb based on its sensory effects—on the taste buds, for instance), Robyn Klein, director of Sweetgrass School of Herbalism, noted that sundew is both acrid and mucilaginous, creating "an irritation not unlike mustard, which then seems to encourage coughing and most

likely a loosening of phlegm. The mucilage would be soothing to the mucous membrane."

British herbalist Simon Y. Mills points out that the bronchial tubes are embryonically linked with the digestive tract and share common nerve roots. Herbs such as sundew that stimulate or soothe the upper digestive mucosa could in theory have a reflex action on the musculature of the bronchial tree. This could explain the expectorant properties witnessed in practice.

New Jersey herbalist David Winston uses sundew clinically "in small amounts for dry, spasmodic, explosive coughing—especially whooping cough (pertussis), bronchitis, measles, or other conditions where the person cannot control coughing spasms. It combines well with bloodroot, wild cherry, mullein, and licorice. I've also used it as part of a cancer protocol but cannot claim any specific activity separate from the overall formula."

New Mexico herbalist Anne-Clement Hill used *Drosera* tincture to calm a dry cough caused by postnasal drip from allergies. Anita Hales of Ketchikan, Alaska, has used sundew mostly "in combination with other herbs for strep and staph infections and bronchitis."

PREPARATION AND DOSAGE

In clinical practice David Winston makes a fresh extract of sundew at 1:2.5, 50 percent ethanol (ETOH)—each ounce of fresh herb is covered with 2 $^1/_2$ ounces of 50 percent alcohol (such as hundred-proof vodka). Steep the herb for two weeks and then strain and rebottle.

Winston advises a therapeutic dose of 1 to 5

drops three times per day, mixed in formula with other herbs. Too much will cause intense irritation, inflammation, and spasmodic coughing.

PROPAGATION AND CULTIVATION

Though tropical species of *Drosera* flourish year-round, dry-climate species tend to be tuberous, dying back in drought conditions and reappearing when it becomes wet. American natives such as *D. rotundifolia* survive cold by shedding leaves and forming hibernacula—tight budlike clusters—as their winter residence.

The Botanique Nursery, one of several sources for sundew plants, recommends "a soil mix of $\frac{1}{3}$ sand and $\frac{2}{3}$ peat moss as a bog garden or container mix. When planting, keep the small crown above the soil surface and firm the soil gently around the plants to reduce splash from the rain. Water transplants well and keep moist but not continuously flooded." If planting from seeds, sprinkle them on the soil surface. Seeds germinate best after exposure to cold (stratification).

When cultivating carnivorous plants, avoid fertilizers and overfeeding. The plants are acclimated to nutrient-poor conditions. As supplementary fare, they will trap small fruit flies and other small insects, luring them with nectar gland secretions, capturing them with adhesives, and digesting them with their enzymes. Sundews are one of the easier carnivorous plants to raise, are self-pollinating, and will generally spread after several seasons. Those desiring in-depth information on cultivation and on terrariums for raising carnivorous plants may contact the following sources:

- Botanique Nursery, 387 Pitcher Plant Lane, Standardsville, VA 22973. Specializes in nursery-propagated carnivorous plants.
- California Carnivores, 7020 Trenton-Healdsburg Road, Forestville, CA 95436; www.californiacarnivores.com. Sells a twenty-six-page growing guide and catalog for $3 and has a wide variety of *Drosera* species for sale.
- A free carnivorous plant seed bank and additional growing tips is accessible on the Internet at www.geocities.com/Rainforest/1150/growinst.html.
- The International Carnivorous Plant Society, c/o Fullerton Arboretum, Box 6850, California State University, Fullerton, CA 92834-6850. Publishes a carnivorous plant newsletter and quarterly journal, as well as operating a seed bank.

HARVESTING

The entire herb is gathered, usually in flower (when it is easiest to locate). Michael Moore, director of the Southwest School for Botanical Medicine, advises cleaning the plant as well as possible. "This sounds easy, but imagine trying to wash off a huge, wet Gummi Bear covered in sand." (And flies!)

UpS RECOMMENDATIONS

• Use only cultivated resources.

• Cultivated echinacea, mullein, and elecampane are good substitutes. Also include spilanthes for respiratory complaints and its antibacterial, antiviral, and antifungal properties. Use sage for sore throats and its antibacterial and antiviral actions. Thyme also has good antibacterial and antifungal properties.

Dr. Earle Sweet, D.C., M.H., describes sundew as "a very noble but rare plant." In the mainland United States (and much of the world), sundews face untold challenges in remaining on the planet. Wherever we live, it is up to us to collectively work to keep this noble herb a native herb, and not a casualty in that thing called progress.

NOTES

1. Those interested in additional information on Sundew Flower Essence may contact the Alaskan Flower Essence Project, P.O. Box 1369, Homer, AK 99603; phone (907) 235-2188; fax (907) 235-2188; email afed@alaska.net.

REFERENCES

Bisset, N. G. *Herbal Drugs and Phytopharmaceuticals.* Stuttgart: CRC Press and Medpharm Scientific Publishers, 1994.

Botanique Nursery. *Care Sheets.* www.bontaniq.com.

Clark, Lewis J. *Wild Flowers of the Pacific Northwest from Alaska to Northern California.* Sidney, B.C.: Gray's Publishing, 1976.

Millspaugh, Charles F. *American Medicinal Plants, an Illustrated and Descriptive Guide to the American Plants Used as Homeopathic Remedies.* 1884–1885. Reprint, New York: Dover, 1974.

Moore, Michael. *Medicinal Plants of the Pacific West.* Santa Fe: Red Crane Books, 1993.

TRILLIUM
Trillium spp.

PAMELA HIRSCH

My first encounter with trillium was many years ago on an herb walk at Sage Mountain, Rosemary Gladstar's education and retreat center in East Barre, Vermont. It was at the end of a hot, muggy July day and I was suffering from a heady mixture of jet lag, fatigue, and nervous excitement at meeting Rosemary. It was the first evening of our apprenticeship and I wanted dinner, not an herb walk. However, wanting to appear an avid gardener (not) and an enthusiastic herbalist, I trekked gamely around the property. I blithely tasted lobelia, violets, comfrey, and mullein—all the while wondering if Rosemary was really someone I could trust. Toward the end of the walk, we were shown trillium. What a plant! A perfect set of three threes. That is, the plant was made up of three leaves, three sepals, and three petals. The symmetry was clean and beautiful. I couldn't help but notice trillium's similarity to the threefold schematic called triskelion, often encountered in Celtic knot designs. I was also struck by the plant's apparent fragility, having only the one stem.

Years later, back on the West Coast, I met trillium again. This occasion was more surreal than the first; I was deep into a vision journey led by Rick de la Tour, wilderness expert and coowner of the Dry Creek Herb Farm in Auburn, California. Our task was to find our plant ally or, rather, allow it to find us. I returned without much medicinal information but had loads of more esoteric content, the foremost being that trillium was a forest mandala as well as "the phoenix rising." This made me wonder if trillium grew well in areas that had been burned at one time, though I have not found any science-based information that would lead me this conclusion. I have been filled, ever since, with a deep connection to the plant.

BOTANICAL FEATURES

There are many species of trillium, hence there are quite a few common names, the most often used being bethroot and birthroot. It is also called American ground ivy, Indian balm, squaw root, and wake robin, the latter attributed to the plant's ability to "wake the robins into song" as the leaves and stem emerge in early spring. A member of the Liliaceae family, trillium is a perennial that grows worldwide, primarily in North America and eastern Asia. On the East

Coast of North America, it grows from as far north as Québec south to North Carolina. On the West Coast, *Trillium ovatum* can be found as far south as the Monterey coast in California and north into British Columbia. Sources disagree on the number of species. The highest number is forty-eight, while most agree that there are approximately twenty to thirty species within the genus. Within California and Oregon alone five to six species are available.

Trillium likes a moist, rich soil such as the kind provided in shaded woodlands. The tuberlike rhizome is barrel shaped, elongates with age, and emits a light turpentine fragrance. While the rhizome has at first a sweet, aromatic flavor, this soon turns to an astringent, bitter taste, causing salivation. The trillium plant has three net-veined, mottled leaves that range in size from 2 to 15 inches and sit on top of a stem 3 to 30 inches high that grows directly out of the rhizome. Erik Jules, an assistant professor of biology at Humboldt State University, has studied trillium in depth and reports having seen individuals with more than one flower. However, most plants bear a single, terminal flower with three sepals and three petals that bloom in May or June in a wide variety of colors—white, pink, maroon, red-brown, green, yellow-green, and bright yellow—depending on the specific species. Jules also notes that *Trillium ovatum* individuals rarely flower prior to their fifteenth year, and then flowering often occurs sporadically, sometimes on alternate years and sometimes consecutively.

HISTORICAL INFORMATION

The Native American Indians, especially those living in Appalachia, made use of trillium to treat female disorders. Likewise, it was employed by the early settlers and Eclectic physicians to allay uterine hemorrhage and lessen the pain of childbirth. The early names squaw root and birth root reflect those usages. In addition, the plant was traditionally used as an aphrodisiac. Rafinesque and his contemporaries (1830) felt the different trillium species could be used interchangeably, although Native Americans generally considered the white-flowering species to be the most potent. In 1892 Charles Millspaugh indicated that only *Trillium erectum* was an effective medicinal. This was met with some disagreement, but most current herbals do list *T. erectum* as the species of use.

MEDICINAL USES

Trillium contains the active constituent trillene and is an astringent, antispasmodic, expectorant, emmenagogue, antiseptic, and uterine tonic. Due to its astringent action, it was often employed in cases of hemorrhage and excessive bleeding, especially in excess menstrual blood loss (menorrhagia). David Hoffmann in *The New Holistic Herbal* notes that trillium "is considered to be a specific for excessive blood loss associated with menopausal changes." Trillium's drying and antiseptic properties caused it to work effectively as a douche for treatment of leukorrhea, a whitish vaginal discharge, and other vaginal infections such as trichomonas or thrush.

Trillium contains diosgenin, which the body seems able to use or disregard depending upon individual need, making trillium a natural uterine tonic. While it is excellent for stimulation of contractions in childbirth, it would be contraindicated in pregnancy for the same reasons.

Trillium was also used as a remedy for dysentery or diarrhea. Made into a poultice or salve, trillium was useful for external ulcers, sores, and chronic skin problems.

PREPARATION AND DOSAGE

Old herbals indicate that for diarrhea or dysentery, 1 teaspoon of powdered root may be boiled in 2 cups of milk. This was drunk throughout the day. Trillium was commonly prepared as a decoction by simmering 1 to 2 teaspoons of the dried rhizome or root in 1 cup of water for ten minutes. Several cups would then be drunk throughout the day.

Trillium may be prepared as an extract, 1:5 in 40 percent alcohol. An easy way to do this is to pour 5 fluid ounces of eighty-proof vodka, rum, or brandy over 1 ounce of powdered, dried herb placed in a jar. Place a tight-fitting lid on the jar (it helps to put waxed paper over the jar first, so that the lid does not rust and stick). Store in a cool, dark place, remembering to shake the jar and its contents once or twice a day. After two to six weeks strain the resulting extract by pouring the contents of the jar into a sieve lined with a clean, thin cotton cloth, placed over a bowl. Squeeze additional fluid from the cloth containing the herbal material. The extract may be stored in a dark bottle in-

definitely. A general dosage is 1 dropperful three times a day.

PROPAGATION AND CULTIVATION

In nature, trillium seeds are dispersed by ants. Each seed has a number of fat bodies, little chunks of fat, which lie on the outside of the seed. Ants are attracted to the fat bodies and they carry them back to their nests. After eating the fat, the ants place the seeds in their trash heap/compost pile, where they await winter and germination.

Trillium may be propagated from seeds produced at the end of the summer. In the fall, place the seeds $1/2$ to 1 inch deep in a good, organic soil, similar to that found in moist forests. In its first spring trillium will put out its root radical (first root), but there will be no aboveground growth. It then requires another winter or cold period prior to the emergence of its first leaf. In the first five to ten years, only a single leaf may be made, and as I noted earlier, the plant may take as long as fifteen years to flower, depending upon the species.

It is also possible to propagate trillium from rhizomes. If you are using this method, it is important to obtain cuttings with a bit of originating soil. The reason for this is quite interesting. Trillium has small, smooth, hairless roots that grow downward from its rhizome. In many species roots have root hairs, which allow the plant to more easily absorb required nutrients. It has been noted, however, that plants without root hairs, such as trillium, often require the presence of a microscopic fungus called mycorrhizae in the soil. The mycorrhizae have a symbiotic relationship with the plant that facilitates the plant's process of obtaining nutrients from the soil, just as root hairs do. It appears that trillium requires these mycorrhizae to grow well. Planting a bare section of trillium rhizome in a soil lacking in mycorrhizae may not result in healthy growth. Ask for some of the earth surrounding the rhizome to take home to mix in with existing soil before planting.

HARVESTING

Wild trillium is protected in most states, so only cultivated trillium should be harvested. As with most medicinal roots and tubers, the trillium rhizome and roots may be dug in late summer to early autumn, when the plant's energy turns downward to the underground portions of the plant. The rhizomes are cleaned and cut, then dried on screens in a dry, well-ventilated structure. The dried rhizome should be stored in well-sealed jars in a dark area to prevent loss of medicinal properties.

Having discussed the proper method for harvesting trillium, it should be noted that it takes many years for the plant to create its prized rhizome. Unlike many of our medicinal plants, it is possible to discover the age of a particular trillium plant. Each year, as the stem emerges from the rhizome, one leaf scar is made on the rhizome. By counting the rhizome's leaf scars, you can determine the number of years the plant has been alive. Erik Jules found one *Trillium ovatum* plant that was seventy-two years old. This particular plant's rhizome was approxi-

mately 1 inch in diameter and only 2$^1/_2$ or 3 inches long. Not very big for seventy-two years of existence! And certainly not appropriate to harvest such a plant growing in the wild.

Unfortunately, the current harvest method—harvesting only a portion of the rhizome and returning the remainder to its earthy bed—is not particularly successful as a way of preservation in trillium's case. Jules specifically does not recommend this procedure, because it appears to significantly disturb the plant.

UpS RECOMMENDATIONS

- Use only cultivated resources.
- Good alternatives are raspberry leaf (as an astringent for the female reproductive system) and motherwort. Use shepherd's purse as antihemorrhagic and astringent.

It has become harder to find trillium in health food and herb stores. In fact, I found only one source (mail order) of dried bethroot and it was, predictably, wildcrafted. In my opinion, this difficulty in sourcing is as it should be for any medicinal that is tricky to cultivate and/or slow growing. At a time in our earth's history when plant species are becoming extinct daily, I would be hard pressed to harvest a wild plant such as trillium that produces only a 3-inch rhizome after seventy-two years of growth. There are other, more abundant plants that should be used instead—yarrow and shepherd's purse for excess bleeding; raspberry leaf, burdock, and motherwort as gentle uterine tonics; and lady's mantle for its astringent and emmenagogue actions.

In addition, there are other means of availing yourself of a plant's healing properties. Kate Gilday, herbalist and coowner of Woodland Essence in Cold Brook, New York, makes flower essences from at-risk North American plants (see pages 55–59, Flower Essences, and the resources at the end of this book). She uses a special process that allows the flower to remain attached and intact, without destroying the plant. Trillium *(Trillium erectum)* is part of her flower essence repertoire. The Woodland Essence brochure states that trillium flower essence is useful for "tender but strong support during times of birth, death and re-birth. Helps one develop the courage and flexibility to flow with life's changes and cycles. Coming home to oneself. Peaceful centeredness, knowing that is enough." This is a wonderful way for us to continue a healing relationship with trillium without sacrificing the plant.[1]

The plants are here willingly to be of service to Earth and all her inhabitants. As with any dear friend, it is our responsibility and right to reciprocate this service. We may do this by admiring and teaching others about these green beings, creating and maintaining a habitable environment—and sometimes by leaving them to stand alone as elegant forest mandalas.

(I am indebted to Erik Jules, who gave me much of his time and information on a plant he knows well, trillium. Much of the information in this chapter comes from years of Erik's study of the plant. Thank you, Erik.)

NOTES

1. For more information on Woodland Essence and its tree, shrub, and forest floor flower essences, contact Woodland Essence, P.O. Box 206, Cold Brook, NY 13324.

REFERENCES

Brown, O. Phelps, M.D. *The Complete Herbalist.* North Hollywood, Calif.: Newcastle Publishing, 1993.

Gilday, Kate, and Don Babineau. *Woodland Essence Brochure.* Cold Brook, N.Y.: authors, 1998.

Hoffmann, David. *The New Holistic Herbal.* Rockport, Mass.: Element Books, 1995.

Hutchens, Alma R. *Indian Herbalogy of North America.* Windsor, Ont.: Merco Publishers, 1973.

Keville, Kathi. *Herbs: An Illustrated Encyclopedia.* Fairfax, Va.: Friedman, 1992.

Kloss, Jethro. *Back to Eden.* Loma Linda, Calif.: Back to Eden Books Publishing, 1994.

McIntyre, Anne. *The Complete Woman's Herbal.* New York: Henry Holt, 1995.

Stuart, Malcolm. *Encyclopedia of Herbs and Herbalism.* New York: Grosset and Dunlap, 1979.

VENUS'S-FLYTRAP
Dionaea muscipula

JAMES GREEN

The peculiarity I appreciate most about Venus's-flytraps is that they put "teeth" in the vegetable kingdom. You don't find these little plants standing around passively vegetating while being grazed or otherwise abused by the animal world. They're green, they're mean, and with deft precision, they take their bites out of life. One must admire the pluck of these prodigious predators. And even though currently it is considered a mere myth by the horticultural elite, the carnivorous plant devas continue whispering into the ears of our human psyche, quite convincingly, that out there somewhere, hiding in a remote jungle of life, there just might be a highly irreverent, very hungry carnivorous plant large enough to eat a human.

Unquestionably, Venus's-flytraps command the same awe and acclaim that we bestow on piranhas, tarantulas, Big Foot, and vampire bats. Deep in my being a tiny balance of righteousness is tipped in favor of the predominantly benign plant kingdom by the sensually wanton lifestyles of these floriferous superstars and the other members of the carnivorous gang. It delights my herbalist spirit to know that there lives in the savory wilds of this planet a family of charismatic plants that has secured the role of harvester in the gastronomic interaction of plant and animal species. I say to them, "Hurrah! Well done!"

And as to certain nitrogenous morsels of their harvest, well, in my opinion, it couldn't happen to a better crop of protein. Mind you, I respect and appreciate most beings on this globe, and certainly almost all life-forms command that respect. Creatures mind their own business, go about their work and play, and, for the most part, let others alone to enjoy their lives. But not the fly! No, the fly has to do its business on naked portions of human skin whenever and wherever it can. How often, during a precious moment of profound contemplation, or upon entering a lazy, delicious slumber, do I find my senses targeted and assaulted by the incessant buzzing and perpetual landings of a merciless Muscidae? The fly, coldly disregarding my wishes to be alone, willfully ignoring my attempts to shoo it away, returns again and again to plague my reveries. "Pick on someone your own size!" I have been heard to shout in crazed frustration.

Well, the flytrap is just that someone . . . and my primordial yearning for retaliation is jubilantly satisfied by the Venus's-flytrap's abiding entrapment and dissolution of its namesake. For this I thank you, my carnivorous green comrades, and I salute you.

In tribute to these self-empowered, though rare little beings, I have created an outdoor home bog in my northwestern coastal herb garden, and with impish delight, I have given a hand to populating it with voracious Venus's-flytraps along with many of their cousin carnivores, the pitcher plants (*Sarracenia* spp.), the sundews (*Drosera* spp.), and the butterworts (*Pinguicula* spp.). The composed, Epicurean demeanor of these insect-eating plants bestows a delightfully curious diversity to my garden—an eccentricity that evades articulation. One can only experience it when in their company. Their intriguing sensuality and dietary preferences occupy a unique position in my family, one that vibrates betwixt flora and fauna. These green beings feel more like pets than garden plants. And once again, dreaming outdoors bogside has become a peaceful, meditative experience, as my attack plants feed nearby. And the best part of all is though these carnivorous plants generate an air of exotic mystery, they can be simpler to grow than many common houseplants.

So it is with avid affection and deep appreciation that I applaud the magnificent manifestation we call Venus's-flytrap, along with all other species of carnivorous plants. In addition, I state forthrightly, that it is my agenda in this chapter to inspire its readers to contribute passionately to the well-being of these rare and precious plant allies. It is my honor and pleasure to introduce to you the one and only *Dionaea*, the beautiful, the sensual, Venus's-flytrap.

BOTANICAL FEATURES

The Venus's-flytrap is a hardy perennial member of the Sundew (Droseraceae) family. The plant is a rosette of highly specialized leaves that are totally or partially reclining and radiate from a central point. The leaves arise from a somewhat elongate, fleshy, white rhizome that is often miscalled a bulb. The rhizome elongates and enlarges annually, producing numerous offshoots including rudimentary fibrous roots that descend 4 to 6 inches. The green leaves grow up to 5 inches long. Each leaf is composed of two parts. There is a narrow to relatively broad leaflike portion (petiole) at the base near the rosette center, which functions as an ordinary green leaf, photosynthesizing organic compounds. Beyond this the leaf is constricted to the midrib, which expands again to form a unique trap measuring up to $1^1/_4$ inches long. The flytrap's white blossoms perch on foot-high stalks, proclaiming their kinship with the Sundew family. After fertilization, tiny, black pear-shaped seeds mature in six to eight weeks. The seeds will germinate promptly when sown on a suitable medium. The plant will mature to flowering age in six to seven years and can live for two to three decades.

Dionaea's traps consist of two clamshell-like halves capable of closing together, with the midrib serving as the "hinge." The free margin or unattached edge of each half is lined with tiny nectar glands and numerous rigid, comblike guard hairs that interlock like fingers when the trap closes. The interior surface of each half is lined with minute glands that have secretory and absorbing functions; in the center of each half lie normally three short, stiff spines (trigger hairs) in a triangular pattern that, when one or more are touched twice, initiates trap closure. The mechanism of the closure remains a mystery. Despite initial appearances, during the initial rapid phase of closure the two halves do not rotate on the midrib to close like a bear trap. It appears that, when open, the outer surface of each trap half is concave or dished outward, as concurrently the inner surface is bulging inward. During closure, these surface conformations are reversed and the free edges are suddenly brought sufficiently close together to interlock the stout guard hairs, entrapping the prey.

The trap does not close tightly right away, however. Darwin surmised that this allowed small insects to escape through the intermeshed teeth, so the plant wouldn't waste time and energy eating an insignificant meal. (Why settle for a light snack when you can swill a satiating *Musca* smoothie?) When a large insect is caught, its struggling stimulates the trigger hairs even further. In a few hours the lobes are slowly pressed tightly together as the trap seals itself closed. During this stage of closure it is suspected that there is, in fact, a hingelike rotation on the midrib of the trap. At this point, glands on the inside surface of the lobes begin to secrete digestive juices. Shortly the insect drowns in the fluid. In the wild ants and spiders are the most frequent prey. While other "carnies" can digest either fresh or pre-expired foods, the flycatcher and its medicinal accomplice, the sundew *(Drosera rotundifolia)*, require the wiggling of live food to stimulate secretion of digestive enzymes.

In the wild *Dionaea* lives primarily in sandy, peat soil in damp areas on the edges of swamps, fens, and pocosins. The plants are typically found growing among wiregrasses, sedges, and native orchids in grasslands between sparsely scattered longleaf pines or in open, sunny, acidic savannas. Their preferred climate is warm, temperate, and humid, where winters are chilly with occasional periods of frost but only rarely snow.

HISTORICAL BACKGROUND

The Venus's-flytrap is unquestionably the most dramatic and famous of all the carnivorous plants. Charles Darwin referred to it as "one of the most wonderful plants in the world."

In 1763 Arthur Dobbs, the governor of North Carolina, directed public attention to the Venus's-flytrap for the first time, calling it the "Fly Trap Sensitive." Soon after that, specimens were sent to England, where it became the first plant ever suspected of being carnivorous. Charles Darwin made it official in 1875 when he published *Insectivorous Plants*, therein reporting observations that some plants, in fact, really do eat insects and larger animals. You can imagine that fauna supremacists everywhere were aghast by this news. Enthralled botanists named the seductive flytrap with reference to Venus, who beguiles and captivates all men. Venus's-flytrap's Latin binomial, *Dionaea muscipula*, refers both to the plant's charming appearance and to the object of its prime passion. Dione is the mother of Venus, who reigns as the most beautiful and sensuous goddess in Greek mythology. *Muscipula* refers to the plant's artistry in catching the elusive flying insects of the Muscidae family (of which *Musca domestica*, the common housefly, is the most renowned). Through the ages *Dionaea* has been known by other common names such as flycatcher, tipitiwitchet, and catch-fly sensitive.

There is only one species in the monotypic genus *Dionaea*, and that is the inscrutable *D. muscipula*. There are, however, several forms and cultivars of *D. muscipula*. Some of these may represent natural varieties found in the wilds, whereas others are artificially bred and named cultivations or mutations that occur in tissue-cultured plants. (Might this be where the cryptic human-eating variety bides its time?)

Worldwide, *Dionaea* is found native only in the United States, in the scattered savannas of the coastal plain of southeastern North Carolina and in the extreme northeast of South Carolina, an approximate landward radius of merely 60 to 75 miles around Wilmington, North Carolina. Few wildflowers occupy such a restricted range. Although introduced with some success in New Jersey and California, it has been naturalized in relatively great abundance only in Appalachicola State Park, a small area on the Florida panhandle. Venus's-flytrap has taken hold in this wild region and is reproducing very well. Fortunately, because of its state park sta-

tus this community is well protected from further predatory acquisitions of a sprawling human civilization.

Although few in numbers and relatively unfamiliar to most people's common experience, *Dionaea* and its carnivorous family's societal impact on the human community is significant. After the botanical scandal instigated by the disclosure of *Dionaea*'s predaceous dietary practices cooled down, the world's first carnivorous plant society convened in Japan in 1948 and continues to thrive today. In 1972 the International Carnivorous Plant Society was founded in the United States, and is currently promoting worldwide interest in this fascinating plant family. Several other societies have germinated and are growing in Europe, Australia, and San Francisco. Who really knows the full extent of these gatherings? In face of these outcrops, it may be noted that an interspecies relationship with carnivorous plants can be more emotionally addicting to humans than either chocolate or shopping.

MEDICINAL USES

Dionaea is a beautifully enchanting plant that freely sets its unique tone in life; its spirit is fascinating and uplifting to behold. From my personal perspective as a health practitioner, this is the cardinal gift this inspirational ally contributes to a human being's health and feeling of well-being.

In the region of human pathology *Dionaea* appears to be equally generous. Dr. Helmut Keller, a German research oncologist, while conducting studies in the treatment of chronic, degenerative illnesses since the 1970s, discovered extensive therapeutic potentials residing in *Dionaea*'s tissues. From this plant's fresh-squeezed juices Dr. Keller developed a product he named Carnivora. He has used this plant extract in the treatment of chronic diseases including most forms of cancer, arthritis, ulcerative colitis, multiple sclerosis, herpes infections, and many immune deficiency states, including AIDS. With cancer patients, it is particularly useful for those individuals who have not been treated previously by chemo- or radiation therapy. In clinical application *Dionaea* extract has been shown to boost immune function and eliminate HIV virus from the blood. In line with its demonstrated ability to reduce the growth rate of tumor tissue, *Dionaea* fresh-plant extract appears to assist a person to decrease suppressor cells, and to increase the number and activity of T-helper cells and other immune system components, thereby helping improve the individual's general condition and sense of well-being. *Dionaea* is an uplifter in many ways.

PREPARATION AND DOSAGE

To prepare *Dionaea* extracts, you normally use the entire fresh, undried plant including the rhizome ("bulb"). However, *Dionaea*'s leaves and traps contain all the constituents that are found in the whole plant; herbalists might consider harvesting only these portions of their cultivated plants, thereby conserving the life of the community. This calls for a large spread of plants, however, for it takes approximately 150 fresh whole plants to accumulate a pound of *Dionaea*;

each mature plant weighs in at about .1 ounce. Eighty-six to 90 percent of this total weight is water.

The standard recipe for preparing *Dionaea* for use as an herbal medicine consists of blending 1 part pure fresh plant juice, 1 part 190-proof ethyl alcohol, and 1 part distilled water. The constituents of this herb are alcohol soluble, however, so you could prepare the extract by making a fresh-plant tincture at a ratio of 1:2 (weight to volume) using 100 percent ethyl alcohol for the menstruum.

In line with Dr. Keller's dosage and treatment protocol, the recommended adult dosage is 30 drops of *Dionaea* fresh-plant extract taken in 8 ounces of water, three to five times daily, preferably before meals. When treating lung and bronchial conditions, in addition to ingestion of the extract you can inhale *Dionaea* by means of a nebulizer or cold vaporizer. Prepare the inhalant by mixing 2 ml of liquid *Dionaea* extract with 2 ml of saline solution (0.9 salt solution). Inhale this up to five times a day.

My herbalist friend and peer Richo Cech, founder of Horizon Seeds in Williams, Oregon, has extensive experience in preparing fresh *Dionaea* extract and has supplied me with the majority of this medicinal information. Richo warns that you need to be cautious when juicing *Dionaea*, for the process unleashes high quantities of proteolytic enzymes that the plant under normal conditions employs to digest animal protein. Human skin is composed of a variety of animal proteins, and *Dionaea*'s fresh juice in contact with skin can and will damage the tissue. Such contact elicits irritation and wounds similar to a burn. Herbal medicine makers best beware of plants with teeth!

PROPAGATION AND CULTIVATION

The flytrap is one of the easiest of all the carnivorous plants to grow. Given any chance at all, like all sprightly weeds, it will survive admirably. Peter D'Amato, coowner of California Carnivores nursery in Forestville, California, told me a story about his recent travels through *Dionaea*'s homeland—Brunswick County in North Carolina. He discovered to his heart's delight that along the roadsides of this county's public highways where the soil is acidic, no herbicides are sprayed, and the grass is routinely mowed, wild *Dionaea* communities are active and thriving.

As you might expect, *Dionaea* is a survivor, providing itself a number of ways to multiply in the wilds. Propagation by seeds, leaf cuttings, rhizome divisions, and aerial sets are the most appropriate methods to discuss. Herbalists and other *Dionaea* fans can quite easily employ these means at home.

PROPAGATING *DIONAEA* FROM SEEDS

The flytrap's white blossoms are pollinated by bees and insects, or by the human hand. After fertilization, the small black seeds mature in six to eight weeks. These seeds will germinate within three weeks when sown on a suitable medium such as very moist peat moss. They respond favorably to strong sunlight, high temperature, and high humidity, making greenhouse (with good air circulation) propagation ideal. Plants mature to flowering age in six to seven years.

PROPAGATING *DIONAEA* FROM LEAF CUTTINGS

Dionaea's widened, bladelike petioles are capable of producing vegetative buds that can generate a mature plant in two to three years. Cut off a mature leaf at the base of the petiole and place it right-side up on a bed of moist sphagnum peat moss. Make sure the lower side of the leaf is lying flat on the surface of the moss. Over several weeks plantlets will appear from the margins and surfaces of the leaves. Let these grow until roots have formed. When they are well rooted, carefully transplant them to separate containers. This procedure is best initiated early in the growing season.

RHIZOME DIVISION

Dionaea often develops rhizome offshoots or bulbils at the base of its leaf rosette. There are sometimes as many as six or seven of these plantlets, which can be squeezed and pulled apart into sets and planted in moist peat moss. They will generate a mature plant in two to three years.

PROPAGATING *DIONAEA* FROM AERIAL SETS

The mature flower stalk of some plants will produce several aerial sets. These are actually miniature flytrap plants. If you will allow these little ones to mature on the stalk, you can then plant them out in moist peat moss. They will grow into mature plants in three to four years. This process pulls energy from the parent plant, so commercial venders trim the flower stalks back to increase the size of plants for market.

PLANT-TISSUE CULTURE

This propagation technique is performed in a lab under sterile conditions, in vitro, using vessels such as flasks. The flask contains the plant tissue, a suitable growing mixture of organic and inorganic salts, and a carbon source (sugar) for energy and hormones to manipulate the cultured cells to perform as needed. The process is remarkably rapid and generates a potted plant within a year or so. The most salient aspect of plant-tissue culture as a propagation tool is its ability to produce literally tens of thousands of plants quickly at a relatively low cost. Several labs in the United States, the Netherlands, India, and Australia have produced millions of Venus's-flytraps for the horticulture industry. This has provided great relief to the dwindling (previously overharvested) populations remaining in the wilds, and is probably the greatest benefit of tissue culture. This process is not ideal for repopulating an area, because its myriad progeny lack biodiversity. Employed creatively, however, it can be a blessing (see Atlanta Botanical Gardens in the resource section at the end of this chapter).

Cultivating the flytrap at home is simple—in fact it is considered one of the easiest of all carnivorous plants to grow. Place the plant into a simple mixture of half sphagnum peat moss and half sterile horticultural sand. The pot used should sit in a shallow saucer of water kept filled with about $1/2$ inch of water, keeping the potted soil wet. It is important to note that tap water and many well waters are ordinarily too high in mineral content, and water from a water soft-ener adds too much sodium to the soil. The water used must be either rainwater collected during the rainy season and stored for later use, or a purified, quality water that has been made available by distillation, deionization, or reverse osmosis. Using these waters is considered by experienced growers to be the secret to successful cultivation. Demineralized waters are required to avoid long-term mineral buildup in the soil. Mineral-rich soil damages these plants, which are native to acidic, mineral-poor bogs and swamps. This is why, with their roots planted in mineral-depleted soil pantries, they have learned to seduce their nitrogen-rich food from the air. In line with this, it is important to avoid fertilizing these plants. Venus's-flytraps like their soil environment to be moist but not flooded for too lengthy a time. The plant requires a sunny area for growth. In winter the plant must experience at least three months of chilly temperature; 40 to 50 degrees is ideal, although they can tolerate temperatures down to the teens briefly. This is required by the plant so it can rest in a semidormant state.

When this dormant period begins, the leaves usually turn black and die back. But it is important to understand that the rhizomes remain healthy. Flowering has a weakening effect on the plant, so clipping flower buds is recommended if you want to promote larger summer traps more quickly. But if you want to promote seed production, it is beneficial to have two or more plants in flower simultaneously, for self-pollination is difficult for these plants. Trimming away old black leaves is helpful, because new leaves are constantly produced during their rapid growing season (April through May). *Dionaea* likes to be transplanted to a new medium every one or two years, and this is best done in February through April.

Practical instructions for building a home bog are furnished in the publication *Carnivorous Plants of the United States and Canada* by Donald E. Schnell. Simple procedures for populating these bogs with a wide variety of carnies are clearly explained in the colorful, award-winning publication *The Savage Garden* by Peter D'Amato.

HARVESTING

In light of the extremely fragile state of *Dionaea*'s native habitats and the fact that this herb is currently listed on the Convention on International Trade in Endangered Species list (which prohibits export without official documentation showing that the plant was legally and sustainably harvested or cultivated), this plant should never be field-harvested or purchased from unreliable sources. Plants that have been propagated for commercial harvest by leaf cuttings and rhizome division are accessible to herbalists, and relatively inexpensive tissue-cultured plants are plentiful and readily available from the commercial wholesalers that supply primarily the horticulture industry.

UpS RECOMMENDATIONS

- This plant is too fragile for wildcrafting. Use cultivated resources only.
- Possible alternatives are cultivated echinacea and red clover.

The government of North Carolina has upgraded its laws and intensified its enforcement efforts in an attempt to safeguard the native plant communities of its wetland regions. Whereas traditionally a fine of $10 was levied on any poacher caught with a truckload of gunny sacks filled with *Dionaea*, this has now been increased to $10 per plant. This reflects a favorable political attitude and is a sincere step in the right direction, although it remains difficult to catch illegal harvesters. What has busted the poachers far more effectively is the recently developed tissue-culture technique for propagating *Dionaea*. This has made available vast amounts of inexpensively propagated Venus's-flytraps, thus reducing their market price to well below what even a mean and odious poacher will work for. While the demand for allopathic herbal medicines and pilfered booty might no longer pose a major threat to the native plant populations due to the availability of cloned plants, the greatest threat to their safety and continued existence in the wilds remains the domiciliary sprawl of the rest of humanity. We find that the native population decline is due primarily to:

- A rapidly growing population and the drainage of wetlands for lumber, agriculture, and residential development. In the 100-mile radius of Wilmington, North Carolina, where at one time it is estimated that over a billion *Dionaea* lived, only 5 percent as many remain. The rest have been covered over by civilization's asphalt and concrete carpeting. This area is now devoted to retirement homes, golf courses, and neighborhood malls. As a matter of statistics, of all the carnivorous plant stands in the southeastern United States, only 5 percent of the natural habitats are left intact. This is approximately the same percentage of virgin forests that remain standing in the Pacific Northwest.

• The prevention of naturally occurring brush fires (most often due to lightning strikes). Venus's-flytraps are choked out by thick scrub that would otherwise be burned back by these fires.

The good news is that the Venus's-flytrap is a resilient and versatile perennial that tends to remain on a deteriorating home site longer than many associated carnivorous and noncarnivorous plants. It will tolerate short periods of drought and flooding. Submerged plants have even been observed supplementing their normal diet of airborne and crawling victuals with small aquatic animals. The underground stem of the *Dionaea* is so well protected that it is among the first plants to sprout back vigorously in a recently burned area. *Dionaea* communities appreciate the benefits of a rapid autumnal surface fire. *Dionaea* is also climatically hardy, which has been demonstrated by successful transplantings that have thrived as far north as New Jersey and the bogs in Pennsylvania.

What can herbalists do to assist the green carnivores? As always, inspire and educate consumers, other herbalists, and members of the herbal community. Encourage them to adopt wide varieties of carnivorous plants, building home bogs for them (noting how fun and easy it is). As a consumer, too, you can insist on zero harvesting of these plants from the wilds. Home propagation and cultivation are simple, and tissue culture is here!

Orchestrate unified efforts of groups such as United Plant Savers (UpS), Atlanta Botanical Gardens, and The Nature Conservancy to direct their focus and vision on the issues and support with "green cash" any judicious government attempts to preserve wetlands and native and introduced carnivorous plant communities.

UpS's Jubilation Committee or the likes thereof might create and sponsor an international carnivorous plant carnival as a magical theater conceived to accumulate enough funds to support appropriate sanctuaries in the Carolinas and other U.S. wetlands. There is a highly successful precedent for such a party. *Allium sativum*, the notorious stink rose, inspires a merry gathering every year known as the Garlic Festival in Gilroy, California. This energetic event has titillated folks' imaginations and playful spirits for years and appears to excite an abundant flow of legal tender as well.

But most important, passionately visualize the vibrant health and well-being of these remarkable carnivorous plant beings. See them thriving as vigorous allies living in abundance with us on this planet. Appreciate their perpetual companionship.

There is much to cherish and learn about the unique environment of the wetlands in this country and the carnivorous plants that embellish them. And most especially, we can learn to appreciate the love bite of *Dionaea muscipula*.

BIBLIOGRAPHY, REFERENCES, AND RESOURCES

The Savage Garden, by Peter D'Amato. Ten Speed Press, P.O. Box 7123, Berkeley, CA 94707, 1998. In full color, a delightfully illustrated 336-page book. It supplies extensive information on the propagation, care, and fascinating lore of carnivorous plants. Peter has been cultivating carnies for more than twenty-five years.

Activity Book for Carnivorous Plants, by Michael Szesze. Michael Szesze is a teacher who has developed a program using carnivorous plants to educate children on a wide variety of topics: general botany, photosynthesis, reproduction, soil chemistry, insect life associated with carnivorous plants, wetlands and the conservation of natural habitats, endangered species, drawing, geography, and more. Write to:

Calvert County Public Schools
Attn.: Michael Szesze
1305 Dares Beach Road
Prince Frederick, MD 20678

Carnivorous Plants of the United States and Canada, by Donald E. Schnell. John F. Blair, Publisher, 1406 Plaza Drive, Winston-Salem, NC 27103, 1976.

A Guide to Carnivorous Plants of the World, by Gorden Cheers (1993). Out of print but can be found in libraries.

Carnivorous Plants, by Adrian Slack (1979). Out of print but can be found in libraries.

International Carnivorous Plant Society, the Fullerton Arboretum, P.O. Box 6850, California State University, Fullerton, CA 92834-6850. The annual membership fee is $20 U.S., $25 foreign. Membership includes a subscription to the informative and colorful *Carnivorous Plant Newsletter*, which is published quarterly.

Bay Area Carniverous Plant Society, 39011 Applegate Terrace, California Carnivores, 7020 Trenton-Healdsburg Road, Forestville, CA 95436, (707) 838-1630, www.californiacarnivores.com. In 1989 Peter D'Amato and his partner, Marilee Maertz, created the California Carnivores nursery, the only nursery in the world devoted to the cultivation of carnivores that is open daily to the public as a retail nursery. More than four hundred plants are on display, with informative signs to help provide a self-guided tour. Their large array of plants are all commercially cultivated. This nursery is one of the plant wonders of California. An excellent source for a remarkably wide variety of carnivorous plants. Packed and shipped worldwide. Call for a free list of plants and price guide.

Atlanta Botanical Gardens, P.O. Box 77246, Atlanta, GA 30357. Crusaders in the U.S. repopulation of natural stands of native plants, and re-creating wetlands on selected sites that have been badly damaged and on land that has been bought by The Nature Conservancy. The staff use tissue-cultured plants for this undertaking, but these reintroduced specimens are cultured from a wide variety of plants in order to help preserve the gene pool and repopulate natural stands with a diversity of plants.

Gublers Nursery, P.O. Box 3100, Landers, CA 92285-0100, 1-800-GUBLERS. Wholesaler of tissue-cultured carnivorous plants.

VIRGINIA SNAKEROOT

Aristolochia serpentaria

DOUG ELLIOTT

A large velvety-black butterfly flashing metallic blue hind wings fluttered past my feet. It was a sunny April afternoon and I was exploring an open woods of oak, hickory, and ironwood near the Broad River in the piedmont of North Carolina. The butterfly was flitting along near the ground. There were no flowers in bloom in the area, yet the butterfly was flying up to every young green shoot—honeysuckle, asters, grasses, and tree seedlings. It didn't land on these plants but rather flew from one plant to another, spending a second or two at each sprout as if it were checking each one out. The butterfly sailed right by taller plants and bushes, pausing only at delicate shoots between about 2 and 4 inches in height. The butterfly was hunting a rare herb.

This was a gravid female pipevine swallowtail *(Battus philenor)*, ready to lay her eggs. She was searching for the one species of pipevine found in this area—*Aristolochia serpentaria*, the famous Virginia snakeroot. As an adult butterfly she can sip the nectar of many different flowers, but her young can only feed on members of the Aristolochiaceae family and in this region, Virginia snakeroot was her only choice. I watched her hover excitedly around one particular delicate sprout with three light green unfurling leaves. No doubt she was receiving chemical and olfactory confirmation. "Yes! Finally I've found it!" her rapidly fluttering wings seemed to say. While her wings kept her airborne, her legs reached out and grasped the plant. The tip of her abdomen briefly touched the stem, and there she placed a glistening golden egg hardly bigger than a poppy seed. Within a few seconds she was on her way again, continuing her plant-by-plant search for the next snakeroot. I followed her (at a respectful distance) for the next half hour or so as she continued her thorough survey of the forest floor. We may have covered as much as 100 yards, and she may have inspected as many as a thousand plants as she zigzagged back and forth along the ground. In the entire time I spent observing her, she found only the one Virginia snakeroot shoot. She eventually flew up into the canopy, and I lost sight of her.

This was the first time I had ever had a butterfly to serve as an herb-hunting guide. Although there were obviously enough snakeroots in the area to support at least a small population of these swallowtails, this confirmed for me something I had long suspected—that even though Virginia snakeroot has a wide range (from Florida and Texas north to Missouri, Illinois, and southern New England), it is rarely abundant. It is an understated, diminutive herb. Any specimen over a foot tall and having more than ten leaves is considered large. The rhizome is rarely over an inch long and weighs a tiny fraction of an ounce. Even in areas of ideal habitat where the plant is relatively common, I never see it growing thickly in beds or patches—just an occasional plant here and there. Even the butterfly I followed, which had dozens of eggs to deposit, seemed to instinctively understand the plant's limited growth habit. She only placed one egg on that single plant she found, for a single plant like this can support only one caterpillar. Up in the higher mountains on *Aristolochia macrophylla*—the huge Dutchman's pipe—I have seen a swallowtail lay more than a dozen eggs on one leaf.

BOTANICAL FEATURES

Virginia snakeroot is part of Aristolochiaceae, the Birthwort family. Members of this group of plants are found in a variety of habitats, from northern forests to deserts and jungles around the world. Other temperate North American members of this family include wild ginger (*Asarum canadensis*, sometimes known as Canada snakeroot), the heartleafs (*Hexastylis* spp.), and the Dutchman's pipe (*Aristolochia macrophylla*, also known as pipe vine).

Virginia snakeroot's strange-shaped, velvety, maroon-brown flower comes into bloom in late spring after the leaves appear. Growing from a short basal stem, the flower is swollen at the base with a narrow curved calyx tube that flares open at the mouth. It usually lies directly on the ground.

HISTORICAL BACKGROUND

As scarce and little used as the plant seems to be now, in the nineteenth and early twentieth centuries Virginia snakeroot regularly found its way into herbal markets in 100-pound bales. Due to this demand, it may have been exterminated in some parts of its range. It was listed as an official drug in the *United States Pharmacopoeia* until 1942, and in the *National Formulary* until 1955. It also was listed in the pharmacopoeias of London, Dublin, and Edinburgh. The 1927 edition of Culbreth's *Manual of Materia Medica and Pharmacology* considers it to be a "stimulant, tonic, diaphoretic, diuretic, emmenagogue, aphrodisiac, antiperiodic, [that was used to] stimulate appetite and digestion, increase bronchial and intestinal secretion, heart action and mental exhilaration. [It was also used] as a stimulating expectorant in typhoid pneumonia, exanthematous diseases, intermittents, dyspepsia, diphtheria. Fluid extract good locally against poison ivy rash."

MEDICINAL USES

I remember once visiting one of my herbal mentors, an older Appalachian mountain man named Theron Edwards. When I complained of a headache, he held out a small jar to me and said, "Smell of this, buddy, it'll he'p ya!" In that jar was a tiny rhizome with a bundle of dry fibrous roots. I took a tentative sniff and noted a distinct balsamic, turpentine-like aroma. "Hit's Virginia snakeroot," he explained, "but you gotta breathe it in deeper than that for it to do you any good." I placed my nose over the jar and inhaled deeply several times. In an hour or so my headache dissipated. These results were neither dramatic nor conclusive, and this was hardly a clinical trial; still, I was intrigued at how a folk practitioner (who had no qualms about gathering considerable quantities of more common roots and herbs for medicines and tonics) had found a way to use this tiny, scarce herb in a relatively nonconsumptive way. In his folk version of aromatherapy, one small root can be used over and over for several years.

In the doctrine of signatures, an ancient system of knowing plants, it was believed that every herb contains a sign or a "signature" that offers a clue to its use. The curved, bulbous shape of the *Aristolochia* flower reminded the ancients of a fetus, hence the name birthwort and the use of some species as an aid to childbirth. The name *Aristolochia* comes from the Greek, *aristos* (best) and *lochia* (delivery), from its supposed value in childbirth.

At least one member of the genus is still used in other ways. I once stayed with a Mexican family in a village tucked in among the foothills of the Sierra Madre Mountains and found myself ailing with a case of "turista," the loose-boweled intestinal distress so common among newly arrived gringos. Once my hosts learned of my condition, one of the youngsters was dispatched into the dry scrub countryside to find *yerba del Indio* (herb of the Indians). Before long he brought back a small creeping vine with narrow heart-shaped leaves and a familiar ruddy, purplish flower much like our eastern species, but with accentuated veins at the mouth of the floral tube. It was none other than *A. watsonii*, a dwarf desert species of *Aristolochia*. They brewed it up into a tea. I drank a cupful and by the next morning my symptoms were gone. "*Es bueno para pegarle*," they assured me: "It's good to stop you up."

Recently, however, the *Aristolochia* genus has been analyzed chemically and a compound known as aristolochic acid isolated from every species that has been studied. This acid has been found to be mutagenic and carcinogenic in animals. According to Norman Farnsworth, professor of pharmacognosy at the University of Illinois at Chicago, "No herbal medicine in the genus *Aristolochia* should be used by humans over an extended period of time." After learning this, I am glad 1 cupful did the job while I was in the Sierra Madre!

In his book *Los Remedios*, contemporary herbalist and director of the Southwestern School of Botanical Medicine Michael Moore calls *Aristolochia watsonnii* "raiz del Indio" and considers it to be highly useful in small doses, in tea or as a tincture to treat "early stages of flu or fever . . . infections and blood poisoning . . . to stimulate digestion" and in powdered form as a wound dressing.

Some of the same chemical compounds that yield medicinal benefits to humans are also used by the butterflies that take their name from these plants. The adult pipe vine swallowtails are reported to have a pungent, penetrating odor and disagreeable taste, which is believed to come from chemical compounds in the pipe vine leaves eaten by their larvae. This is similar to the mechanism in monarch butterflies that lets them derive a protective chemistry from compounds in the milkweeds that their larvae feed upon.

PROPAGATION AND CULTIVATION

Aristolochia serpentaria is a woodland herbaceous perennial. The root consists of a short, knotted rhizome with numerous wiry rootlets. The plant grows best in rich forest soils, shaded by mixed hardwood trees, or in the shade garden.

To propagate by root cutting, cut the rhizome with a sharp knife into two or more pieces, then replant them just under the soil surface and cover with a mulch of decomposing leaves. In the wild these small plants tend to live in colonies, and in cultivation may be spaced as closely as 1 foot apart. All transplanting should be accomplished in the fall, so that the plants can become used to their new location and "dig in" over the winter, sending up new stems in the spring.

The seeds of Virginia snakeroot are quite rare and difficult to collect. As in many forest-dependent species, the seeds have short longevity after drying, so they should be planted in moist soil as soon as possible after maturation. If the newly harvested seeds are to be stored, they should be placed in moist, sifted peat moss in a plastic bag and kept under refrigeration until they can be planted. Sow them shallowly in a prepared bed in the forest or a shade garden. The area should be well marked, because germination times are extensive, and once germinated the young plants must be watched carefully to protect them from foot traffic, weeds, and slugs. The plant is a hypogeal germinator: that is, the shoot arises from the seed, emerging from the ground as a single, vining stem without cotyledon leaves. The first true leaf develops in the fifth week after germination. Fresh seeds sown in the fall will begin to exhibit germination in the spring as the soil warms. Some seeds will remain dormant for up to two years, germinating in the spring of the second year after planting. Seedlings may be grown out at close spacing for a year or two. Once they develop a palpable rhizome, they may be separated and transplanted to 1 foot apart. Although the plants withstand dry woodland conditions, they will grow more quickly and robustly if given a moist, shady location.

HARVESTING

The aromatic and camphoraceous root and rhizome (the root) of Virginia snakeroot is traditionally harvested from mature plants in the fall, when the characteristically elongated, heart-shaped leaves begin to turn bright yellow. However, this plant is too rare in the wild to be harvested. Use the following information for harvesting cultivated roots.

The roots are most potent in the fall, after the plant has stored its energy reserves for the winter. Both the knotty rhizome and the hairy rootlets are equally potent medicines. As with all rare forest-dependent species, it is important to wait until the seed is ripened and disseminated, either by natural vectors or by human hand, prior to digging the mother plant. Given that the seed is very difficult to germinate, it makes sense to wait until a healthy generation of young plants is well established before harvesting seed-bearing plants. After digging, the portion of the knotty rhizome bearing the nascent bud should be broken free and replanted immediately.

UpS RECOMMENDATIONS

- Use only cultivated resources.
- Both blessed thistle and burdock are good substitutes.
- Yucca may be used instead for joint conditions.
- Use dill, fennel, or ginger as substitutes when treating digestive concerns.
- For ingested poisons, poisonous bites, and snakebite, cultivated echinacea may be substituted.

I didn't know what I was seeing the first time I laid eyes on a large pipe vine caterpillar. It was like a weird, purplish-brown sea slug with rubbery tentacles sticking out on all sides and two rows of yellow-orange spots running down its back. It was calmly munching its way down the stem of our prize Virginia snakeroot plant, which grew wild at the edge of our orchard. The larva had already eaten all the terminal leaves on the stem and was now in the process of finishing off the rest of the lower leaves.

What was I to do? I had been able to find very few of these special plants in our area. And here this prize specimen (the only one I'd found near the house) was being completely devoured by the larva of a magnificently beautiful and special butterfly. Should I consider the caterpillar a pest and simply squash it like a bean beetle or a cabbage worm in my garden?

Pondering this, I gave the critter a tentative prod, and the caterpillar responded immediately with a pair of what looked like slimy yellow horns that seemed to ooze out from behind its head. Suddenly the air was filled with a strange bitter odor. In a few seconds the horns were pulled back into the head and the odor dissipated. What an awesome display! These horn-like appendages are actually a gland called the osmaterium, and the odor serves as a repellent to parasitic wasps and other predators.

Suddenly, a few feet away, something caught my eye. It was another caterpillar just like this one, munching away on another Virginia snakeroot! And then I saw another, and another, and another. Each caterpillar was on a separate plant. With the help of these eye-catching caterpillars I ended up finding eight more snakeroot plants in the orchard—plants that I might have never seen and probably would have mowed over if the caterpillars hadn't called my attention to them.

So I left those caterpillars alone and over the next few days watched as they ate my plants right to the ground. Then they crawled away to pupate. With the caterpillars out of the picture, the snakeroots soon sent up new shoots with new leaves, and these lasted the rest of the summer.

Now each of those snakeroots is protected by a circle of stones. I spend a fair amount of time with the plants, and I keep them weeded as well as I can. Some years the butterflies appear and we can witness their entire cycle. We have even watched a swallowtail emerge from its chrysalis before our eyes and fly away.

The pipe vine swallowtail in its various life forms has taught me a great deal, not only about the Virginia snakeroot plant but also about the miraculous interconnectedness of life. Above all

I am reminded that the key to our survival on this tiny blue-green sphere we call Mother Earth is in using her healing resources in a sustainable way.

REFERENCES

Culbreth, David. *A Manual of Materia Medica and Pharmacology*. Philadelphia: Lea and Febriger, 1927.

Farnsworth, N. R. "Relative safety of herbal medicines." *HerbalGram* 29 (spring/summer 1993): 36D.

Moore, Michael. *Los Remedios, Traditional Herbal Remedies of the Southwest*. Santa Fe: Red Crane Books, 1990.

WHITE SAGE
Salvia apiana

JANE BOTHWELL

Eat sage in May and you'll live for aye.

Old English saying

The young sow wild oats, the old grow sage.

Winston Churchill

Salvia apiana, a member of the Lamiaceae family commonly known as white sage, is a Native American medicinal plant indigenous to southwestern California and northern Baja. This desert shrub can be found growing in the foothills, on slopes and canyon walls, in desert washes, and on mountain hillsides. White sage is a highly aromatic evergreen shrub growing to a height of 5 feet or more. Along the many sticky stems grow sparsely spaced silver-white leaves, which form a beautiful rosette at the end of the stem. It sends up many graceful wands of silver-white flowers. Small plants or plants suffering severe drought may simply present a bunch of clustered rosettes.

White sage holds a place dear in my heart, as many plants do, for plants are one of my most passionate relationships. They nourish and enliven my spirit and help make sense out of a sometimes confusing world. As I burn a leaf of white sage, I am reminded of the power of the open spaces and the adaptability of a plant that grows in the canyon washes and stands vibrant and radiant, glowing silver-white above a fresh winter snow. During our yearly pilgrimage to visit our family in the Anza-Borrego desert of southern California, we hike up Cahuilla Mountain to be with the desert plants. Along the trail are lush ripe manzanita berries on bushes with solid, thick, voluptuous red branches. We eat the berries and fill our pockets with more to be prepared into a festive tea back in the bustling holiday kitchen. The earth is slippery under our feet with newly fallen snow, but now the sun shines and the clouds part, exposing the brilliant blue of the desert sky. Around each bend we wonder if this will be the glorious hillside that we remember is covered with white sage. As so often happens on the trail, it's a few more switchbacks farther than we remembered, but at the next turn there she is, shining brilliantly among the mountain landscape. We just sit with

247

her awhile, admiring. We then begin to chant and pray and ask permission to harvest and gather. We are cautious with every snip of her branches to take a little and leave a lot, moving from plant to plant so our impact is possibly unnoticed. We are full, we say our thanks and begin our journey down the mountain.

Salvia apiana has been used historically as a purifying smudge or incense and recently has become quite popular for the healing qualities of its smoke. In some localities it is being over-harvested and is thus a plant to harvest conservatively; do what you can to encourage its abundant regeneration. Rather than bundling it into smudge sticks, as is done so often in present times, traditional Native American ways suggest burning only single leaves. Historically, this has been the suggested way of burning white sage, with recognition of its scarcity. Adoption and continuation of this simple act would help in the preservation of this Native American medicinal plant. It is also suggested that you burn herbs that are abundant and local to you. There are many other sacred healing incense plants that can be used in place of the increasingly scarce white sage.

BOTANICAL FEATURES

Salvia apiana is found in the semi-arid mountains and foothills of southern California and northern Baja California. Its range extends from Santa Barbara County to the west and north to Imperial County to the east and Rosario, Baja California, to the south. It is a native North American plant growing within this limited range. It inhabits various soils, including sandy loam, granite scree, and loamy clay.

This perennial evergreen boasts smooth silver-white leaves and white flowers touched with lavender or blue. Its flowering spike, as noted, grows to 5 feet. The flowers are prodigious nectar producers, but the tiny flowers, which grow in pairs, are known to bedevil bees by being a bit too inaccessible. The frequent presence of bees around the plant gives the plant its botanical name *apiana*, or "attractor of bees."

The plant has many thick stems, each of which carries opposite paired leaves. The leaves are 1 to 4 inches long and form a rosette at the end of the stem.

The plant is fairly frost resistant and thrives in hot, dry climates. Hot, sunny days help create the volatile oils that keep the leaves supple and provide the plant's most valuable characteristic. These oils include camphor and eucalyptol, which are released when the leaves are burned as incense.

HISTORICAL BACKGROUND

White sage has a rich history as a spiritual and medicinal plant. From ancient times, *Salvia* species have been associated with wisdom, longevity, and strength. The root of the name *Salvia* comes from the Latin verb *salvare*, meaning "to heal or save," another indication of its powerful medicinal and spiritual purposes. Historically, the Dutch used sage to barter with the Chinese, bringing as much as three times its weight in tea.

In divination sage is said to invoke wisdom,

give protection to the user, and help dreams come true. For this purpose, you can carry sage and a clear intention of your desires along with you. You can also bathe with sage and keep it in a place of reverence in your dwelling. Being anointed with sage as a powder, tea, or smoke brings clarity, protection, and wisdom. Planting sage in your garden will draw in and enhance powerful male energy and is a beautiful complement to the strong female energy of rosemary. When sage and rosemary grow together, the male and female energy are equally represented and in balance.

White sage is considered a sacred plant to many Native American tribes and has traditionally been burned for its healing smoke. The method of burning herbs for their healing qualities is often referred to as smudging. Native peoples throughout time have used sacred smoke in their spiritual healing traditions. The herbs are either tied into bundles or kept loose and then burned. White sage is traditionally burned as a single leaf, rather than as a bundle, because of its scarcity. When burned, different herbs emit different healing qualities. The smoke of white sage has been used to drive away evil spirits and to clear negative thoughts and feelings. The smudge of white sage is also used to keep negative entities away from areas where ceremonies are taking place. Sacred ceremonial objects are protected and kept safe by bundling them with sage. The aromatic and spirit powers of the plant can also be released by simply warming and rubbing the plant or placing it in a pot of water on the top of your woodstove.

During the sweat lodge ceremony, white sage tea is often splashed on heated stones when more steam is required. Also during the sweat lodge, people rub their bodies with sage for further purifying. Often sage is added to the fire, too.

There are many ways that white sage can be eaten. It gives of itself in so many ways that we may be both physically and spiritually nourished. The seeds, raw or cooked, can be mixed with cereals such as oats or wheat, ground into a powder and used as a mush, toasted then powdered and eaten dry, or used as a spice in cooking. Soaking seeds overnight makes them usable as a drink in water or fruit juice. The leaves can be used to flavor soups, stews, sauces, and other dishes. Use it sparingly, because white sage has a stronger flavor than garden sage, which is what recipes generally call for. The young stalks can be eaten raw, as can the peeled ripe stem tops.

The abundance of uses for white sage is not limited to food, medicine, and ceremony. A tea of white sage can be used as a hair shampoo and hair straightener. Powdered sage alone or in combination with white clay or cornstarch makes an excellent deodorant.

MEDICINAL USES

Salvia apiana is one of the most highly valued of the traditional ceremonial plants. Its rich, transforming smoke has been used for centuries to purify and cleanse.

White sage is antispasmodic and astringent. It is used to slow secretions, such as night sweats and milk flow, and to treat dysentery. It is also antibiotic and antiseptic and aids in treatment of mouth sores, burns, insect bites, and bleeding gums. Pharyngitis can be treated with tea used as a gargle. The tea can be used as a blood tonic.

In *Medicinal Plants of the Pacific West*, Michael Moore describes the tincture as being effective against staph, *Candida*, and *Klebsiella pneumoniae*. The tea and tincture are used for chest colds, as are the vapors from steamed leaves. Effectiveness is increased if used at the early onset of a cold or flu. The douche is effective for acute *Candida vaginitis*. Moore also recommends alternating tea with a hydrogen peroxide wash to treat skin abrasions and injuries.

White sage contains a volatile oil whose chief chemical constituent is thujone, which is contraindicated for epileptics and pregnant women.

PREPARATION AND DOSAGE

Tinctures should be 1:2 for fresh or 1:5 for dried herbs. The menstruum is 50 percent alcohol. The dosage is 20 to 60 drops up to five times per day. Because of the thujone content the tincture should not be used internally for more than seven to ten days.

A douche may be made with 1 teaspoon tincture per cup of warm water (you can also use this as a simple tea). Douches should be limited to once a day for no longer than a week.

A tea is prepared by steeping 1 ounce of herbs to 1 quart of water for an hour. Drink 2 to 4 ounces up to four times a day. The tea contains very little thujone.

Gargles are made with 3 parts water to 1 part tincture or as a simple infusion. Gargling often— every three hours—will expedite your healing.

Sitz baths can be prepared by adding $1/2$ ounce of the herbs to your tub.

The powder is useful as a topical dressing.

Steams may be prepared with $1/2$ ounce of crushed herbs added to a pot of simmering water.

PROPAGATION AND CULTIVATION

White sage can be cultivated, if care is taken. It prefers a well-drained, rich, sandy soil that is not overly wet. If your area is not warm and dry, it may be best to cultivate the plant as an annual or bring it indoors for winter.

Sow seeds in very sandy soil and water daily. The average germination time is fourteen days. Fire treatment will increase the likelihood of germination; otherwise, germination rates are low. This treatment consists of planting the seeds in a wooden flat and burning a small pile of dry kindling above them. Allow the seedlings to rise through the ash. In the wild *Salvia apiana* is a dominant recovery plant after fires and helps reclaim the scorched earth.

Cuttings may be successfully taken of half-ripe wood in the spring and early summer.

HARVESTING

Collect the leafing stems or the leaf rosettes. To optimize plant regeneration, harvest only by pinching off the tops of the leafy shoots. They may be used fresh or can be dried on a drying rack or in a paper bag. Because of its strong and powerful characteristics, white sage may be harvested at any time of the year. However, according to Michael Moore, its strength is highest in early summer and midsummer, but the difference is minimal. The best time for harvesting is after the plant has seeded and is somewhat dormant. This is usually between May and November.

UpS RECOMMENDATIONS

• Use only cultivated plants or wild-harvest sparingly and only for personal use.

• Possible substitutes are garden sage (*Salvia officinalis*), sagebrush (*Artemisia tridentata*), and mugwort (*Artemisia vulgaris*).

White sage is a plant with a long history of wide and varied uses, ranging from a topical astringent to a purifying and healing smudge. As with many plants, the more time you spend with it, harvesting it, preparing it, and concocting with it, the more you will learn and deeply understand its many gifts. At this time in our history, it is important to help protect and preserve all our native plant species. Optimally, white sage should only be harvested from cultivated plants. If these are not available, wild-harvest sparingly from the tops of the leafy shoots of summer. The plant will produce two more new shoots. Harvest only what you need for personal use, remembering to choose analogs (see UpS Recommendations) when appropriate.

REFERENCES

Facciola, S. *Cornucopia—A Source Book of Edible Plants*. Vista, Calif.: Kampong Publications, 1990.

Hickman, James C., ed. *The Jepson Manual: Higher Plants of California*. Berkeley: University of California Press, 1993.

Kunkel, G. *Plants for Human Consumption*. Koenigstein, Germany: Koeltz Scientific Books, 1984.

Moerman, D. *Native American Ethnobotany*. Portland, Oreg.: Timber Press Oregon, 1998.

Moore, Michael. *Medicinal Plants of the Pacific West*. Santa Fe: Red Crane Books, 1993.

WILD INDIGO
Baptisia tinctoria

DAVID BUNTING

Wild indigo, often referred to by the generic name *Baptisia* in herbal medicine, was once a well-known and popular medicine. It was used by "regular" doctors, traditional herbalists, Eclectic physicians, physiomedicalists, and homeopaths. The classic Eclectic text *King's American Dispensatory* notes that while wild indigo was "a favorite drug of the early Eclectics, it has fallen into unmerited neglect." Little has changed in this respect; wild indigo continues to be greatly overlooked as an herbal remedy. The neglect is still unwarranted because wild indigo is as relevant a remedy today as it was 150 years ago.

BOTANICAL FEATURES

Wild indigo is a member of the genus *Baptisia*, one of about six hundred genera in the Fabaceae or Pea family. The genus contains about thirty to thirty-five species native to North America. Other common names include shoofly, horsefly weed, and rattleweed. *B. tinctoria* grows mainly in the southeastern United States but can range north to New England and west to Minnesota. This species prefers dry soil, growing in drier woodlands and especially the dry,

sandy, coastal areas of the Southeast. Associated with poor soil in general, it is rarely encountered in rich, loamy conditions.

A hardy perennial herb, wild indigo grows from 2 to 4 feet tall with alternate leaves, consisting of three leaflets up to 1 inch long. Blooming in summer, the flowers are bright yellow and papilionaceous—which means "resembling a butterfly"—a form typical of the Pea family. Flowers are born in racemes, each with ten stamens that are separate. The fruit is a short, inflated legume.

HISTORICAL BACKGROUND

Wild indigo is indigenous only to North America, so our knowledge of traditional use comes entirely from North American Indians. The Penobscot, of what is now Maine, used a decoction of wild indigo in combination with six other herbs for treatment of gonorrhea. In the Southeast, the Creek used a decoction externally and internally for children who seemed drowsy, lifeless, and on the verge of becoming sick. The Mohegan, of the southern New England coastal area, steeped the root and used the infusion as a wash for cuts and wounds. A related species, *Baptisia leucantha*, was used by the Meskwaki in combination with other plants for treatment of eczema, sores, and snakebite.

Along with medicine, wild indigo has several other traditional uses. Both the common and botanical names allude to some of these. The generic name *Baptisia* is derived from the Greek *baptizo*, meaning "to dip under water." The specific name *tinctoria* is derived from the Latin *tinctorius*, "belonging to dyeing." The common name wild indigo is derived from the use of the leaves as a dye substitute for true indigo *(Indigofera tinctoria)*. Dyeing with wild indigo was generally abandoned in favor of the superior blue color obtained from true indigo. The flowering tops have also been used to repel flies and other insects. Bunches of the plant were fastened to harnesses to keep flies off draft horses.

The young shoots have been eaten like asparagus, particularly in New England. As with young pokeweed *(Phytolacca americana)*, wild indigo shoots can become increasingly toxic as they mature, especially given the amounts consumed when eaten as a food. James Thacher comments that those eating the vegetable have doubtlessly observed its drastic "evacuating powers."

In 1830 wild indigo was included as *Baptisia* in the first revision of the *United States Pharmacopoeia (USP)*, published in New York. It was dropped in 1840 and did not appear in the second *USP* revision, published in 1842. Wild indigo was never reinstated as an official drug of the *USP*.

Eclectic physicians during the 1800s and early 1900s held wild indigo in very high esteem. John Scudder, a prominent Eclectic elder, calls wild indigo one of the most valuable remedies we have for sore mouth and sore throat. Harvey Felter, who contributed to some of the finest Eclectic medical writings, also found wild indigo distinctly useful for septic conditions such as putrid forms of sore throat and tonsillitis. Professor Locke, professor of materia medica at the Eclectic College in Cincinnati, taught that wild indigo always be given internally and applied locally.

Scudder recommends wild indigo for all cases of enfeebled capillary circulation with a tendency to ulceration, to be used internally and externally and in all cases of softening or breaking down of tissue. Felter found wild indigo most useful when tissues are swollen, dusky, or blanched with free secretions and active sloughing of tissue. Lloyd Brothers Pharmacy of Cincinnati manufactured a specialty line of extracts used by most of the later Eclectic physicians. The label for its Specific Medicine Baptisia began, "This is one of our most important remedies." Indications included purplish, reddish, or dusky coloration of the mucous membranes. Tissue discoloration, degradation, and sepsis were the classic indications used by Eclectic physicians.

Wild indigo was probably best known as an epidemic remedy, especially for typhoid-related epidemics. In typhoid, typhoid-related conditions, and epidemic dysentery, Felter gives the somewhat horrifying indication of stools resembling "prune juice or fetid meat washings." Locke found wild indigo to be the best remedy to protect the groups of lymph nodules in the intestines, known as Peyer's patches, from the degradation common in typhoid.

Many of the historical indications and uses for wild indigo are very similar throughout Western medicine. John King, one of the grandfathers of Eclectic medicine, recognized wild indigo as a remedy for the entire glandular system. It has been found to increase not only intestinal secretions but also those of the liver, useful in hepatic derangement. Of special interest are the peripheral observations regarding wild indigo made by the brilliant Eclectic diagnostician Finley Ellingwood. He states that it reinforces the blood, exerts a pronounced tonic effect, and, very similar to the Creek Indian use, overcomes weariness and "produces a sense of vigor and general improved tone and well-being."

MEDICINAL USES

Wild indigo acts as a metabolic stimulant, accelerating expulsion of waste and speeding repair of tissue. Antiseptic, alterative, and immune enhancing, this remedy is especially effective in conditions related to deficient, weak, or enfeebled states. Wild indigo combines well with echinacea for any alterative or immune system applications.

Tincture of the root is useful in atonic states when depressed vitality is suppressing immunity. It is highly effective in adverse reactions to inoculations, congested or enlarged lymph nodes, spongy gums, gastric or duodenal ulcers, ulcerative colitis, septic sore throat, and many other conditions that are still seen today. Wild indigo is applicable in most conditions that involve putrid discharges, ulceration, or infection.

In Naturopathic medicine, wild indigo is recommended for ulcerative colitis, amoebic dysentery, and intestinal toxemia, often in combination with myrrh when putrescence or offensive secretions are present. For tonsillitis and quinsy (inflammation of the throat), it has been recommended together with poke fruit as a gargle. For eroded cervix, wild indigo is used with calendula on a tampon for local application. Kuts-Cheraux recommends an oral wash of wild indigo for gingivitis. In mammitis and cracked nipples, he uses a compress of the decoction or infusion in conjunction with witch hazel and glycerine. All topical treatments are given in conjunction with internal wild indigo.

Several species of wild indigo have been the subject of research into the immune activity of plant constituents. Investigations into the activity of glycoproteins in *Baptisia tinctoria* by Beuscher and other researchers have shown positive results. H. Wagner has led investigations into the activity of polysaccharides and glycosides from *B. tinctoria* and M. Udayama into the triterpenoidal saponins in *B. australis*.

Wild indigo contains polysaccharides, glycoproteins, quinolizidine alkaloids, hydroxycoumarins, and various glucosides. It acts as an antiseptic, stimulating, and astringent alterative, a circulatory stimulant and discutient, reducing swollen tissues. The ethanolic extract of wild indigo has been shown to stimulate the immune system. It has a significantly positive effect on the phagocytic action of human erythrocytes; it has been found to raise leukocyte count and improve immunity. Wild indigo is also mildly estrogenic.

PREPARATION AND DOSAGE

The whole plant *Baptisia tinctoria* was originally official in the *USP*. By the time wild indigo was included in the *National Formulary*, the dried root was the officially recognized drug. Fresh root is also used as medicine and is more active than the dried root. Here, there were differences of opinion among various schools of medicine. Cook's *Physio-Medical Dispensatory* claims that fresh wild indigo should never be used, because it is too strong. The seminal Eclectic work *King's American Dispensatory* states that wild indigo "loses much of its activity when dried or boiled" and that the "dried plant is almost worthless." Thacher also notes that the effects of the root are greatly diminished by long storage.

Wild indigo is a remedy that is best used locally, as well as internally, whenever possible. This is seen in traditional Native American medicine as well as the various schools of more recent medicine. Locke emphasizes the use of wild indigo locally as an antiseptic wash, especially in cases of ulceration of mucous membranes with a tendency toward putrescence. The numerous methods of local application proposed by Kuts-Cheraux attest to the flexibility and range available in using wild indigo.

Preparations include infusions, decoctions, tinctures, and fluid extracts. Infusions and decoctions are generally made from dried root, since fresh is not usually available. The infusion, made with 1 ounce of root to 2 cups of water, is given in doses of 1 tablespoon every one, two, or four hours as required. The dose of dried root is 1 gram or the equivalent. Therefore, the fluid extract, which was the official preparation, is given in average doses of 1 ml.

Alcohol extracts allow the use and preservation of the fresh root and its activity. Fresh root tincture at a strength of 1:2 may be given in doses up to 1 ml, two times daily. The equivalent would be approximately $1/4$ to $1/2$ gram of fresh root twice daily. The tincture may be applied topically full strength or diluted with a small amount of water or glycerine where appropriate.

In large doses wild indigo is emetic and cathartic, and any preparation should be reduced or discontinued if these symptoms occur. Large doses may also cause increased and thickened saliva, insomnia, restlessness, ocular disturbances, and a general soreness in the body. In excessive doses wild indigo can be toxic and reportedly accelerates respiration reflex activity, eventually leading to paralysis of respiration and death.

PROPAGATION AND CULTIVATION

Wild indigo thrives in poor, sandy, and dry soil, which is not a common garden scenario. This is in contrast to related species, such as *Baptisia australis*, that enjoy common garden conditions. Planting on hillsides may help in providing the excellent drainage this plant requires. Seeds should be started in sandy soil after they have been scored with sandpaper. They can be sown directly or started in individual pots in the spring, grown out for the summer, and planted in the fall. Seeds sown in the summer greenhouse should be set out the following spring. Once established, plants may be propagated from root divisions. Plants can be lifted and divided in the early fall, which can be incorporated as part of harvest.

HARVESTING

At the time of Thacher's writing, wild indigo was apparently "growing in great abundance in almost every barren pasture, and in the woods." The commonness of the plant was echoed by Stille and Maisch in 1887. Unfortunately, populations have declined and this is no longer the case. Most supplies of wild indigo are harvested from the wild, which is an unacceptable practice at this time.

The root crowns should be split at harvest, with a healthy section replanted to assure the continuance of the population. The root is very twisted and knotty, requiring thorough washing to remove pockets of dirt. At this point, the roots should ideally be processed into medicine while fresh. If dried material is required, expect the roots to take on a blackish coloration during the drying process.

UpS RECOMMENDATIONS

• Use primarily cultivated resources.

• Boneset and cultivated echinacea are good alternatives, as well as spilanthes for its antimicrobial, fever-reducing, and antiseptic properties.

Why has wild indigo remained in near-obscurity for so many years? This may be partly due to its reputation for treating typhoid and related epidemic diseases. Its association with these diseases when they were rampant in the United States may have pigeonholed its use. Now that typhoid is not the concern it once was in North America, the many other uses of wild indigo may be overlooked.

In addition, opinions differed greatly among the various schools of medicine on the question of fresh versus dried wild indigo. It may well be true, as *King's American Dispensatory* claims, that wild indigo is nearly worthless when dried. If so, the advocates of dried plant material may have done a disservice both to wild indigo and to herbal medicine in general by promoting the use of an inferior drug.

If we choose to resurrect this plant as a regular member of our materia medica, we must explore two paths. First, we must learn how to cultivate *Baptisia tinctoria*. For the sake of continuity, our supplies of this botanical will need to come from cultivated rather than wild sources. Second, we should further examine the medical application of other species of *Baptisia*, such as *B. australis*. The species that are more readily adaptable to the garden may also serve as suitable therapeutic substitutes for *B. tinctoria*.

In this way, our healing will be twofold. We will be assured of keeping this cherished medicine in our herbal repertory, available for treating illness. Moreover, there is the healing we will derive from helping preserve this amazing plant in the wild lands.

REFERENCES

Bailey, L. H. *The Standard Cyclopedia of Horticulture*. Vol. 1. London: MacMillan, 1925.

Beuscher, N., et al. "Stimulation of immunity by the contents of Baptisia tinctoria." *Planta Medica* 57 (5): 381–84 (Oct. 1995).

Beuscher, N., K. H. Scheit, C. Bodinet, and L. Kopanski. "Immunologically active glycoproteins of Baptisia tinctoria." *Planta Medica* 51 (4): 358–63 (Aug. 1989).

Boericke, W. *Pocket Manual of Homeopathic Materia Medica*. New Dehli: B. Jain Publisher, 1975.

Boyle, W. *Official Herbs: Botanical Substances in the United States Pharmacopoeias 1820–1990*. East Palestine, Ohio: Buckeye Naturopathic Press, 1991.

Cech, R. *Horizon Herbs, Strictly Medicinal Growing Guide and 1998 Catalog*. Williams, Oreg.: author, 1998.

Claus, E. P., and V. E. Tyler. *Pharmacognosy*, 5th ed. Philadelphia: Lea & Febiger, 1965.

Ellingwood, Finley. *American Materia Medica, Therapeutics and Pharmacognosy*. 1898. Reprint, Portland, Oreg.: Eclectic Medical Publications, 1983.

Felter, Harvey Wickes, M.D., ed. *Syllabus of Eclectic Materia Medica and Therapeutics*. Cincinnati: John M. Scudder's Sons, 1985.

Felter, Harvey Wickes, M.D. *Eclectic Materia Medica, Pharmacology and Therapeutics*. Cincinnati: John K. Scudder, 1922.

Felter, Harvey Wickes, M.D., and John Uri Lloyd. *King's American Dispensatory*. 1898. Reprint, Portland, Oreg.: Eclectic Medical Publications, 1983.

Flemming, T., chief ed. *Physician's Desk Reference for Herbal Medicines*. Montvale, N.J.: Medical Economics, 1998.

Hedrick, U. P. *Sturtevant's Notes on Edible Plants*. Albany: State of New York Department of Agriculture, 1919.

Henkel, A. *American Root Drugs*. Washington, D.C.: United States Department of Agriculture, 1907.

Hocking, G. M. *A Dictionary of Natural Products*. Medford, N.J.: Plexus Publishing, 1997.

Homeopathic Materia Medica, Vol 1. 8th ed. Falls Church, Va.: American Institute of Homeopathy, 1979.

Hughes, R. *A Manual of Pharmacodynamics*. New Dehli: B. Jain Publishers, 1988.

Jaeger, E. C. *A Source Book of Biological Names and Terms*. Springfield, Ill.: Charles C. Thomas, 1955.

King. J. *The American Dispensatory*. Cincinnati: Moore, Wilstach, Keys and Co., 1859.

Kutz-Chereaux, A. W., ed. *Naturae Medicina and Naturopathic Dispensatory*. Des Moines: American Naturopathic Physicians and Surgeons Association, 1953.

Lloyd Brothers. *Dose Book of Specific Medicines*. Cincinnati: Lloyd Brothers, 1907.

Merck Index, 12th ed. Whitehouse Station, N.J.: Merck, 1996.

Millspaugh, Charles F. *American Medicinal Plants, an Illustrated and Descriptive Guide to the American Plants Used as Homeopathic Remedies*. 1884–1885. Reprint, New York: Dover, 1974.

National Formulary, 5th ed. Easton, Penn.: American Pharmaceutical Association, 1926.

National Formulary, 4th ed. Philadelphia: American Pharmaceutical Association, 1921.

Priest, A. W., and L. R. Priest. *Herbal Medication*. London: L. N. Fowler, 1982.

Scudder, John M., M.D. *Specific Medication and Specific Medicines*. Cincinnati: John K. Scudder, 1913.

Smith, E. *Therapeutic Herb Manual*. Williams, Oreg.: author, 1999.

Staff of the L. H. Bailey Hortorium. *Hortus Third*. New York: MacMillan, 1976.

Stille, A., and J. Maisch. *The National Dispensatory*. Philadelphia: Lea Brothers, 1887.

Thacher, J. *The American New Dispensatory*. Boston: Thomas B. Wait, 1821.

Udayama, M., et al. *Phytochemistry* 48 (7): 1233–35 (Aug. 1998).

Uphof, J. C. *Dictionary of Economic Plants*. New York: J. Cramer Stechert-Hafner Service Agency, 1968.

Vogel, Virgil J. *American Indian Medicine*. Norman: University of Oklahoma Press, 1970.

Wagner, H., et al. *Arzneimittelforschung* 34 (6): 659–61 (1984).

———. *Chem Ber.* 102 (9): 3006-08 (1969).

AMERICAN WILD YAM

Dioscorea villosa and *Dioscorea quaternata*

❦

RICHO CECH

As I entered the greenhouse, the humidity and heat enveloped me in a familiar embrace. I bent to push aside the stoneroot plants that surrounded the central bench, and was treated to a deep, lemony fragrance emanating from their yellow flowers. An old calendula plant was inadvertently jiggled and sprayed seeds at my feet. Going down on my knees and peering into the dark, weed-protected recesses under the bench, I found the huge pot of wild yam with its upright vines. Early that spring these vines had tendriled their way up through the slats in the benches, now creating over my bent back a giant plume of heart-shaped leaves and hanging, three-winged fruits.

I was ready to harvest wild yam rhizomes for autumn replanting, but was having a hard time moving the pot. In fact, restricted in this mousehole of a space between the central pole of the greenhouse and a wooden side leg of the bench, I couldn't gain enough leverage even to budge the pot. Then as my pupils widened in the half-light, I noticed why this pot was so immobile. A large branching rhizome had pushed its way through the drainage hole and solidly anchored itself into the sandy loam and stones

of the greenhouse floor. I had to smile at the tenaciousness of this plant, strongly identifying with its urge to find freedom from the confines of a plastic pot. Wielding my trusty snips, I trimmed the vines off above the pot, then with some difficulty snipped the rhizome at the point where it entered the dirt.

Next spring, the new vines would emerge from this remaining piece of rhizome, becoming another permanent feature of this old greenhouse where ginkgo trees, hawthorns, and legions of celandine, larkspur, thistles, grasses, wild lettuce, catnip, clover, buttercups, purslane, plantain, and vervain had already escaped in uncontrolled riot. You get the picture. As someone once said upon entering: "Weedy." I guess a lot of it comes from my relative respect for weeds and my reticence to demolish good medicine, but the rest of it comes from my own inability to keep up with pulling weeds. They always win.

Turning the wild yam pot on its side, I rolled it out past the stoneroots and over the calendula, noticing as I did so that the alligator-shaped seeds were now being pressed into the eclectic soil mix of the floor, assuring that the yellow and orange flowers would again usher in the spring. I dumped out the pot, revealing a contorted mass of light brown rhizomes, and began to separate and break them into lengths for replanting. The wholesome smell of wild yam, which my friend John once likened to "your mom's good cooking," arose in the heat. More potting soil spilled from the tough rootball and covered the calendula seeds with a nice, cushy layer as I continued to wrench away piece after piece of the rhizome. In this fresh state the rhizomes of the wild yam could be broken with effort, but I knew that once they dried, they would be immutable and as hard as bone. The cuttings, carrying their load of fine root hairs and potting soil, were plunked into a bucket and eventually carried into the seed house to weigh. They tipped the scales at more than 5 pounds.

That's what I like about wild yam. Among the forest-dependent species, it increases the fastest. In the wilds I've seen big ones at the edge of the woods climb 20 feet into a poplar tree. Working there in the Kentucky shade, poking around after the rhizomes, I found that they covered a prodigious subsurface expanse, gnarling their way among tree roots and through the roots of grasses and other herbs. In its native habitat and under cultivation as well, wild yam is big medicine.

BOTANICAL FEATURES

The wild yam root of commerce is actually the entire underground structure of the wild yam, technically a rhizome (thickened, underground stem) and the associated wiry roots. These native American species are herbaceous perennial climbing vines. They are dioecious, having separate male and female plants. The female plants of both species bear distinctive, three-celled fruits that are held curiously upright from the drooping spike by means of a short, hook-shaped stalk. When the fruit dries, it turns from bright green to a papery brown and, upon breaking open, reveals a silvery, mother-of-pearl interior. Each pod contains up to six seeds, which are chocolate brown, flat, and winged for transport by the air.

DIOSCOREA VILLOSA

The plant grows in colonies or clumps at the edge of the forest, where it can find purchase to climb among trees and bushes and where it receives plenty of light. The multiple smooth, green stems bear prominently veined, heart-shaped leaves, sometimes occurring in a whorl at the base of the plant, sometimes not. Progressing upward, the leaves attach alternately up the stem, diminishing in size as they reach the tip of the vine. The underside of the leaves may demonstrate a very short pubescence, but apparently this feature has become less prominent since the 1800s. There is regional variation within the species and a possible intergrading of types. The rhizome runs parallel to the ground surface, with wiry roots underneath and short, blunt branches on the sides. The stems strike up from the top of the rhizome. The rhizome grows from the leading tip, and tends to increase its mass by running out, not by becoming thicker.

DIOSCOREA QUATERNATA

The plant tends to grow singly in the deep forest or at the edges of the forest. It is not a very inspired climber and tends to be single stemmed; many plants may be found demonstrating only a single whorl of leaves without a vine. Older plants or, perhaps more accurately, plants that receive more nutrients and light will become multiple stemmed and vine up from the forest floor, draping over small brush, young trees, and fallen limbs. The leaves generally occur as two sets of whorls at the base of the plant, followed by an upper vining portion where the leaves occur alternately. The leaves are completely smooth, prominently veined, and heart shaped, and tend to be larger than those of *D. villosa*, perhaps indicating an adaptation to growing in darker areas. The rhizome is heavy and knuckled like the back of a fist. Wiry roots extend from every portion, and when these break off from the dried rhizome, the nubs can be quite prickly. The rhizome gets heavier by increasing its girth, growing out from the leading tip, and by branching out at the sides. I have seen specimens reach a length of 2 feet and grow as thick as my thumb (pretty thick).

Wild yam prefers moist, humid, mixed deciduous forests. The current distribution of both species encompasses most of the central and eastern states, from Minnesota south to Texas and across to the eastern seaboard, excluding the states of northern New England. However, wild yam can be expected to grow most prolifically in the South.

HISTORICAL BACKGROUND

There is scant evidence of the use of American wild yam among the Native Americans, perhaps because it is too hard to be eaten as food. There is, however, one ethnobotanical reference indicating that the Meskwaki tribe used the root to relieve pain at childbirth. This is consistent with the current use of the root extract as an antispasmodic for smooth muscles and demonstrates again that the Native Americans had a most accurate feel for the uses of the plants that grew around them. In my opinion, the most interesting historical reference to wild yam is found in *King's Dispensatory*. The authors mention that from the 1830s (when the Eclectic physicians first began to use the plant) up to the year 1850, the wild yam root of commerce was obtained solely from what they called true wild yam, a plant that was then and is now correctly identified as *Dioscorea villosa*. Between the years 1850 and 1860, druggists began to notice another type of root mixed into their raw material shipments, which at first they rejected as an adulterant. This new root was much thicker and appeared knuckly, or "knotted." The diggers, however, insisted that the vines associated with this new root, which came to be called false wild yam, were essentially identical, and eventually the druggists were compelled to accept this new root, especially since the true wild yam was becoming *"very scarce."* The false wild yam was named *Dioscorea villosa* var. *glabra* due to the smoothness of its leaves. This plant is today correctly identified as *D. quaternata*. However, the rhizomes of these two species of wild yam are still used interchangeably in commerce, and although most of the wild yam employed by herbalists these days is *D. quaternata*, it is almost without exception labeled as *D. villosa*. I find it most fascinating that a tradition of adulteration first accepted in 1860 prevails into the year 2000. I find it doubly interesting that issues of overharvest and insufficiency of herbal materials challenged the Eclectic physicians in the mid-1800s just as the increasing scarcity of native medicinal herbs challenges herbalists to this day.

MEDICINAL USES

As indicated by its alternate common names—colic root and rheumatism root—wild yam is generally used for allaying pain. Most especially, it has an antispasmodic influence on the gastrointestinal tract and the uterus. It is an old and well-respected treatment for acute abdominal pain, pain caused by gallstones, flatulence, spasmodic hiccups, menstrual cramps, pain and nausea during pregnancy, and rheumatic pain arising from liver and intestinal malfunction. Priest and Priest classify wild yam as a "general relaxant" and recommend the following combinations: wild yam, valerian, and black cohosh for dysmenorrhea and uterine pains; wild yam, cramp bark, and partridgeberry for nervousness, restlessness, and pains of pregnancy.

Wild yam contains a molecule known as diosgenin, which is used for the manufacture of progesterone and steroidal drugs. In fact, birth control pills were first manufactured from components derived from wild yam. However, wild yam does not contain human hormones, but rather the chemical precursors to these hormones. There is an ongoing debate among herbalists as to whether the human body is able to use wild yam, for instance, to assist in manufacture of increased levels of progesterone. There is no known physiological pathway for this synthesis, yet many women find relief from premenstrual syndrome and menopausal symptoms by taking wild yam in the form of a tincture, tea, or "cream." The creams are most popular. Some commercially manufactured products are made with concentrated extracts of the actual herb, while others contain as their active ingredient synthetically derived progesterone, which is readily absorbed through the skin. I have also noticed that, regardless of whether these creams contain botanical ingredients or not, they are with few exceptions called "Wild Yam Cream."

At Herb Pharm's analytical laboratory, an unpublished chromatographic study was performed comparing the chemistry of *Dioscorea villosa* and *D. quaternata* rhizomes. The purpose of this experiment was to investigate the impact of the industrywide practice of using *D. villosa* and *D. quaternata* interchangeably. First of all, the qualitative comparison of the two plants showed a high degree of similarity on the basis of all ten prominent compounds. This immediately put my mind at ease. The best kind of adulterant is one that does not differ in substance from the plant it resembles. In addition, a quantitative analysis was performed, testing the relative concentration of total saponins and diosgenin in the rhizomes of the two plants. The *D. villosa* contained only 71 percent of the concentration of total saponins found in *D. quaternata*. Additionally, the *D. villosa* contained only 77.5 percent as much diosgenin as the *D. quaternata*. So on the basis of this study at least, it appears that there is no major chemical difference between the two plants, and in fact the plant that the Eclectics named false wild yam may be even stronger than the true wild yam.

PREPARATION AND DOSAGE

Finely sliced and recently dried wild yam rhizome (root) can be made into a decoction or a tincture. To make a strong decoction (basically a simmered tea), put $1/2$ ounce of the dried root pieces or coarsely powdered root in 2 cups of cold water. Bring this slowly to the boiling point, then simmer for ten minutes, remove from the heat, and allow to return to room temperature. Then strain the decoction through a cheesecloth or tea strainer. The dosage is $1/4$ to $1/2$ cup twice daily or as circumstances require. The tea should not be held over for the next day, but rather made anew.

The tincture is made by combining 1 part by weight (in grams) of finely sliced or ground dried root with 5 parts of liquid (in ml). This liquid, which is known as the menstruum, consists of 50 percent distilled water and 50 percent grain alcohol (190 proof). Using this recipe, 100 grams of the dried root would be combined with 500 ml of menstruum, composed of 250 ml distilled water and 250 ml grain alcohol. The menstruum is added over the dried root in a jar, which is tightly capped and shaken. Then it is stored in a cool and dark place and shaken daily

for at least five weeks. The long maceration period is due to the fact that this very hard herb, especially if not thoroughly ground, takes a long time to fully extract. After maceration, the herb and liquid are poured off through cheesecloth and thoroughly squeezed into a bowl. The remaining herb, now divested of its medicinal virtues, may be composted. The light yellow liquid is poured back into a jar and allowed to sit overnight; it may then be filtered by pouring slowly through at least four layers of clean cheesecloth, in order to remove any remaining particulate matter. The resulting finished tincture should be stored in an amber glass bottle, in a cool place and out of the light. The dosage is 30 to 60 drops up to five times per day.

The correct dosage of any wild yam preparation is dependent on individual body weight, personal sensitivity, the degree of activity desired, and the urgency of the problem being addressed. Overdose of wild yam can cause nausea, so it is best to start with the lower dosage in order to assure that the herb is well tolerated. In acute conditions, it is not necessary to take any more of this herb than will do the job, but it may be necessary to continue dosage for an extended period of time in order to realize any hormone-regulating effects.

PROPAGATION AND CULTIVATION

Wild yam grows very well in warm, humid climates. If you live in the North, it makes sense to grow it in the greenhouse. If you live in South Carolina, grow it outdoors.

The seeds tolerate dry storage. They should

be sown in the fall, midwinter, or very early spring, outdoors in pots, flats, or directly in a shaded woodland nursery bed. Germination occurs in the spring as the ground warms up. The cold conditioning period, natural rain, snowfall, and oscillating temperatures afforded by sowing the seeds outdoors is a good stimulus to efficient germination. The seedlings are quite sensitive and should be left undisturbed for two years, except (of course) to keep them weeded and watered. Then, once the rootlet begins to swell into a rhizome, the seedling may be transplanted to its final location. The plant prefers open woodlands, partial shade at the edge of the forest, a shaded spot in the garden, or a moist and shady location right in the greenhouse. Because this is a vine, a suitable trellis should be erected, or the plant may be allowed to climb up into bushes and trees. Raising wild yam from seeds takes four years from sowing to harvest of a good-sized root.

It is easy to grow the plant from a piece of the rhizome. Cuttings are usually made in the fall, after the parent plant has matured its fruit and started to die back. Choose the young, vigorous, and growing portions of the rhizome, which are covered with many root hairs, then cut or break the piece to at least 2 inches in length. The cuttings can be planted out immediately, thereby allowing them to become accustomed to the new environment before the growing season. Spring transplanting is possible, but disturbance at this time of year can damage the newly emerging vines. Planted in a good spot in the woods, a nice cutting will grow into a harvestable-sized plant in two or three years.

Planted in shaded beds or pots in the greenhouse, the plants will attain harvestable size in a single season, with significant added yield if the plants are allowed to grow for a full two years.

HARVESTING

As with most roots, the best time to dig wild yam is in the fall, after the plant has stored nutrients to carry it through the winter. The roots do not strike very deeply in the soil, but rather crawl around just beneath the surface. The vines are cut back and the rhizome is popped up out of the ground with a spade or trowel and shaken free of clinging dirt or debris. Then the growing tip, attached to at least 4 inches of solid rhizome, is replanted back into the loosened dirt and covered with leaf mulch. This will assure the resurgence of a plant in this spot the following year. The harvested rhizome, with its many wiry rootlets, is thoroughly washed, cut up into small pieces with snips, then dried in the shade on screens. Once dried, these smaller pieces can (with difficulty) be ground to a coarse powder in a coffee grinder or hammer mill. If you forget to snip the fresh root into pieces before drying, you will find that it is *impossible* to snip it into small pieces after drying. I once watched an apprentice try to break up dried wild yam roots on the front porch using a cold chisel, a brick, and a sledgehammer. He had on a pair of protective goggles and had set up a box to try to catch the pieces, which were ending up almost everywhere but in the box. I picked up several, about the size and hardness of ivory dice, from the middle of the driveway . . . wild yam root is the hardest substance known to the herbalist, and large pieces eat hammer mills alive.

Fresh wild yam root, on the average, has a water content of 64 percent. This means that every 10 pounds of fresh root harvested will dry down to 3.6 pounds of dried root. The rhizome should *always* be dried before use, because ingesting the fresh root may induce vomiting or other unpleasant symptoms. The roots should be thoroughly dried before storage; incompletely dried root will mold in closed storage. The dried root should be stored in sealed containers, in a cool place and out of the light. According to *King's American Dispensatory*, the root prepared in this manner is stable for only a year in storage, after which time any remaining herb should be discarded and replaced by recently harvested and dried material.

UpS RECOMMENDATIONS

- Choose cultivated resources if at all possible.
- Good alternatives include chamomile, licorice, and catnip. Peppermint is a good substitute for digestive issues.

Wild yam lives in a climax hardwood forest and its fate in the wilds rests with the future of this forest ecosystem, upon which it is dependent. As long as the forest is there, wild yam regenerates vigorously by means of clonal division, also spreading to previously uninhabited areas by disseminating its seeds. The rhizome is not subject to rot, and it is hard enough to withstand the onslaught of almost any insect—with the possible exception of highly industrious termites wearing goggles, wielding bricks and cold chisels. Disease does not seem to touch the plant, perhaps due to the presence of saponins, which serve to further protect it from insect predation. How old is wild yam? Counting stem scars on single-stemmed rhizomes of *Dioscorea quaternata* gives us an approximate age, and in so doing I have found healthy individuals that are at least sixty years old. As long as the forest prevails and we learn to fulfill our herbal needs through cultivation, this wild plant will continue to outlive us all. May it be ever so.

REFERENCES

Amarguaye, Ambrose, and Richard A. Cech. "Comparison of American Wild Yam Species." Williams, Oreg.: Herb Pharm Analytical Laboratory (Ed Smith, director), Nov. 1998.

Felter, Harvey Wickes, M.D., and John Uri Lloyd. *King's American Dispensatory*. Vol. 1. 1898. Reprint, Portland, Oreg.: Eclectic Medical Publications, 1983.

Priest, A. W., and L. R. Priest. *Herbal Medication*. London: L. N. Fowler, 1982.

Smith, Huron H. "Ethnobotany of the Meskwaki Indians." *Bulletin of the Public Museum of Milwaukee* 4 (1928): 175–326.

YERBA MANSA
Anemopsis californica

TIM BLAKLEY

Like so many other herbalists in the United States, I was first introduced to yerba mansa by Michael Moore. One year when he was teaching at the California School of Herbal Studies, where I resided for more than thirteen years, he was talking about several plants native to the southwestern United States. He began talking about one plant and suddenly became quite animated. I figured if he liked this herb, then it was a good one to get to know. He spoke about its various medicinal uses and how it grew in wet areas of the desert. Soon I became a firm believer in the merits and benefits of this plant.

Interestingly enough, the first time I encountered yerba mansa as a living, growing species was at my friend Kathy Krezak-Larson's garden in Iowa. She had dug up a couple of small plants while on a desert plant trip with Feather Jones and brought them back to her garden in the icy northern plains where, to the surprise of many, they thrived. I took a couple of divisions from those plants, and they also thrived at my home on the Iowa-Minnesota border. Since then I have raised more than a thousand plants from those original two that Kathy had brought back from the desert. I have grown them in five dif-

ferent growing zones and have passed on numerous plants to other herb growers. To say that yerba mansa is a hardy plant would definitely be an understatement. It is truly one of my most favorite herbs to grow and use.

BOTANICAL FEATURES

Yerba mansa is a member of the Saururaceae family, commonly known as the Lizard's-Tail family. This is a small family with only five genera. Seven species are found only in North America and East Asia. Yerba mansa is the only member of the genus *Anemopsis*. Other common names for it are Apache beads, yerba del manso, manso, lizard tail, and swamp root. Yerba mansa is a low-growing plant that sends out long runners that root along the way, forming large patches or stands of the plant. Its basal leaves are round to ovate, somewhat succulent, and grow from 3 to 8 inches in length. They often turn a reddish brown color during the growing season and become very red in the fall before dying back at severe frost. They will reappear in the spring from the established root crowns. The flowers are white and quite beautiful, rising

266

about 12 inches above the ground. Though several references list the plant as growing up to 2 feet in height, I have never measured one taller than 16 inches when in full flower. The flowers turn brown as the seeds mature. The entire plant is aromatic; Moore describes it as smelling like a cross between camphor and eucalyptus, and I agree. I find the smell very appealing.

Yerba mansa is native to the southwestern United States and Mexico. It is found in California, Nevada, Utah, Arizona, New Mexico, and Texas. In California it grows as far north as the delta region east of San Francisco. It grows well into Texas, following the Rio Grande nearly to the Gulf. It thrives in the wet areas of the region—which are somewhat rare. It will grow both in fresh water and in boggy or low sink areas of the dry valleys. From personal experience, it appears to be hardy from Zone 4 to Zone 9. In both Zones 4 and 5, I recommend mulching to protect it from extreme winter cold.

HISTORICAL BACKGROUND

This plant has a long history of use among the people who have lived in its native region. It was and is still used by both the Native American and Hispanic populations of the Southwest. There is a reference to it being used by the Ohlone Indians in central California as a root decoction for alleviating menstrual cramps. The Eclectic physicians of the late nineteenth and early twentieth centuries used it for a variety of conditions. It appears to have been introduced into Eclectic use by Dr. W. H. George of California in 1877, though Bergner mentions that

it was mainly used in the western states. It was also used in homeopathic formulations and is still used today by several companies.

Yerba mansa is not commonly used in the rest of the United States. I travel about the country from region to region for better than half the year talking to natural food store workers, and by far the majority of those people have never used, recommended, or even heard of yerba mansa. The areas where I do find familiarity with the herb are in the Boulder-Denver region, the Southwest, and California. Only a few herbalists have been major proponents of yerba mansa in this country, and only a few companies sell much of it.

MEDICINAL USES

Yerba mansa has many medicinal uses, most relating to its actions on the mucous membranes. It is used as a mucous membrane tonic and intestinal tonic; it is good for skin ulcers, staph infections, and other bacterial infections both internally and externally. It is astringent, diuretic, antibacterial, and antifungal. Somewhat similar to goldenseal in its actions on the mucous membranes, it has been touted in recent years as a goldenseal substitute. It does not contain any berberine, hydrastine, or the other alkaloids that goldenseal or its more common substitutes do. It appears to have a significant percentage of essential oil, and its actions may be primarily or at least partly due to its volatile constituents.

Herbalists who use yerba mansa tend to love it and speak very highly of it. It gives a very warm sensation when swallowed, which in my opinion

Yerba Mansa

is quite pleasing. It also creates a soothing feeling. In talking with several herbalists, I've discovered that many have strong feelings about the plant. Daniel Gagnon, an herbalist from New Mexico, uses it to strengthen connective tissue and for skin ulcerations, gastrointestinal ulcerations, urinary problems, and some forms of gout. He uses it extensively for sore throats and other inflamed mucous membrane tissues, especially when the inflammation has become chronic. Feather Jones, an herbalist from Colorado, uses it in respiratory congestion if the mucus is hard to cough up, for herpes, *Candida* formulas, skin ulcerations, hemorrhoids, urinary tract infections, arthritis formulas, diaper rash, and subacute mucous membrane infections. Tammi Hartung, grower and herbalist from Colorado, uses it mainly for bacterial infections, staph infections, and for "stuck" conditions in which a "kick in the pants" is needed. Michael Moore lists it as beneficial for boggy, poorly healing infections that have reached the "cold," or nonrepairing congestive conditions. He considers it of benefit for slow-healing conditions of the mouth, intestinal and urinary tracts, and lungs; as a diuretic that stimulates uric acid secretion for potential arthritis benefit; and as an external antibacterial and antifungal.

PREPARATION AND DOSAGE

Both the leaf and the root have been and are used for medicinal purposes, though the root is by far the most often-used part of the plant. Using the dried plant material is most common, though the fresh plant has been utilized as both a tea and a tincture. Because the plant is aromatic and its volatile constituents are very active, the drying technique is critical. Many growers and wildcrafters dry herbs at high temperatures to facilitate a quick turnaround of material and to reduce chances of fungal or bacterial contamination. However, with yerba mansa or any plant with significant volatile constituents, it is imperative to use lower temperatures for drying. I suggest temperatures of between 80 and 100 degrees. As with burdock, the root should be sliced to facilitate drying at these temperatures.

Yerba mansa can be used as a tea or tincture (extract), dried in capsules, or as a homeopathic preparation. I do not recommend it as a bulk herb, because the volatile components will degrade relatively rapidly.

As a tea it is best used as a dried herb. Volatile components seem to be much more readily soluble in water when dried first. Still, as a fresh tea it has a subtle but delightful flavor and goes down smoothly with a refreshing aftertaste. The leaf is easy to use in the fresh state, and I recommend it over the root because it is easy to harvest and use. As a dried tea it is even more effervescent, but I recommend the root for extra strength.

As a tincture or extract, it can be prepared from fresh or dried material. Most herbalists recommend a ratio of 1:2 for a fresh tincture and 1:5 for a tincture made of dried material. This ratio represents the percentage of the herb to the menstruum, or liquid portion. The menstruum should have an alcohol percentage of approximately 60 percent, with distilled water

268

making up the other 40 percent. The tincture, after being mixed, should sit for a minimum of three weeks and should be shaken daily. After that, it should be filtered through an appropriate medium to eliminate any solids. At home, cheesecloth and strong hands are usually utilized, while in a laboratory a press and filter combination can be used.

The dosage is based somewhat on the condition it is being used for. For a nonacute condition use 30 to 60 drops of tincture, or 1 to 2 dropperfuls, one to three times daily. For a severe sore throat or gum disease, gargling with the tea or extract every hour is beneficial. For external use as an antibacterial or antifungal, it is best to apply it frequently. Remember that the dosage is always based on a variety of factors, such as purpose of use, weight, type of product you are consuming (tea versus tincture), and personal needs or sensitivity.

PROPAGATION AND CULTIVATION

As noted earlier, yerba mansa is hardy from Zone 4 to Zone 9. I've seen several references that restrict its hardiness to Zone 7 or Zone 8, but it is easily hardy to Zone 5 and, I think, to Zone 4 with mulch applied for winter protection. It will grow in virtually any type of soil, and its fertility needs seem minimal. We have much more to learn about what fertility levels will enhance its production; perhaps in the future we will have answers for growers as to the conditions it will produce best in.

Yerba mansa is very easy to propagate from divisions taken from the spreading stems that root at each node. To facilitate this, you could more or less layer the stems by intentionally burying selected stems. You can also make cuttings of the stem using two nodes, one under the rooting medium and one above. Whether there are leaves present or not is not critical. It will take approximately three weeks for rooting to occur. Keep the cuttings moist. Propagation from seeds is not as easy. For several years I had zero success in germinating the seeds. I discovered the secret accidentally when I took several seed trays and put them on my heat bench, which I normally use for cuttings. The seeds germinated in about four weeks. They obviously need heat to germinate, and they prefer extreme heat. I suggest temperatures of close to 100 degrees during the day with slightly lower temperatures during the night. Germination should occur in three to four weeks and will be close to 75 percent. Plants are ready for transplanting in approximately eight weeks. As I write this, I'm looking out my window to my greenhouse where an entire table of baby yerba mansa plants (several thousand) are growing. These were started in late summer and will be held over until spring for planting. A fall planting in a cold climate is not advisable.

I suggest planting on 12-inch centers in rows. Set row spacing to best utilize any cultivation equipment you might have. Weed control is crucial in the early stages. The plants like full sun but will grow in partial shade, especially in the hot and dry Southwest. Though a desert plant, yerba mansa needs water. Depending on the soil type, humidity levels, and moisture levels in the soil, it will need from one to several major waterings during the dry part of the growing season. At this point, I'm not aware of any major disease problems associated with yerba mansa.

HARVESTING

Up until this past year, virtually 100 percent of the yerba mansa crop came from wildcrafted material. The root has traditionally been harvested in the fall after the foliage has died back. The age of the roots has really not been an issue. After harvesting, as mentioned before, it must be carefully dried at between 80 and 100 degrees with adequate airflow. As I often mention when giving a presentation on drying, the three most important things to remember are "airflow, airflow, and airflow." The material will take several days to dry depending on temperature, humidity, amount of airflow, and the original moisture content of the root. Make sure the dried material is stored in dark containers and not exposed to high temperatures or moisture after storing.

While you can get a reasonable harvest after one growing season, I don't believe that this is the ideal time to harvest in order to maximize profit. Yerba mansa is primarily a second-year crop that can be extended to three years. Currently, we have a trial under way that will give us the data we need to determine the best time to harvest. Harvesting can be done either with a shovel or a spade (if you're growing only a small amount). If the crop is significant, than a root digger would be preferable. There is no accurate data yet on yields, though that information should be available within two or three years.

UpS RECOMMENDATIONS

- Use cultivated resources only, if you can find them.
- Possible alternatives are tormentil (*Potentilla tormentilla*) and self-heal (*Prunella vulgaris*).

At this time yerba mansa is a minor herb in terms of the amount of material being consumed. However, I believe it has the potential to become a major herb due to its many beneficial and multifaceted medicinal actions. At present, virtually the entire supply comes from wildcrafted material. It grows in wet areas of the desert, and in many cases these areas are depositories for liquid farm runoff. I believe that some of the yerba mansa harvested today is probably tainted with these chemicals—and that percentage will only increase as the herb becomes more popular. In addition, it has the potential to be overpicked to the point where wild populations will begin to shrink. This has an impact on its natural environment, because yerba mansa is a key ingredient in the health of many of the muddy bogs in which it grows. The solution to the problem is, of course, cultivation. We can easily meet the needs of the market by simply growing all of our yerba mansa. Within three or four years nearly all the yerba mansa consumed in the United States could, and should, come from cultivated plants, preferably certified organic. This would eliminate any potential population pressures on the plant and ensure good-quality herbs for the long run.

REFERENCES

Bergner, Paul. *The Healing Power of Echinacea and Goldenseal and Other Immune System Herbs.* Rocklin, Calif.: Prima Publishing, 1997.

Heywood, V. H. *Flowering Plants of the World.* New York: Mayflower Books, 1978.

Moore, Michael. *Medicinal Plants of the Desert and Canyon West.* Santa Fe: Museum of New Mexico Press, 1989.

YERBA SANTA
Eriodictyon californicum

SHATOIYA AND RICK DE LA TOUR

Named by the early Spaniards as the "holy herb," yerba santa was one of the most important herbs to all the Native tribes who shared an environment with it. It is also known as mountain balm, wild balsam, gum leaves, and miner's tobacco. The Indians' lexicon had many names for this beneficial plant. Uses for this plant extend from the physical realm to the emotional and spiritual.

Matthew Wood refers to yerba santa as the "portable temple." Burning it as a smudge is said to clear any psychic toxins from the area. The smell is sweet and most pleasant. It occasionally grows sporadically along side roads but more often is found on lonely ridgetops surrounded by guardian poison oaks. While researching this chapter we found a lovely patch, but to get to it we had to brave poison oak, various stickers, and a rattlesnake. When we did make our way to the cluster of yerba santa bushes, we were rewarded with a beautiful view of the American River canyon and found a beautifully formed hummingbird nest with a solitary egg resting in the branches of the most prominent of the yerba santa bushes.

Sitting in this grove of yerba santa gave us a very strong connection to the history of this land. It was as if the plants could recall the days of the Forty-Niners—and those recollections weren't all happy. Remembered was the disrespect for the land and the raping of entire mountainsides for the recovery of some perceived precious metal. We both received the message that this is a plant that demands respect—that if used wisely its rewards are great, but if used disrespectfully its dangers are equally great. "Use me and I will ground you," the plant said to us. "Use me improperly and I will ground you to a pulp." This is a plant that wants you to earn its lessons.

Once prolific in our area, patches of yerba santa have succumbed to urban sprawl. Perhaps that is why local old-timers now come into our shop to buy it instead of picking it in the wild. These hardy foothill folk are the ones who first piqued our interest in this herb. "When I was a kid, if I caught a cold, my mama would make me drink this tea. I still use it to this day," was a common statement we heard.

BOTANICAL FEATURES

E. californicum, while considered the "official" yerba santa, is only one of several species of *Eriodictyon* that goes by that name. *E. trichocalyx* is found in southern California and the central coast, up to the Salinas valley; *E. angustifolium* grows in California's Mojave Desert and has also spread into southern Utah and Arizona.

Yerba santa is an evergreen, aromatic, resinous, leafy shrub that grows in the oak savanna and chaparral of the foothills and canyons of California, southern Oregon, Baja California, and parts of Arizona and Utah. It can grow to 8 feet tall but is usually found at a height somewhere between 3 and 6 feet. The alternately arranged leaves are lanceolate with serrated edges. Mature leaves are typically found to be 3 to 4 inches long. The upper sides of the leaves are dark green and shiny while the undersides are yellowish and slightly fuzzy. Visible on the underside is a distinctive mosaic vein pattern. The leaves that are overly mature occasionally become black due to a fungus that often attacks the older leaves. Yerba santa is found growing between the elevations of 500 and 5,500 feet, usually in dry sites. Often growing among the native grasses, poison oaks, and ceanothus, it is distinctive due to the shiny upper surface of its leaves, and also because the leaves are often found clustered at the ends of the branches. The bark—which is light brown in color—tends to have a shredded appearance. The short-lived flowers are purple to white.

HISTORICAL BACKGROUND

Native Americans, then Spaniards, and then gold miners learned the healing properties of this plant. During the California Gold Rush of 1849 many of the miners took to smoking this herb due to the difficulty of getting tobacco to the mine fields. Smoking yerba santa does have an effect that's similar, though more subtle, to smoking tobacco. The taste is slightly sweeter, but the sensation as the smoke enters the lungs is much like what is felt when smoking tobacco. Modern herbalists on the western side of the United States recognize it as an effective respiratory herb.

MEDICINAL USES

All varieties of yerba santa may be used medicinally. They are most often used for severe or chronic respiratory problems. The plant is recommended in many herbals for bronchitis, asthma, hay fever, and any wet, phlegmy condition. As a tea it is often combined with other respiratory herbs—mullein, nettle, grindelia, and coltsfoot. By itself, or in combination, it is an effective decongestant and expectorant. Toward this end it was also smoked in the belief that the smoke went exactly to the place it was needed—the lungs. We use it in combination with grindelia in the tincture form as a "kick butt" cold and cough remedy when gentler herbs don't seem to do the job. A tincture of equal parts nettle, horseradish, and yerba santa is very effective for sinus congestion and infection.

We don't generally recommend smoking herbs for respiratory problems, although yerba santa was used this way by Native Americans and root doctors, and some modern herbalists as well. We have mentioned it to people trying to transition off tobacco cigarettes. Not wanting to offer something we haven't tried ourselves, we decided to roll one up and take a few tokes. Neither of us is a cigarette smoker but from recollections of our youthful attempts to be "cool" we can tell you that the yerba santa wasn't as harsh as tobacco. The smoke has a sweet, minty flavor. It did make both of us feel a little dizzy and out of it, very much as our pubescent tobacco experiences left us. If you do intend to use the herb in this way, use the dried herb and make sure you get good-quality papers. Never mind the look you get from the clerk when you buy them. If you've been an herbalist for any length of time, you should be used to getting funny looks.

We did have a student who helped her boyfriend transition off tobacco chew by using a yerba santa blend. She combined dried yerba santa, mullein, coltsfoot, mint, a dash of lobelia, and honey. Lobelia contains lobeline, very similar to nicotine, and helps withdrawal from that deadly stuff. The herbal chew was a hit, and eventually he became chew-free.

Although we have not used this with out clients, old herbals speak of drinking the tea to clear up hemorrhoids. Perhaps this is because it has a reputation for strengthening fragile membrane capillaries.

It has been cited for use in urethral irritation and catarrh. The water infusion has a beautiful gold color, like the urine of someone who's taken a lot of B vitamins. Perhaps that's the doctrine of signatures at work here.

Internally and externally, it is recommended for rheumatic pain. Local Native Americans used it as poultices, fresh or dried, for their own broken skin as well as that of their animals. Its sticky nature makes it a good adhesive bandage. They also used poultices for sore muscles and skin inflammations. We can personally attest to the muscle-relaxing effects of a bath with yerba santa and eucalyptus.

PREPARATION AND DOSAGE

To make a tea, use 1 tablespoon per cup of water and decoct for ten to fifteen minutes. If you are combining it with leafier herbs such as mullein, coltsfoot, nettle, or comfrey leaf, go ahead and make it as an infusion, steeping the whole mixture for twenty minutes. Add a little honey, mint, or apple juice, if you wish to enhance the flavor.

Michael Moore recommends tincturing the fresh herb 1:2, the dried herb 1:5, in 65 percent alcohol. The home herbalist can make an effective tincture by using Bacardi or Myers 151 rum, which tends to bring out the sweetness in the herb.

For coughs and colds, combine with other lung herbs (as above). Make 2 to 4 cups of tea and sip on it all day. For stubborn coughs or colds, add 2 dropperfuls of tincture of either straight yerba santa or the herb in combination with grindelia, licorice, wild cherry bark, and/or thyme, to 1 cup of yerba santa tea.

For asthma and hay fever, yerba santa combines well in a tincture with skunk cabbage, skullcap, nettle, wild cherry bark, mullein, and coltsfoot. For hay fever, eyebright may be added. Take 2 dropperfuls as needed.

For a muscle-soothing bath, combine five or six whole yerba santa leaves with the same number of eucalyptus leaves. Place them in a muslin bag, or tie them up in a bit of cheesecloth. Fasten the bundle to the water faucet and let the hot water run through it as the tub fills. Let the bundle of herbs float around as you relax in the healing waters.

Yerba santa leaves may be used in a compress or poultice. In an outdoor emergency, fresh leaves work best. Find the stickiest ones to use and chew them slightly. Place them on the wound. Tie gauze around it if you have some. At home, make a strong tea with dried leaves and apply cloths soaked in the tea to sore muscles, wounds, and the like.

PROPAGATION AND CULTIVATION

California University libraries have a plethora of documents with opinions about the proper way to start the seeds of California's native plants. Although the details vary, most subscribe to the idea of starting them in charate, an ashy substance obtained by burning and grinding a variety of native plants.

Yerba santa is considered a fire-following plant, and in the wilds, it often needs a fire if the seeds are to successfully germinate. Gardeners can duplicate this by putting the seeds in a 200-degree oven for five minutes. If you know someone who lives with a posse of yerba santa plants in the backyard, it would be much easier to carefully dig up some babies in the fall. Try not to disturb their roots. Transplant them into the worst possible soil in your garden (a dry, red clay is perfect). Barely give them enough water to establish, and never water them again, unless you are experiencing a seven-year drought. Put them near their dearest friends—ceanothus, poison oak, and any kind of thistle. They should settle in quite comfortably. New England gardeners will have as much fun trying to grow this as California Central Valley gardeners have trying to grow bloodroot.

HARVESTING

Generally, late spring and early summer are when the plant is at its stickiest, full of its rich resin. If there is a hillside of beautifully abundant plants, you can gather a few full clusters of leaves off a few plants. Cut the branch above a joint on the stem at a 45-degree angle. If you are taking a small amount, just pinch off one or two leaves out of a few clusters.

I hang up clusters of branches or dry individual leaves on a screen. They will be crunchy when dry, but still maintain a somewhat leathery texture.

> ## UpS RECOMMENDATIONS
> - Some limited wild harvest is permissible, but only when absolutely necessary.
> - Possible alternatives include pine, elecampane, thyme, sage, and grindelia.

Much of American Indian culture and tradition have been lost. The uses of yerba santa that were passed from one generation to the next for centuries are in jeopardy if we let this plant follow the path of the dinosaur. We can't afford to lose any of our history, especially elements that offer benefits for society. Do what you can to preserve this wonderful, helpful plant.

REFERENCES

Balls, Edward K. *Early Uses of California Plants*. Berkeley: University of California Press, 1962.

Clarke, Charlotte Bringle. *Edible and Useful Plants of California*. Berkeley: University of California Press, 1977.

Emery, Dara E. *Seed Propagation of Native California Plants*. Santa Barbara, Calif.: Santa Barbara Botanic Garden, 1988.

Grieve, Mrs. Maude. *A Modern Herbal*. 1931. Reprint, New York: Dover, 1971.

Hutchens, Alma. *Indian Herbalogy of North America*. Windsor, Ont.: Merco Publishers, 1973.

Moore, Michael. *Medicinal Plants of the Pacific West*. Santa Fe: Red Crane Books, 1993.

———. *Medicinal Plants of the Mountain West*. Santa Fe: Museum of New Mexico Press, 1979.

Storer, Tracy I., and Robert L. Usinger. *Sierra Nevada Natural History*. Berkeley: University of California Press, 1963.

Tilford, Gregory L. *Edible and Medicinal Plants of the West*. Missoula, Mont.: Mountain Press Publishing, 1997.

Wood, Matthew. *Seven Herbs, Plants as Teachers*. Berkeley, Calif.: North Atlantic Books, 1986.

SEA VEGETABLES

RYAN W. DRUM, Ph.D.

Seaweeds—or sea vegetables, as they are also called—are those large macroalgae that any of us who have been to the ocean can see growing on rocks, on the seafloor, and even on each other, in shallow seawater and the intertidal zones. The term "seaweeds," however, is a bit misleading. With a few notable exceptions, seaweeds are actually saltwater-tolerant, land-dependent plants growing almost exclusively at the narrow interface where land and sea meet. Because they are photosynthetic, unlike the truly "pelagic" seaweeds (able to live and grow at sea, independent of land), such as sargasso weed, most seaweeds must be firmly attached to something to stay in the "photic zone," where they can receive sufficient sunlight.

This proximity to land has meant that sea vegetables have been consumed regularly by all coastal peoples for a very long time. The worldwide awareness of healthy living has, in the past twenty years, initiated a very deliberate increase in our dietary seaweed consumption, especially in the developed postindustrial nations where voluntary vegetarian and macrobiotic diets have become increasingly popular. Most East Asian populations (those of Japan, Korea, and China) continue to eat large amounts of seaweed per capita, with Japan having the highest per capita dietary sea vegetable consumption.

In the most developed countries, the amount of sea vegetable consumed unknowingly by the average person probably far exceeds that consumed knowingly. This is a result of the widespread use of several phycocolloids (carageenan from the red algae *Chondrus crispus*, Irish moss, and *Gigartina* spp., grapestone) as food additives to lend bulk to a number of foods. These phycocolloids enable large amounts of water to be controlled as a semisolid gel, making for an even texture and distribution of flavor and coloring in frozen semidairy confections and for stable, semisolid structure in foods such as ice cream. The brown seaweed extract algin is found in the huge eastern Pacific kelp, *Macrocystis* spp., harvested by large automated harvesters from square-mile leases off the coasts of California and Mexico. One pound of algin is used to stabilize a ton of ice cream. A careful reading of labels on most food products that require a stable emulsion or suspension of materials, such as ice cream, will usually show carageenan (from red algae) or sodium alginate (from brown algae) listed as an ingredient.

Enormous quantities of raw seaweeds are harvested worldwide to feed a world market increasingly hungry for phycocolloids used in tens of thousands of food products, beauty products, and industrial applications. Large coastal areas have been vacuumed clean of seaweeds with huge suction harvesters. Broad beaches in the eastern Canadian maritime provinces of Nova Scotia and New Brunswick have been denuded for several years, and there have been attempts by the harvesters to expand their harvests into Maine. Two major Canadian federal departments, Environment Canada and Fisheries, are trying to halt or at least control such egregious waste of intertidal seaweed stands. Much of the harvest in eastern Canada supports the huge market for dried seaweed meal as a soil and veterinary/agricultural enhancer, and provides an excellent source of minerals for poor soils and malnourished livestock. For instance, the agricultural product Ag Kelp is primarily composed of the brown algae *Ascophyllum* and *Fucus* spp., although the exact species composition may vary considerably. In addition to direct soil and animal feed applications, seaweed extracts are sprayed directly onto crop plant leaves to facilitate foliar feeding. Irish moss is also vacuum-harvested; such harvesting is a serious threat to both intertidal and subtidal ecosystems. The bycatch of other seaweeds and fauna is horrific. Another red alga, an agarophyte (produces agar), *Gracilaria* spp. has been mostly eliminated by aggressive harvesting on several Caribbean islands to support a booming industry for male virility tonic (basically flavored hot water extracts) for both local and export consumption.

From Belize (where I purchased a quantity for personal delights and consumer testing) to the Virgin Islands, "seaweed drink" is popular.

Frankly, what once thrilled me now saddens and worries me: my doctoral work was in phycology, the study of algae. For me, it was a combination of cell biology and ecology. Although I started out in freshwater algae, once I had taught in the algae course at Woods Hole and had gone out collecting (among phycologists, "harvesting" is an extremely perjorative term, unacceptable to serious scholars and friends of the seaweeds) the gorgeous huge marine algae and seaweeds growing on the rocky stretches of the Massachusetts' coast, I became an instant fan of these exquisite plants. In truth, I was thrilled at their many industrial, medicinal, and culinary uses. Back in 1967 I did not envision the realities of imminent overharvesting.

I left the University of Massachusetts at Amherst to be a visiting professor at the University of California at Los Angeles, where I taught the Marine Botany class, an advanced class on marine algae, large and small. I was totally excited by the lush growths of huge kelps, enormous greens, bountiful reds, and of course my special friends, the diatoms, solitary and colonial unicellular algae living inside fantastically ornamented glass cell walls, all thriving on the rocky shores of California. Within a month of my arrival at UCLA, controls on drilling rig Number 3 offshore from Carpinteria, California, failed and a huge quantity of sticky, black, viscous petroleum began to coat the coast repeatedly as surge after surge of crude oil spewed into the sea and washed ashore on the breakers, killing the entire intertidal zone for hundreds of miles. Not only were the extant seaweeds killed, but the perfect rock surfaces were filled and coated with tar, renedering them unfit for seaweed growth for a year or more. This was not an isolated one-time event; perhaps more than aggressive harvesting, crude oil from shipping disasters and the accepted customary spillage as it is loaded on and off oil tankers is probably the greatest environmental hazard for seaweeds worldwide. Onshore and nearshore pollution from both sewage and industrial wastes also makes large areas unsuitable for further seaweed growth. I have observed steady, and sometimes abrupt, decline in the total area and biomass and species diversity in all three of the coastal locations where I have lived. As a result I believe that there is a great future in pelagic sea vegetable farming with huge floating artificial substrates in the open seas if sufficient capital became available.

WHICH SEAWEEDS ARE EDIBLE?

All seaweeds are edible. Many are unpalatable. Some are very tasty after drying, roasting, or lightly steaming. Most are not very tasty fresh, wet, and alive. Powdered or flaked sea vegetables are often best. For those who are especially resistant, they can be introduced gradually in cooked foods. Real powdered kelp (not rinsed, de-salinized, reconstituted flakes) is a delicious high-potassium salt replacement in most cooked foods and on popcorn.

Nori (several species of the red alga genus *Porphyra*) is probably the most popular seaweed for eating, both historically and today. Nori was eaten abundantly by native peoples. It is tasty used in soups and, re-wetted, in salads, dried as a snack, toasted lightly in a dry iron skillet, deep-fried with cooked, rolled oats as the Celtic laver bread, and used as a food wrap for sushi. It tends to have a sweet, meaty flavor pleasant to most palates. Dulse, another red alga, is another easy-to-eat snack but quite salty and often a little fermented in the marketplace. Its relatively high fatty acid content results in rancidity after a year or more in storage. The large brown "kelps" (kombu, or, *Laminaria groend-landica*; sugar kelp, or, *Laminaria saccharina*; wakame, or, *Alaria* spp.) can be eaten dried but are usually easier to eat when cooked with grains, legumes, or miso soup broth. The bright green dried fronds of the giant bull kelp *(Nereocystis luetkeana)* are a great snack, salty and high in vitamins and minerals (up to 50 percent dry weight), particularly potassium, protein, and free amino acids. Other brown algae, such as hijiki *(Cystceria geminata)*, sargassum *(Sargassum mutica)*, and sea palm, are usually best cooked with wet food as in soups, miso broth, grains, legumes, vegetable pies, and stews. Sea lettuce (*Ulva lactuca* and *Monostroma* spp.) has a strong seafood taste and odor but is easy to eat as a snack or in salads since it is quite delicate after drying and crumbles easily into tiny, tender pieces.

HARVESTING SEAWEEDS

My personal and professional rules for seaweed harvest are very basic: choose the cleanest waters you can find and verify this by talking to locals and calling ecology and health agencies before harvesting sea vegetables. Cut the seaweeds from rocks using stainless steel scissors, leaving the holdfasts and some plant material for regrowth. As Evelyn McConnaughey indicates in *Sea Vegetables* and Eleanor and John Lewallen state in *Sea Vegetable Cookbook and Forager's Guide*, each specific seaweed has its own special harvesting and processing requirements. Harvest only what you will actually be able to process and use. Try harvesting on cloudy cool days at low tide, when the individual plants are not heat- or drying-stressed, which means they will transport better and tend to yield a much tastier product. I try to dry my seaweeds outside in the full sun for four to ten hours in one day. If this is not possible, I dry them inside at 80 to 100 degrees, using wood heat and small fans for air circulation. Place them in airtight opaque containers immediately after they are totally dried.

In proper storage most dried sea vegetables stay nutritionally and medicinally secure indefinitely. The minerals do not degrade; the phycocolloids slowly fragment over years; the pigments slowly fade, especially the chlorophylls; fats slowly become rancid; proteins fragment slowly to polypeptides and amino acids. "Proper storage" ideally means that the sea vegetables are stored in completely airtight and waterproof opaque containers (not paper or plastic bags) at temperatures less than 70 degrees, and in the dark. Do not store dried sea vegetables in a refrigerator or near sources of strong odors; they readily absorb odors and tend to be aggressively hydroscopic (they absorb water from the air), which is why dry storage is essential. Some sea vegetables, such as nori, improve in taste and texture for at least twenty years in dry storage, becoming sweeter as complex carbohydrates fragment to simple sugars, and meatier as proteins fragment to amino acids.

Bladderwrack and sea lettuce are two exceptions to indefinite storage; they seem to easily discolor and develop unsavory tastes and odors if stored for more than a year. In addition, any dried seaweed that has any trace animals hidden in its folds will tend to putrefy with just a small amount of ambient moisture, releasing amines, such as putrecine and cadaverine, not favored by most.

WHEN ARE SEAWEEDS NOT SAFE TO USE FOR FOOD AND MEDICINE?

Although all seaweeds are innately safe to eat, they can become dangerously contaminated where they grow by sewage and industrial, mining, agricultural, and radioactive wastes. Infectious microbes and parasites are usually absent on seaweeds in cold northern waters. In warm tropical seas, cholera is transmissible via topical seaweed contamination by feces from cholera-infected humans. A few seaweed-sourced cholera deaths were reported in the 1990s after the victims ate raw tropical seaweeds in salads.

Palytoxin, the most deadly marine neurotoxin, has killed some seaweed consumers after the seaweeds came in contact with *Palythoa* sea anemones during harvest in tropical waters. The genus *Palythoa* does not occur yet in northern waters.

In the mid-1980s, Australia and New Zealand banned importation of dietary sea vegetables from Japan due to unacceptably high contents of lead, cadmium, and arsenic. Japanese products dominate much of the wordwide prepackaged commercial sea vegetable market. These seaweeds could have originated anywhere; the packages sold in North America are labeled "Product of Japan" and do not indicate country or site of origin. Most North American dietary sea vegetable harvesters are very proud of their harvest places and practices (see the list of reliable harvesters at the end of this chapter; they all harvest by hand and in small amounts). In England, radioactive medical waste contaminated laver (nori) used abundantly in laver bread and other dietary seafoods and caused radiation sickness in coastal villagers who consumed those products. The lesson: know your sources!

WHAT NUTRITIONAL BENEFITS CAN SEAWEED PROVIDE?

Iodine is the essential element in most thyroid hormones, natural and synthetic, and is essential for the maintenance of normal mammary gland architecture and saliva composition. No land plants are reliable sources of dietary iodine. Seaweeds, eaten regularly, are the best natural food sources of biomolecular dietary iodine, and, unlike marine animals, do not seem to collect fat-soluble pesticides and industrial wastes such as PCP, PCB, and dioxin.

What exactly does "eaten regularly" imply? To me it means eating 5 to 15 grams of dried seaweeds at least twice a week. An ounce (29 grams)

a week is slightly more than 3 pounds a year. My personal consumption is around 10 pounds a year. I usually suggest consuming brown seaweeds and red seaweeds at a 2:1 ratio; roughly 2 pounds of brown algae and 1 pound of red algae. Regular consumption of sea vegetables in the diet encourages resident intestinal microflora to develop enzymes capable of digesting sea vegetables; most of us can so adapt in 4 to 6 weeks. Prolonged or heavy intermittent antibiotic use can severely reduce a human's seaweed digestive capacity. Just eating sea vegetables is only a beginning; for optimal health effects, one must also digest the sea vegetables and absorb nutrients from them.

DIETARY MINERALS

Sea vegetables are excellent sources of most minerals, especially potassium, sodium, calcium, magnesium, sulfur, nitrogen, iron, zinc, boron, copper, manganese, chromium, selenium, bromine, vanadium, and nickel. They are often better sources than meat, whole milk, or eggs and usually better than any land plants. This means that high-quality sea vegetables can be used to compensate for the frequent low mineral content of food plants and animals grown "factory-style" on mineral-depleted soils. See Paul Bergner's *The Healing Power of Minerals* for more information.

VITAMINS

Most sea vegetables are excellent sources of the known vitamins (A, Bs—especially B_{12}—C, D, E, and K) as well as essential fatty acids. Powdered bladderwrack has been mixed with olive oil as a safe effective alternative to cod liver oil. Nori is very rich in vatamins A and C.

Active Removal of Radioactive and Heavy Metal Toxic Cations

The phycocolloids—algin in all brown algae, and carageenan and agar in many red algae—aggressively trap metallic ions. The isolated colloids and the seaweeds containing them can be used to remove heavy metals from our food and bodies and carry these metals out in the stool. Although many seaweeds contain some radioactive elements, careful research indicates that these elements are usually not released into our food or bodies. Powdered kelp, algin, even sodium alginate, are effectively used to move radioactive and heavy metals from the body. The metabolic process is slow and deliberate. In 1954 the Swedish government first recommended a 5 gm/day dose of powdered kelp, algin, or sodium alginate as both a detox treatment and a protective treatment against radioactive fallout. The United States Atomic Energy Commission made a similar recommendation around 1956; this was later rescinded around 1960, so as not to alarm the public unduly. Unfortunately, we are regularly taking in radioactive isotopes from the total world contamination by continual radioactive fallout from all nuclear power plants, weapons facilities, and past nuclear tests. All of our food, air, soil, and water is contaminated. As S. Schecter indicates in his book *Fighting Radiation and Pollution*, any way we can reduce our total body burden of radioactive isotopes will help our health by reducing our personal exposure to ionizing radiation from radioactive isotope decay within our own bodies.

Dietary phycocolloids also bulk and soften the stool, soothe the gastrointestinal tract, and help relieve chronic constipation. However, be advised that red seaweeds high in carageenan can irritate the inner bowel lining in patients with irritable bowel syndrome (IBS), Crohn's disease, or ulcerative colitis.

WHAT THERAPEUTIC BENEFITS CAN SEAWEED PROVIDE?

Respiratory Problems

Phycocolloid carageenan gel, boiled out of red algae, notably Irish moss (*Chondrus crispus*), grapestone (*Gigartina* spp.), and iridea, is partially digested and absorbed as small globular polymeric masses. This gel is effective long-term treatment for damaged lungs, particularly after one has had pneumonia, effects from smoking, emphysema, chronic bronchitis, and possibly mycoplasma and chlamydia. In addition, regular consumption of hijiki and sargassum, brown algae, seems to aid respiratory function, improving lung capacity and gas exchange efficiency. Hayfever and asthma are also helped by 3 to 5 gm of powdered kelp daily.

Herpes Outbreak

The red alga *Dumontia* is dried, powdered, encapsulated, and used as a genital herpes suppressant. *Prionitis lyallii*, an abundant tidepool red alga found from California to Alaska, is used similarly.

SHINGLES OUTBREAK

Three different red algae harvested in southeast Alaska by R. Ellis and Natasha Calvin are also dried, powdered, and encapsulated, and taken in prescribed dosages regularly to suppress outbreaks of shingles, or herpes zoster. Together these three algae are called Alaska dulse.

DAMAGED TISSUE

I use a broth of powdered *Sagassum muticum* (a large local brown alga) and unpasteurized three-year-old barley miso paste for all cancer radiation, chemotherapy, postsurgical, and whole-body-impact (acute auto crashes, falls) trauma patients. I recommend its consumption twice daily, A.M. and P.M., mixing 15 ml of miso paste with 5 gm of sargassum powder in about 300 ml of hot (120 degrees) nonchlorinated water. Japanese studies show very positive clinical and preventive antitumor and antimetastatic success using seaweeds, especially *Sargassum*. For cancer patients, I also recommend 15 ml fresh pressed sheep sorrel (*Rumex acetosella*) juice from live plants twice daily with food. For trauma patients, I recommend 20 to 40 Hawthorn berries (*Crataegus oxycantha* or *C. monogyna*) or 5 ml Hawthorn tincture three times daily with food.

NERVOUS DISORDERS

Attention deficit disorder (ADD), hyperactivity, insomnia, depression, hostility, and schizophrenia are often markedly improved, if not resolved, by regular daily consumption of 3 to 5 gm powdered kelp, especially bull kelp (*Nereocystis*), based on the assumption that these conditions can be exacerbated by long-term malnutrition, especially mineral deficiency. Regular consumption of bladderwrack can improve sleep.

CARDIAC TROUBLES

Regular consumption of kombu (*Laminaria* spp.) tends to result in lowered blood pressure and plaque removal from arteries. Regular consumption of bladderwrack can also lower chronic high blood pressure.

BREAST CANCER

Regular dietary consumption of wakame and other brown algae may prevent breast cancer.

ENLARGED PROSTATE

Regular consumption of bladderwrack, 3 to 5 gm daily, can normalize a swollen prostate, especially in early stages. I find the best results occur when small pieces of the whole plant are eaten with food. The next best way is ingestion of encapsulated, powdered, dried bladderwrack. Alcohol and hot water extracts seem to be the least effective.

MUSCLE AND JOINT DISCOMFORT

An external poultice of bladderwrack or soaking in bladderwrack baths, the hotter the better, can relieve sore joints and achy muscles; it may also stimulate cartilage regrowth.

THYROID DISORDERS

Much of the iodine in bladderwrack presents as di-iodotyrosine (DIT), an immediate precursor of the thyroid hormones thyroxine and tri-iodothyronine. This makes *Fucus* spp. the sea vegetables of choice for treating thyroid disorders by providing the immediate precursors for both hormones. Indeed, *Fucus* seems particularly effective in treating early stage hypothyroidism. Positive results have been obtained in both hypothyroidism and Graves' hyperthyroidism cases.

FUCOIDAN—THE THERAPEUTIC FUTURE FOR SEA VEGETABLES

Fucoidan is a sulfated polysaccharide extracted from many brown algae. It is a potent antiviral that acts by inhibiting virus attachment onto host cells, cell penetration, and viral intracellular replication. As such, it shows strong activity against herpes simplex 1, HIV 1, and H-cytomegalovirus. It also inhibits lung metastases and shows strong antitumor activity by enhancement of inflammatory responses and upregulation of leukocytic phagocytosis. It suppresses cancer cell replication more effectively than comparable doses of Heparin. All human cells studied are found to have receptor sites for fucose, the end-group sugar on fucoidan. This molecule is perhaps most important in the therapeutic future for seaweeds. Pretreatment with fucoidan significantly reduces postsurgical complications. Research continues. Eat your sea vegetables today!

REFERENCES

McConnaughey, Evelyn. *Sea Vegetables*. Happy Camp, Calif.: Nature Graph, 1985.

Lewallen, Eleanor, and John Lewallen. *Sea Vegetable Cookbook and Forager's Guide*. Navarro, Calif.: Mendocino Sea Vegetable Co., 1983.

Rhoads, Sharon. *Cooking With Sea Vegetables*. Cambridge, Mass.: Autumn Press, 1978.

Shannon, Sara. *Diet for the Atomic Age*. n.p.: Instant Improvements, 1993.

Bergner, Paul. *The Healing Power Of Minerals*. Rocklin, Calif.: Prima Publishers, 1997.

Schecter, S. *Fighting Radiation and Pollution*. Encinitas, Calif.: Vitality Link, 1997.

Drum, R. "Thyroid Dysfunction." *Medicines from the Earth*. (1999): 72–75.

SEAWEED SOURCES

Nature Spirit Herbs, P.O. Box 150, Williams, OR 97544

Mendocino Sea Vegetable Co., P.O. Box 1265, Mendocino, CA 95460

Larch Hansen, Maine Seaweed Co., P.O. Box 57, Steuben, ME 04680

Louise Gaudet, P.O. Box 2472, Sidney, B.C. V8L-3Y3 Canada (bull kelp only)

Carla Jo Larmore, Tidewater Herbs, P.O. Box 27, Waldron 98297

CONCERN FOR EUROPEAN MEDICINAL PLANTS

CASCADE ANDERSON GELLER

Medicinal plants around the globe are at risk due to many complicated factors. Though United Plant Savers is stepping up to speak regarding North American herbs, other organizations are beginning to bring similar concerns to the forefront in their own regions. The indigenous European herbs, which have had a long history of use in Europe, North America, and all other European-colonized areas, have been experiencing pressure from overharvest and loss of habitat for many years now. The fact that some of these famous species, such as yellow gentian (*Gentiana lutea* or *Arnica montana*), are still found in mountain meadows of Europe at all is quite amazing considering the many centuries these plants have been used in the herbal pharmacy. The diminishing reserves of these herbs in Europe can cause further harvest pressure on related wild American species. Protection of native stands worldwide coupled with continued efforts at domestication and cultivation are therefore of paramount importance.

A special report prepared by TRAFFIC, a branch of the World Wildlife Fund (WWF), known in Europe as the World Wide Fund for Nature, and the World Conservation Union (IUCN) that monitors wildlife trade, has laid out specific goals for countries both in and outside of the European Union. Their goal is to establish the Medicinal Plant Task Group, which will create a database for monitoring species in trade and allow dialogue among specialists. Their plans also include efforts to aid more sustainable cultivation, as well as the creation of refuges for medicinal plants, seed storage banks, guidelines for sustainable harvest, and monitoring programs by every European nation involved in the trade of wild medicinal plants. TRAFFIC supports strict adherence to the Convention on International Trade of Endangered Species (CITES) treaty.

In June 1998 TRAFFIC hosted the First International Symposium on the Conservation of Medicinal Plants in Trade in Europe at Kew

Gardens in the United Kingdom. The special reports with lovely photographs of their top fifteen species of concern are on the Web. Interesting to note is the inclusion of such commonly used herbs as uva-ursi (*Arctostaphylos* spp.), all species of thyme (*Thymus* spp.), and licorice *(Glycyrrhiza glabra)*. The UpS list and TRAFFIC's list contain some of the same genuses, such as *Drosera*, *Arnica*, and *Gentian*. Both organizations are concerned about various species of orchids. TRAFFIC is particularly interested in removing salep, a mucilaginous blend of various species of orchid tubers, from the required ingredients list for the manufacture of ice cream in Turkey.

Though we face a new millennium full of major environmental challenges, we can find some solace in the fact that people in every nation are challenging old assumptions that the earth is here for the sole purpose of administering to the needs of human beings over and above all other species. As United Plant Saver herbalists, we join the ever growing circle of those endeavoring to better understand and preserve life in all its glorious forms.

On the Web see http://www.traffic.org/news/medicinal_plants.html. TRAFFIC has a host of sites, all of them very interesting; this one features lovely color photos along with monographs on most of the species below. If you have trouble with the address, try searching for TRAFFIC sites.

TRAFFIC's Current Species of Concern

Adonis spp.

Arctostaphylos spp.

Arnica montana

Cetraria spp.

Drosera spp.

Gentiana spp.

Glycyrrhiza glabra

Gypsophila spp.

Menyanthes spp.

Orchids (various)

Paeonia spp.

Primula spp.

Ruscus spp.

Sideritus spp.

Thymus spp.

PLANTING GUIDES
AND RESOURCES

The most frequently asked questions we receive in the United Plant Savers' office are: "I have land and want to grow medicinal herbs. How do I grow these plants? And where to do I get the planting stock?" UpS's Nursery Directory (at the end of this appendix) is a good place to start obtaining nursery-grown stock of at-risk plants. Another source for plant material is local plant rescue teams. Several states already have plant rescues in place, but in most areas it's still a novel idea; you may have to be the one to initiate it. Whenever a housing development, mall, or highway is under construction, get permission to evaluate the plant scenario at the site. Are there plants that that should be rescued and replanted? Enlist your local wildflower societies, herbal organizations, or school programs to help. Or contact the UpS office, and we'll let you know if there are any members in your area to help with the rescue. Many people have written in telling us that they have successfully transplanted at-risk plants from development areas.

Knowing how to plant at-risk medicinals is another challenge. Though several of the at-risk and to-watch plants are very sensitive and have not yet been successfully cultivated, many seem to thrive with minimal care and in a greater variety of habitats than was originally assumed. The following guides and books are excellent resources and will provide planting guidelines and resources for your planting projects.

BOOKS AND PUBLICATIONS

Growing Guides by Richo Cech
Richo Cech, UpS board member and seed man extraordinaire, has written an informative series of small booklets that help growers or gardeners interested in plant conservation get started.

- *Cultivating a Garden for Diversity*. Describes Richo's unique cultivation system. He tells how to successfully grow a few plants in a wide range of species, serving as a basis for home herbal medicine or expansion into large-scale farming. $2.50.

- *Domestication of Wild Medicinal Plants*. An in-depth essay on seed germination theory, directed toward cultivation of medicinal plant species. $4.

- *Echinacea—Native American Tonic Roots*. Complete information on germination, cultivation, harvesting, and marketing of *Echinacea purpurea* and *E. angustifolia.* $3.

- *Finding Your Niche—Making a Living with Medicinal Plants.* Discusses the peculiar medicinal herb market. Lists herbs of economic importance by bioregion. In-depth discussion of cultivation requirements for ginseng, goldenseal, black cohosh, echinacea, Saint-John's-wort, hawthorn, and valerian. $4.

- *Forest Roots.* Gives full cultivation and harvesting directions for black cohosh, ginseng, goldenseal, and wild yam. $3.

To order the entire series of twelve publications on the cultivation of medicinal herbs send $26.50 plus $2.50 shipping. When ordering individual booklets include $2.50 shipping and handling.

Horizon Herbs
P.O. Box 69
Williams, OR 97544
(541) 846-6704
Web site: www.chatlink.com/~herbseed

Medicinal Herbs in the Garden, Field and Marketplace

Written by Lee Sturdivant and Tim Blakley, and published by San Juan Naturals, Friday Harbor, Washington. Coauthored by two experienced herbalists, farmers, and gardeners, this is simply one of the best guides available on the cultivation of medicinal herbs. The information is fully practical, easy to read, and invaluable for the farmer of medicinal plants. Tim Blakley, one of the authors, is the farm manager and steward of the Center for the Preservation of Medicinal Plants in Rutland, Ohio.

Seed Germination: Theory and Practice

Written by Norman Deno. This is the best book on seed germination specifics for many of the at-risk species. It's available by writing the author:

Norman Deno
139 Lenor Drive
State College, PA 16801

From Earth to Herbalist: An Earth Conscious Guide to Medicinal Plants

Written by Gregory Tilford, and published by Mountain Press, Missoula, Mont. (1998). This practical, full-color guide to the sustainable cultivation, harvest, and use of North American medicinal plants profiles fifty-two species. The book highlights UpS at-risk and to-watch herbs and offers alternatives or adjuncts as well as propagation techniques. An excellent resource guide highly recommended by UpS.

How to Grow American Ginseng

Written by Scott and Sylva Harris. A publication of Sylvan Botanicals/American Ginseng, this small pamphlet was written by two successful ginseng farmers. Write to:

Sylvan Botanicals
P.O. Box 91
Cooperstown, NY 13326
(607) 264-8455

Educational Resources for Growing Ginseng and Goldenseal

Produced by the North Carolina Ginseng and Goldenseal Company. These resources include audio tapes, on-site evaluations, and start-up kits for growing ginseng and goldenseal. Write to:

Robert Eidus
North Carolina Ginseng and
    Goldenseal Company
148 Anderson Branch Road
Marshall, NC 28758

American Ginseng: Green Gold

Written by W. Scott Persons, and published by Bright Mountain Books. This is the book that many current ginseng growers started with and is considered by many the bible on ginseng cultivation. It has been fully updated and includes information on growing ginseng in other countries as well. Write to:

Bright Mountain Books
138 Springside Road
Asheville, NC 28803

Ginseng and Other Medicinal Plants

Written by A.R. Harding. This may be the real bible of ginseng growing. Written in 1908, this book is full of information from the pioneers of ginseng and goldenseal farming. Both *Green Gold* and A. R. Harding's books are available through:

Sylvan Botanicals
P.O. Box 91
Cooperstown, NY 13326

Eco-Herbalist Fieldbook

Written by Greg Tilford and published by Mountain Press, Missoula, Montana (1993). This was one of the first herb books to address the issues of medicinal plant conservation and the role herbalists play in the conservation and cultivation of native medicinal species. It provides excellent eco-sensitive guidelines for wildcrafting medicinal herbs.

How to Create and Nurture a Nature Center in Your Community

Written by Brent Evans and Carolyn Chipman-Evans, and published by the University of Texas Press. This excellent and inspiring book provides proven models for creating natural sanctuaries within a variety of communities. Step-by-step instructions for creating and maintaining a nature center are also included. This practical handbook is an essential resource for anyone wishing to create a nature center and/or botanical sanctuary.

Principles and Practice of Plant Conservation

Written by David R. Given, and published by Timber Press, Portland, Oregon (1994). Commissioned in a joint effort by the World Wide Fund for Nature and The World Conservation Union, this work elucidates the concepts that underlie successful conservation efforts. Chapters are devoted to the ethical, educational, and economic aspects of plant conservation.

Native American Ethnobotany

Written by Daniel E. Moerman, and published by Timber Press, Portland, Oregon (1998). An essential reference for all those interested in medicinal uses of North American plants. This book is an important scholarly compendium and lists the use of 4,029 native plants—a total of 44,691 uses!

MAGAZINES AND JOURNALS

Wild Earth
P.O. Box 455
Richmond, VT 05477
Wild Earth is a quarterly journal melding conservation, biology, and wildlands activism. The journal provides a forum for regional wilderness groups and collations and serves as a networking tool for wilderness activists.

Native Plants Journal
http://www.its.uidaho.edu/nativeplants/
A journal providing a forum for dispersing practical information about the planting and growing of North American native plants for conservation, restoration, reforestation, landscaping, highway corridors, and more.

WEB SITES

TRAFFIC: www.traffic.org
United Plant Savers: www.plantsavers.org

ORGANIZATIONS

Native Plant Society and The Nature Conservancy
Your local chapters of the Native Plant Society and The Nature Conservancy are good resources for keeping track of what plants are threatened. They are also good sources of information on harvesting nonnative invasive types of plants during weed pulls.

New England Wildflower Society and Garden in the Woods
180 Hemenway Road
Framingham, Ma 01701
(508) 877-7630

The National Wildflower Research Center
2600 FM 973 North
Austin, TX 78725
(512) 929-3600

Trust for Public Lands
National Office:
116 New Montgomery, Fourth Floor
San Francisco, CA 94105
The Trust for Public Lands is a national organization dedicated to improving the quality of life in our communities through protection of our natural and historic resources. It can furnish information about local land trusts and how to start a land trust in your area.

Land Trust Alliance
1319 F Street NW, Suite 501
Washington, DC 20004-1106
The Land Trust Alliance is a national organiza-

tion of local and regional land trusts. LTA promotes voluntary land conservation and strengthens the land trust movement by providing information and resources needed to conserve land.

UNITED PLANT SAVERS NURSERY DIRECTORY

Abundant Life Seed Foundation
P.O. Box 772
Port Townsend, WA 98368
(360) 385-5660

Arrowhead Nursery, Inc.
870 West Malaga Road
Williamstown, NJ 08094
(609) 697-6045

Aurora Farm
3492 Phillips Road
Creston, BC VOB 1G2 Canada
(250) 428-4404

Bison Belly Futures
S11793 Hazelnut Road
Spring Green, WI 53588
(608) 588-2048

Boothe Hill Farm
921 Boothe Hill
Chapel Hill, NC 28514
(919) 967-4091

Companion Plants
7247 North Coolville Ridge Road
Athens, OH 45701
(740) 592-4643

Crimson Sage Nursery
P.O. Box 337
Colton, OR 97017
(503) 824-4721

Enchanter's Garden
HC 77, Box 108
Hinton, WV 25951
(304) 466-3154

Enders Greenhouse
104 Enders Drive
Cherry Valley, IL 61016
(815) 332-5255

Fedco Seeds
P.O. Box 520
Waterville, ME 04903
(207) 873-6411

Garden in the Woods
180 Hemenway Road
Framingham, MA 01701

Garden Medicinals and Culinaries
P.O. Box 320
Earlysville, VA 22936
(804) 973-4703

Good Scents
1308 North Meridian Road
Meridian, ID 83642
(208) 887-1784

Goodwin Creek Gardens
P.O. Box 83
Williams, OR 97544
(541) 846-7357

Great Basin Natives
75 West 300 South P.O. Box 114
Holden, UT 84636
(435) 795-2303

Healing Spirits
9198 Rt. 415
Avoca, NY 14809

Heirloom Seed Project
Landis Valley Museum
2451 Kissel Hill Road
Lancaster, PA 17601
(717) 569-0401

The Herbal Exchange
P.O. Box 429
Frazeysburg, OH 43822
(740) 828-9968

Horizon Herbs
P.O. Box 69
Williams, OR 97544
(541) 846-6704

Johnny's Selected Seeds
Foss Hill Road
Albion, ME 04910
(207) 437-9294

Land Reformers Nursery and Landscape
35703 Loop Road
Rutland, OH 45775
(740) 742-DIRT (3478)

Legendary Ethnobotanical Resources
16245 Southwest 304 Street
Homestead, FL 33033
(305) 242-0877

Longevity Herb Company
1549 West Jewett Boulevard
White Salmon, WA 98672

Mountain Gardens
3020 Whiteoak Creek Road
Burnsville, NC 28714
(828) 675-5664

Mountain Top Farms
P.O. Box 231
Oswego, NY 13827
(607) 658-9501

Munchkin Nursery and Garden
323 Woodside Drive
Depaw, IN 47115-9039
(812) 633-4858

Native Gardens
5737 Fisher Lane
Greenback, TN 37742
(423) 856-0220

NC Ginseng and Goldenseal Company
300 Indigo Bunting Lane
Marshall, NC 28753
(704) 649-3536

New England Wetland Plants
800 Main Street
Amherst, MA 01002

Nichols Garden Nursery
1190 North Pacific Highway Northeast
Albany, OR 97321
(541) 967-8406

Perennial Pleasures Nursery
P.O. Box 147
East Hardwick, VT 05836
(802) 472-5104

Pinetree Garden Seeds
P.O. Box 300, 616A Lewiston Road
New Gloucester, ME 04260
(207) 926-3400

Prairie Moon Nursery
RR 3, Box 163
Winona, MN 55987
(507) 452-1362

Prairie Oak Seeds
P.O. Box 382
Maryville, MO 64458-0382
(660) 582-4084

Prairie Ridge Nursery
9738 Overland Road
Mount Horeb, WI 53572
(608) 437-5245

Redwood Seed Company
P.O. Box 361
Redwood City, CA 94064
(650) 325-7333

Seeds of Change
1364 Rufina Circle #5
Santa Fe, NM 87501

Southern Exposure Seed Exchange
P.O. Box 460
Mineral, VA 23117
(540) 894-9480

Sylvan Botanicals
P.O. Box 91
Cooperstown, NY 13326
(607) 264-8455

Synergy Seeds
P.O. Box 323
Orleans, CA 95556
(916) 321-3769

Tuckasegee Valley Ginseng
P.O. Box 236
Tuckasegee, NC 28783
(704) 293-5189

Underwood Gardens
4N 381 Maple Avenue
Bensenville, IL 60106
(630) 616-0232 (fax)

Well-Sweep Herb Farm
205 Mount Bethel Road
Port Murray, NJ 07865
(908) 852-5390

Wild Earth Native Plant Nursery
49 Mead Avenue
Freehold, NJ 07728
(732) 303-9777

Zack Woods Herb Farm
278 Mead Road
Hyde Park, VT 05655
(802) 888-7278

ABOUT THE AUTHORS

BABINEAU, DON

Don Babineau has spent his life in the forests and on the shoreline of the Northeast. His family's roots stretch back more than 350 years to Acadia, Nova Scotia. From winter camping in the White Mountains to sailing the coast of Maine, Don has studied the spirit of this land. As a woodworker of many years, he also enjoys primitive skills and crafts of the woodlands. Don lives with his wife, Kate, and their children in the Adirondacks where they grow and wildcraft medicinal plants and run an educational center.

BLAKLEY, TIM

Tim Blakley is the land manager of the National Center for the Preservation of Medicinal Herbs, established by Frontier Natural Products Co-op. He also travels extensively as Frontier's national educator, teaching people about the benefits of using medicinal herbs. Previously, he was a gardener, teacher, staff member and eventually, a co-owner at the California School of Herbal Studies in Forestville, California, and the land manager for Herb Pharm in Oregon. Tim has a degree in botany and horticulture, but his study of plants and herbs began in his youth and has remained one of his passions. He is one of

the country's foremost educators on herbal medicine and an authority on growing medicinal herbs. Tim is the coauthor of *Medicinal Herbs in the Garden, Field, and Marketplace*.

BLUMENTHAL, MARK

Mark Blumenthal is the founder and executive director of the American Botanical Council, a leading nonprofit research and education organization founded in 1988. He is also the editor of *HerbalGram*, an award-winning, peer-reviewed quarterly journal on herbal research, regulation, market trends, and related issues. He has been actively involved in the American herbal movement since the early 1970s as a former herb wholesaler and manufacturer, and then as a researcher, educator, and advocate for a rational regulatory framework for the manufacture and sale of quality herbal products. He is also an adjunct associate professor at the College of Pharmacy at the University of Texas at Austin, where he teaches a course on herbal medicine.

BOTHWELL, JANE

Jane Bothwell is a practicing herbalist, educator, hypnotherapist, and flower essence practitioner. She is the director of the Dandelion

Herbal Center in northern California, which is dedicated to preserving herbal traditions and teaching ecological ways to cohabit our world. Jane is an active member and former board member of United Plant Savers and a former teacher and administrator at the California School of Herbal Studies in Sonoma County, California.

BUHNER, STEPHEN HARROD

Stephen Harrod Buhner is the award-winning author of five books: *Sacred Plant Medicine, One Spirit Many Peoples, Sacred and Herbal Healing Beers, Herbal Antibiotics*, and *Herbal Healing for Hepatitis C and the Liver.* Stephen specializes in crosscultural religious practices, herbal medicine, and alternative psychotherapies. He is an adjunct instructor at the Rocky Mountain Center for Botanic Studies, a guest lecturer at the California School of Herbal Studies, and a regular speaker at Iowa's Herbfest and Boston's International Herb Symposium.

BUNTING, DAVID

David Bunting's study of ethnobotany led him to pursue the practical use of medicinal plants in daily life. In the early 1980s he attended and later taught at the California School of Herbal Studies. He has since worked for fourteen years in various facets of herbal liquid extract production, quality assurance, and product development. Along with herbal medicine, David also enjoys gardening and plant photography. David joined Herb Pharm in 1999 as staff herbalist, blending his commitment and dedication to exceptional quality herbal pharmacy with his love of photography.

CECH, RICHO (RICHARD A.)

Born in Iowa City, Iowa, Richo early demonstrated a fascination for nature and plants, although his plantain soup was generally spurned by his fellow Boy Scouts. He began his professional work as an archaeologist and lay ethnobotanist in East Africa. Upon his return to the United States in 1978, he began cultivating and saving the seeds of medicinal plants. Over the years, this living collection has become the basis for Horizon Herbs, a business dedicated to disseminating the seeds of medicinal plants, both common and rare. A practicing herbalist, Richo is the author of several guides on herb cultivation. He lectures internationally and currently serves on the executive board of directors of United Plant Savers.

DATTA, TANE

Tane has a B.S. in geology with a minor in environmental studies and alternative energy. He has been farming organically in Kona, Hawaii, for nineteen years. Through his company, Adaptations, Inc., he and his wife Maureen have organized growers to supply the local market with culinary herbs, vegetables, and edible flowers. Adaptations supplies herbalists across the Unites States with organically grown and wildcrafted medicinal herbs.

DE LA TOUR, RICK AND SHATOIYA

Rick and Shatoiya de la Tour are the owners of Dry Creek Herb Farm and Learning Center, nestled in the beautiful Gold Country of the Sierra foothills. A thriving education center and working farm established in 1988, Dry Creek also has display gardens and an herb shop open to the public. An herb, flower essence, and Aura Soma consultant, Shatoiya is also the author of *The Herbalist of Yarrow*, a fairy tale about plant wisdom. Rick specializes in teaching wilderness skills.

DRUM, RYAN W., PH.D.

Ryan W. Drum, Ph.D., began his successful career as an academic research scientist. He has been a professional wildcrafter, herbal educator, and practicing medical herbalist for more than twenty years. He studied herbal medicine with Ella Birzneck at Dominion Herbal College for twelve years and has taught at their summer seminars for more than twenty years. He was recently the clinic supervisor at the New Mexico Herb Center in Albuquerque. He has been an adjunct instructor in the Botanical Medicine Department at John Bastyr University since 1985 and has taught at both the Rocky Mountain Center for Botanical Studies and the National College of Phytotherapy. He believes passionately in true patient autonomy and that pleasure is the driving force of the universe.

ELLIOTT, DOUG

Doug Elliott is an herbalist, naturalist, and storyteller. He has traveled from the Canadian North to the Central American jungles in search of useful plants and the lore surrounding them. He has conducted workshops and programs at the American Museum of Natural History in New York, the Royal Ontario Museum in Toronto, and the Smithsonian Institution. He has conducted ranger training sessions for the National Park Service and guided people on wilderness experiences from down-east Maine to the Florida Everglades. He is the author of four books about wild plants and other aspects of the natural world as well as a number of award-winning recordings of stories and songs.

FOSTER, STEVEN

Steven Foster is an author, photographer, and lecturer specializing in medicinal plants. He is the author of twelve books, including *101 Medicinal Herbs* (winner of the 1999 Independent Book Publishers Award as the Best Title in Health and Medicine), *A Field Guide to Medicinal Plants and Herbs* (with James A. Duke), and *A Field Guide to Venomous Animals and Poisonous Plants* (with Roger Caras). He is a frequent contributor to *The Herb Companion, Herbs for Health*, and *HerbalGram* magazines. For more information, see his Web site: www.stevenfoster.com.

GELLER, CASCADE ANDERSON

As an herbalist with roots reaching back to the southern mountains of Appalachia, Cascade believes that herbal medicine has always represented the powerful connection of people and plants. Her emphasis is on making herbal medicine available to anyone who is interested—from parents to health practitioners. She believes that eveyone can learn to use and create medicines from nature. On her own herbal path Cascade has been a wildcrafter, medicine-maker, practitioner, educator, world traveler, and student of traditional peoples.

GILDAY, KATE

Kate Gilday is an herbal practitioner and teacher who lives in the woods of the Adironacks with her family. She and her husband, Don Babineau, are the founders of Woodland Essence Teaching Center and Flower Essence Company. They offer At Risk Woodland Flower Essence kits. Kate brings her love of the wild places, plants, song, and healing to her work and teachings.

GLADSTAR, ROSEMARY

Rosemary Gladstar is the founder and president of United Plant Savers and cofounder of Sage Mountain Herbal Retreat Center and Botanical Sanctuary and founder of the California School of Herbal Studies. She is the author of several popular herb books, including *Herbal Healing for Women* and *Rosemary Gladstar's Herbal Remedies* series. Rosemary's experience includes more than twenty-five years in the herbal community as a healer, teacher, and organizer of herbal events.

GREEN, JAMES

James Green is an herbalist, director of the California School of Herbal Studies, and founder of Simpler's Botanical Company. He is a founding member and past executive council member of the American Herbalists Guild and is currently on the advisory board of United Plant Savers. He is the author of a number of books, including the bestselling *The Male Herbal.*

HIRSCH, PAMELA

Pamela Hirsch, owner of Rowan Mountain Herbals, an herbal body care business specializing in natural soaps, has worked with medicinal herbs for nearly a decade. Growing up in the Middle East, Asia, and Europe, Pamela was exposed to different healing modalities at an early age. Her grandfather's love of the plant world (and his "old time" medicine cabinet) inspires her work with herbs. She is a frequent contributor to several herbal newsletters.

HOBBS, CHRISTOPHER

Christopher Hobbs is a fourth-generation herbalist and botanist with more than twenty years of experience with herbs. Founder of Native Herb Custom Extracts (now Rainbow Light Custom Extracts) and the Institute for Natural Products Research, Christopher writes and lectures internationally on herbal medicine. He is also a consultant to the herb industry.

KATZ, SARA

Sara Katz was studying to be a chiropractor when her interest in natural healing turned to herbal medicines. Sara and her partner, Ed, moved to the pristine countryside of southern Oregon in 1978, where she has ever since dedicated her waking hours to Herb Pharm. In the early years she collected wild herbs, helped to garble and grind them, bottled and shipped out extracts, and staffed the one-woman office. Now she oversees the running of the company, focusing on teamwork and honoring and supporting employees, customers, and suppliers.

KEVILLE, KATHI

Kathi Keville has worked with medicinal herbs for more than thirty years. She has written hundreds of herb magazine articles and is the author of eleven books, including *Herbs for Health and Healing; Women's Herbs, Women's Health* (with Christopher Hobbs); and *Aromatherapy: The Complete Guide to the Healing Arts* (with Mindy Green). She also teaches herb and aromatherapy seminars throughout the United States and is director of the American Herb Association and editor of their quarterly newsletter. Kathi is a founding member of the American Herbalists Guild and an honorary member of the National Association of Holistic Aromatherapy.

KLEIN, ROBYN

Robyn is a professional member of the American Herbalists Guild. She reviews herb books and journals in the periodical, *Robyn's Recommended Reading*, and teaches herb and plant identification classes at the Sweetgrass School of Herbalism. She thrives in Bozeman, Montana, along with a couple thousand plant species.

LIEBMANN, RICHARD, N.D.

Richard Liebmann graduated with honors from the National College of Naturopathic Medicine in 1977. Since that time he has been a college administrator, had an active practice of naturopathic medicine on the big island of Hawaii, cofounded Equinox Botanicals, Inc., in 1983, and has led outdoor adventures in Hawaii. For the past four years, Dr. Liebmann has served as the executive director of United Plant Savers. Presently, much of his energy is going toward operation of United Plant Savers first Botanical Sanctuary, a 380-acre site located in the Appalachian foothills of southeastern Ohio.

MARS, BRIGITTE

Brigitte Mars is an herbalist and nutritional consultant from Boulder, Colorado, who has been working with natural medicine for nearly three decades. She teaches herbology through the Rocky Mountain Center for Botanical Studies, the Boulder School of Massage Therapy, and Naropa Institute. Brigitte has a weekly Boulder radio show called "Naturally" and is the formulator for UniTea Herbs. Her articles have appeared in numerous magazines, and she is the author of several books, including *Elder, Natural First Aid*, and *Dandelion Medicine*. She is a professional member of the American Herbalist Guild.

MONTGOMERY, PAM

Pam Montgomery is an herbalist and plant spirit practitioner as well as the cofounder and consultant of Green Terrestrial, an herbal product business. Through Partner Earth Education Center, her southern Vermont home and educational center, she teaches a seven-month herbal apprenticeship program and spiritual ecology intensives. Pam organizes the annual herbal conference, Green Nations Gathering, participates on the Board of Directors of United Plant Savers, and is the author of *Partner Earth: A Spiritual Ecology*.

PHILLIPS, NANCY AND MICHAEL

Nancy, Michael, and daughter, Grace, live on Heartsong Farm in northern New Hampshire. Nancy teaches and practices herbalism in her community and assists Rosemary Gladstar with the Sage Mountain herbal apprentice program.

A dedicated organic gardener, Michael is the author of *The Apple Grower: A Guide for the Organic Orchardist*. Nancy and Michael have embarked on a second book project, *The Village Herbalist*, which will serve as a guide for community herbalists everywhere.

SCHOFIELD, JANICE J.

Herbalist Janice Schofield, author of *Discovering Wild Plants*, lives in Homer, Alaska, where she works as a freelance writer and photographer. Janice travels and teaches herbalism internationally.

SNOW, JOANNE MARIE

Joanne Marie Snow is an herbalist, botanist, consultant, writer, teacher, and botanical researcher. With more than fifteen years of experience in the health field, she has lectured at both national and international symposiums. She is the author of *Everything You Need to Know About Menopause* as well as several herb monographs.

SOULE, DEB

Deb Soule is the author of *A Woman's Book of Herbs*. In 1985 she started Avena Botanicals, an herbal apothecary in West Rockport, Maine, that specializes in organically grown herbal remedies, and later she founded Avena Institute, a nonprofit education center that includes a lovely half-acre medicinal herb garden open to the public. Deb is a full time organic gardener, teaches in her gardens, and consults with women and health care providers around the country.

STRAUSS, PAUL

Paul Strauss is the land steward of the United Plant Savers Botanical Sanctuary. An Ohio farmer, herbalist, and beekeeper, Paul emulates the life of the Green Man. From seed to harvest to product, he works intimately with the plants. The owner of Equinox Botanicals, a small herb business, Paul grows most of what is used in his products. He has lived on his farm for twenty-seven years and as he says, "it's a good marriage."

THIE, KRISTA

A medical botanist, Krista Thie lives near White Salmon, Washington. She holds a B.S. degree in botany from the University of Washington. She has been a student of Cascade Anderson Geller, numerous other herbalists, and, of course, the plants. Since 1979, she and her husband (and now her son) have made their living by contracting to build trails and trail bridges, mostly in the old-growth forests of the Pacific Northwest. At home, they build and sell tincture presses through their business, Longevity Herb Company, as well as research and write about herbs. Passionate about native plant preservation, Krista is an active member of United Plant Savers and the Native Plant Societies of Washington and Oregon.

TILFORD, GREGORY L.

Greg Tilford is well known for his unprecedented work in the field of ecoherbalism—the ecological stewardship of wild medicinal plants. He is co-owner with his wife, Mary, of Animals Apawthecary, a company that produces high-quality herbal products for animals. He is the author of *The Ecoherbalists Fieldbook*, *Edible and Medicinal Plants of the West*, and *From Earth to Herbalist* and coauthor with his wife of *All You Ever Wanted to Know about Herbs for Pets*.

WALL, MARTIN

Martin Wall is an herbalist and botanical photographer who lives with his wife, Deetra Thompson, and daughter, Avery, in his home state of North Carolina. Martin and Deetra codirect the Southeastern School of Herbal Studies in Greensboro. His interest in medicinal plants began during college in the early 1980s. He spent a number of years studying the plants of the southern Blue Ridge Mountains before graduating from Appalachian State University with a degree in physics. After graduating, he moved to the Piedmont where he has continued to study and photograph the medicinal plants of North Carolina and elsewhere. Martin's photography has appeared in many publications in the United States and abroad, including *HerbalGram*, *Herbs for Health*, and *Natural Pharmacy*. Photographing plants gives him an opportunity to spend time with them up close and observe them in great detail, which constantly renews his awe of the green world.

WEED, SUSUN S.

Susun S. Weed, a wise woman and green witch, is perhaps best known for her Wise Woman Herbals (*Healing Wise*, *Menopausal Years the Wise Woman Way*, *Breast Cancer? Breast Health!* and *Wise Woman Herbal for the Childbearing Year*), is an extraordinary teacher with an encyclopedic knowledge of herbs and health. Susun runs the Wise Woman Center and Ash Tree Publishing. She is a devoted goat keeper, a Peace Elder, a high priestess of Dianic Wicca, and an advisor to many health magazines and organizations.

WINSTON, DAVID

Trained in Cherokee, Chinese, and Western/Eclectic herbal traditions, David has thirty years of experience as a practitioner and educator. A founding member of the American Herbalists Guild, he serves as an herbal consultant to physicians and industry. He is president of Herbalist and Alchemist, a manufacturer of high-quality herbal extracts, author of *Saw Palmetto*, and Dean of the Herbal Therapeutics School of Botanic Medicine in New Jersey.

WOOD, MATTHEW

Matthew Wood has been a practicing herbalist for fifteen years. He lives and works at Sunnyfield Herb Farm Minnesota. He is a professional member of the American Herbalists Guild and has authored numerous herb books, including *The Book of Herbal Wisdom* and *Seven Herbs: Plants as Teachers*.

JOIN UNITED PLANT SAVERS

Become an Advocate for the Plants

United Plant Savers (UpS) is a nonprofit, grassroots organization dedicated to the conservation and cultivation of at-risk native medicinal plants. As an organization for herbalists and people who love plants, our purpose is to ensure the future of our rich diversity of medicinal species. Formed in the spirit of hope by a group of herbalists committed to protecting and preserving at-risk species and to raising public awareness, United Plant Savers reflects the great diversity of American herbalism. Our membership includes wildcrafters, seed collectors, herbal product manufacturers, growers, botanists, educators, practictioners, and plant lovers from all walks of life. We recognize that environmentally responsible cultivation, land stewardship, habitat protection, and sustainable wild harvesting are of critical importance to ensure an abundant renewable supply of medicinal plants for future generations. We invite you to join United Plant Savers. For more information, please write to UpS, P.O. Box 98, East Barre, VT, 05649.

INDEX

abutilon, 46
acne, 61, 212
adaptogens, 107
Aesculapis, 199
Alaskan Flower Essence Project, 225
alcoholism, 42, 107, 114, 124
algae, 277, 278, 279, 282–84
ambrosia, 103
American Extra Pharmacopoeia
    (AEP), 41–54
American Herbal Products Associa-
    tion (AHPA), 117
anemia, 51
angelica, 164, 179, 180
anxiety, 54, 133–34
aphrodisiacs, 142–42, 227
Apollo, 199
appendicitis, 50
aralia hispida, 70
arborvitae, 164
arnica, 29, 60–63
    harvesting, 63
    lifespan, 34
    medicinal uses, 61–62
    side effects, 62
    substitutes for, 63
    on To-Watch list, 12
arrow-leaved balsamroot, 35
arthritis
    and club moss, 48
    and cocklebur, 48
    and Hercules' club, 50
    and Japanese knotweed, 42
    and Venus's-flytrap, 235
    and yerba mansa, 268
ashwagandha, 109
aspirin, 153, 194
aster, 46, 139
asthma
    and black cohosh, 70

and bloodroot, 74
and ganoderma, 49
and lobelia, 154
and mulberry, 51
and sea vegetables, 282
and spicebush, 44
and spikenard, 212
and sundew, 222, 223
and whitlow grass, 54
and wild radish, 54
and yerba santa, 273, 275
astralagus, 98, 109
At-Risk List of plants, 9–10, 11, 13,
    26–28
attention-deficit disorder (ADD), 54,
    283
Ayurvedic medicine, 4, 39, 66
Babineau, Don, 125, 294, 297
Bach, Edward, 55–56
Baker, Jeannine Parvati, 185
balsamroot, 33
baneberry, 40
barberry, 46, 118, 126, 167, 174
Barton, Benjamin Smith, 67, 113
beach almond, 130
bead lily, 33
beggarsticks, 47
Bell, Jane, 222–23
Bergner, Paul, 113, 153, 155, 162,
    267, 281
Bermuda grass, 47
bethroot. See trillium
Beuscher, N., 254
Bierzychudek, Paulette, 25
Bioforce, 93
birch, 47, 195
birth control pills, 262
Birzneck, Ella, 296
black cohosh, 1–2, 6, 27, 64–71, 94,
    111

on At-Risk list, 11
B & B formula, 70
flower essence, 57
harvesting, 70–71
medicinal uses, 65–69, 262
and replanting programs, 9
side effects, 69
substitutes for, 71
blackberry, 187
bladderwrack, 280, 281, 283–84
Blakley, Tim, 218, 288, 294
Blanchan, Neltje, 145
blessed thistle, 245
bloodroot, 1–2, 6, 27, 72–77
on At-Risk list, 11
flower essence, 57
harvesting, 76–77
medicinal uses, 73–76, 223
and replanting programs, 9
side effects, 74, 76
substitutes for, 77
blue cohosh, 6, 27, 78–83
on At-Risk list, 11
flower essence, 57
harvesting, 81–83
medicinal uses, 70, 80–81, 179
and replanting programs, 9
side effects, 81
substitutes for, 83
blue vervain, 70, 86
bluebells, 47
Blumenthal, Mark, 294
body painting, 73, 75–76
boneset, 98, 256
botanical sanctuaries
    creating, 15, 18–23, 289
    and United Plant Savers, x, 10, 19, 20
Botanique Nursery, 224
Bothwell, Jane, 294–95
Braunschweig, 142–43

breast-feeding, 184, 185, 187, 188, 254
breath freshener, 86
Brekhman, I.I., 107
Brinker, Frances, 169
British herbal tobacco, 102
bronchitis
  and aster, 46
  and bloodroot, 74
  and catalpa, 47
  and Japanese knotwood, 42
  and lomatium, 161–62
  and osha, 178–79
  and pleurisy root, 197–98, 199, 200
  and sea vegetables, 282
  and slippery elm, 206
  and spikenard, 212
  and sundew, 223
  and trillium, 41
  and Venus's-flytrap, 235
  and yerba santa, 273
Brounstein, Howie, 163
bruises
  and arnica, 61, 62
  and loosestrife, 43
  and smartweed, 52
  and stoneroot, 217
  and trillium, 41
buckthorn, 92
bugleweed, 47, 139
Buhner, Stephen Harrod, 295
Bunting, David, 295
bur marigold, 47
bur reed, 47
Burbank, Luther, 139
burdock, 15, 98, 212, 229, 245
burnet, 47
burns, 85, 206, 249
butterfly weed, 29
butterwort, 232
Cain, Michael, 25
calamus, 29, 84–87
  harvesting, 86–87
  medicinal uses, 85–86
  side effects, 85
  substitutes for, 86
  on To-Watch list, 12
calendula, 63
California Carnivores, 222, 236
California poppy, 136, 148

California School of Herbal Studies, 266
Calvin, Natasha, 283
Canadian fleabane, 47
cancer
  and birch, 47
  and bloodroot, 73, 74–75
  and chaga, 48
  and ginseng, 107
  and goldenseal, 113
  and Japanese knotweed, 42
  and sea vegetables, 283, 284
  and self-heal, 44
  and slippery elm, 205
  and sundew, 223
  and turkey tails, 53
  and Venus's-flytrap, 235
Candida. See vaginal infections
Carnivora, 235
carnivorous plants, 221, 224, 231–34, 239
carrots, 160
cascara sagrada, 88–92
  harvesting, 90–91
  medicinal uses, 88, 89
  substitutes for, 92
  on To-Watch list, 12
cassia, 47, 92
catalpa, 47
catnip, 136, 189, 265
cattail, 48
caulophylum, 70
cayenne, 144, 152, 155
Cech, Richo, 76, 162, 163, 172, 213, 235, 287–88, 295
celandine, 77
celery, 160
centaury, 86
chaga, 48
chamomile, 136, 265
chaparral, 25, 33
chaparro, 12, 29
chervil, 160
chicken pox, 49, 68
chickory, 32, 48
chickweed, 22, 213
childbirth. *See also* pregnancy
  and black cohosh, 65
  and blue cohosh, 80

  and cattail, 48
  and kava, 133
  and lobelia, 154
  and osha, 178, 179
  and partridgeberry, 185
  and pipsissewa, 194
  and slippery elm, 205
  and snakeroot, 243
  and spikenard, 212
  and trillium, 227, 228
  and wild yam (American), 261
Chinese coptis, 103
Chiron, 199
cholera, 205, 280
cholesterol, 47, 54
Christmasberry, 130–31
Christopher, John R., 70, 143, 144, 170, 186–87, 188
chronic fatigue syndrome. *See* fatigue
Churchill, Winston, 247
cilantro, 160
Clark, Lewis, 221–22
cleavers, 22, 213
club moss, 48
Clusius, 85
Clymer, R.S., 185
Cochran, Margaret E., 31
cocklebur, 48
cockscomb, 48
Coffey, Timothy, 142
Coffin, Albert, 153
cold sores, 124–25, 249
colds
  and calamus, 85
  and echinacea, 97
  and eyebright, 100, 102
  and goldenseal, 114, 119
  and kudzu, 42
  and lobelia, 154
  and lomatium, 161–62, 165
  and mulberry, 51
  and pipsissewa, 194
  and pleurisy root, 197–98
  and sage, 51, 250
  and self-heal, 44
  and trillium, 41
  and yerba santa, 272, 274
colic, 154, 216
Collinson, Peter, 216

coltsfoot, 212, 273, 274, 275
comfrey, 32, 63, 208
concussion, 61
constipation
  and abutilon, 46
  and cascara sagrada, 88, 89
  and cassia, 47
  and partridgeberry, 185
  and pleurisy root, 199
  and sea vegetables, 282
  and slippery elm, 206
  and velvet leaf, 53
Cook, James, 133
Cook, William, 69, 70
corydalis, 34
cow parsnip, 48
Cowan, Eliot, 72
cramp bark, 186, 262
croup, 74
Cullina, Bill, 146
Culpeper, Nicholas, 101
Currim, Fara, 163
cypripedium, 70
cystitis. *See* urinary tract infection
D'Amato, Peter, 236, 238
daffodil, 33
Damman, Hans, 25
Dana, Mrs. W.S., 141, 142
dandelion, 22, 162, 174, 187, 212
Darwin, Charles, 144, 222, 233
Datta, Tane, 295
Davis, Jeanine, 116
Davis, Richard, 93
dayflower, 48
de L'Obel, Matthias, 153
de la Tour, Rick, 226, 295
de la Tour, Shatoiya, 295
Dean, Nance, 75
Densmore, Frances, 184
deodorant, 249
depression, 65, 68, 283
diabetes, 45, 49, 107
diaper rash, 268
diarrhea
  and Canadian fleabane, 47
  and cascara sagrada, 89
  and goldenseal, 113, 115–16, 120
  and hawkweed, 49
  and loosestrife, 43

and partridgeberry, 185
and pleurisy root, 199
and purslane, 52
and self-heal, 44
and snakeroot, 243
and sumac, 45
and sweet gum, 53
and trillium, 228
Dietz, H., 32
digestion
  and calamus, 85
  and goldenseal, 114
  and goldthread, 125
  and Oregon grape, 170
  and partridgeberry, 184
  and spicebush, 44
  and slippery elm, 206
  and snakeroot, 243
  and stoneroot, 217
  and trillium, 41
dill, 86, 160, 245
Dione, 234
divination, 248–49
Dobbs, Arthur, 233
doctrine of signatures, 101, 243
dodder, 48
dogwood, 48, 49
Donovuolo, April, 146–47
drug use, 70, 118, 154
Drum, Ryan W., 296
Dry Creek Herb Farm, 226
duckweed, 49
Duke, James, 22, 74, 185
dulse, 279
Dutch elm tree disease, 203–4, 207, 208
dysentery
  and beggarsticks, 47
  and Canadian fleabane, 47
  and Japanese knotweed, 42
  and lion's-foot, 50
  and loosestrife, 43
  and pleurisy root, 199
  and sage, 249
  and smartweed, 52
  and sweet gum, 53
  and tree-of-heaven, 53
  and trillium, 228
  and wild indigo, 253–54
ear infections, 51, 70, 85

echinacea, 27, 35, 93–99, 111, 238
  on At-Risk list, 11
  harvesting, 97–99, 287–88
  medicinal uses, 96–97, 164, 225,
    245, 254, 256
  substitutes for, 98
Eclecticism, 39, 67, 101, 113, 114,
  252, 253–54
eclipta, 49
ecosystems, 3
eczema, 73, 170, 253
Edwards, Theron, 242–43
elder, 162
elecampane, 180, 201, 212, 225, 275
elephant tree, 12, 29
Ellingwood, Finley, 152, 254
Elliott, Doug, 112, 127, 128, 296
Ellis, John, 112
Ellis, R., 283
Ellner, Stephen, 31
epilepsy. *See* seizure disorders
Epstein-Barr, 162
Erichsen-Brown, Charlotte, 184
Essiac formula, 74, 205
eucalyptus, 274
euonymus, 49
Euphrosyne, 101
European horse chestnut, 219
eyebright, 27, 100–104
  on At-Risk list, 11
  harvesting, 103–4
  medicinal uses, 100, 101–3
  substitutes for, 103
eyes
  and eyebright, 101–3
  and goldenseal, 113, 114
  and loosestrife, 43
  and partridgeberry, 184, 187
false hellebore, 34
Farnsworth, Norman R., 73, 243
fatigue, 51, 85, 161
Fells, Dr., 73
Felter, Harvey Wickes, 80, 113–14,
  128, 143, 154, 253
fennel, 86, 102, 160, 177, 179, 245
Fielder, Mildred, 187
First World Congress on Medicinal
  and Aromatic Plants for Human
  Welfare, 3

fishing, 161
Fletcher, Robyn, 218
flower essences, 55–59, 222, 225, 230. *See also* individual plants
food poisoning, 51, 52
forests, old-growth, 18, 191
Foster, Steven, 3, 22, 118, 184, 185, 296
foxtail grass, 49
fraxinus, 70
Frontier Herbs, 116
fungal infections, 44, 73, 74
Funk, Judy, 10, 20
Funk, Michael, 10, 20
Gagnon, Daniel, 268
Gaia, 116
gallstones, 52
ganoderma, 49
Garden in the Woods, 129
garlic, 219
Garlic Festival, 239
gayfeather, 34
Geller, Cascade Anderson, 296, 299
gentian, 12, 24, 29, 32, 33, 40, 85, 285
George, W.H., 267
Gerard, John, 85
Gerarde-Johnson, 193
germander, 33, 40
Giardia, 169, 172
Gibson, William Hamilton, 149
Gilday, Kate, 75, 125, 230, 297
Gilmore, Melvin R., 96
ginger, 25, 34, 57–58, 245
gingivitis
    and bloodroot, 75
    and loosestrife, 43
    and Oregon grape, 172
    and pipsissewa, 194
    and sage, 250
    and sumac, 45
    and wild indigo, 254
ginkgo, 33
ginseng (American), 1–2, 6, 27, 32, 94, 105–10, 111, 211, 213
    on At-Risk list, 11, 40
    flower essence, 56, 57–58
    harvesting, 108–9, 288–89
    lifespan, 33, 36
    medicinal uses, 107

side effects, 107
    substitutes for, 109
Giono, Jean, 14
glacier lily, 24
Gladstar, Rosemary, 21, 56, 226, 297
Glum, Gary, 74
glycerine, 187, 254
goldenrod, 195
goldenseal, 1–2, 6, 27, 40, 64, 94, 111–22
    on At-Risk list, ix–x, 11
    flower essence, 56, 57, 58
    harvesting, 116–17, 288–89
    medicinal uses, 102, 113–16, 124, 144, 187
    side effects, 115
    substitutes for, 118, 124, 267
goldthread, 29, 118, 123–26
    harvesting, 125–26
    medicinal uses, 124–25
    substitutes for, 126
    on To-Watch list, 12
gonorrhea, 113, 133, 193, 252
Good, Peter, 74
gotu kola, 130
grape leaf, 49
grapestone, 277, 282
gravel root, 195
Green Nations Gathering, 8
green tea, 103
Green, James, 297
Grieve, Maude, 43, 81, 101, 102, 184
grindelia, 162, 172, 273, 274, 275
ground cherry, 49
ground ivy. *See* trillium
hair growth, 49, 61
Hales, Anita, 223
Harding, A.R., 106, 289
Hartung, Tammi, 268
hawkweed, 49
Hawthorn, 283
hay fever, 102, 215, 273, 275, 282
headache, 133, 143, 161, 243
heart disease
    and arnica, 61
    and bloodroot, 74
    and goldenseal, 113
    and kudzu, 42
    and lobelia, 154

and pleurisy root, 199, 200
    and sea vegetables, 283
    and stoneroot, 217
    and sweet gum, 53
    and tree-of-heaven, 53
helionas, 27, 32, 40, 127–29
    on At-Risk list, 11
    harvesting, 129
    lifespan, 33, 35
    medicinal uses, 128–29
    substitutes for, 129
hemlock parsley, 177
hemorrhoids
    and cascara sagrada, 89
    and cockscomb, 48
    and grape leaf, 49
    and partridgeberry, 185
    and stoneroot, 215, 217
    and yerba mansa, 268
    and yerba santa, 274
Hemple, C.J., 67
hepatitis, 42, 50, 124, 169. *See also* jaundice
Herb Pharm, 8, 93, 216, 262
herbal medicine. *See also* individual diseases and plants; plants, medicinal
    American rediscovery of, 5, 39–41
    and flower essences, 55–59, 222, 225, 230
    Native American, 39, 40
    worldwide use of, ix
Herbs for Kids, 117
Hercules' club, 50
Heroic medicine, 152–53
herpes
    and bloodroot, 73
    and Oregon grape, 169, 170
    and sea vegetables, 282, 284
    and sweet gum, 53
    and Venus's-flytrap, 235
    and yerba mansa, 268
hiccups, 51, 70
hijiki, 279, 282
Hill, Anne-Clement, 223
Hippocrates, 5
Hirsch, Pamela, 297
HIV, 124, 161, 235, 284
Hobbs, Christopher, 114, 297

Hoffman, David, 5, 189, 227
Homer, 5
honeysuckle, 50
Horizon Herbs, 76, 162, 179, 181, 213, 235, 288, 295
horse medicine, 161
horseradish, 32, 103, 273
Hoyne, Temple, 69
Hutchens, Alma, 182, 187
hypertension
  and beggarsticks, 47
  and black cohosh, 68
  and cassia, 47
  and mulberry, 51
  and olive leaf, 51
  and osha, 178
  and persimmon, 52
  and puncture vine, 52
  and sweet goldenrod, 49
hyssop, 54, 157
immune stimulation
  and echinacea, 97, 254
  and ganoderma, 49
  and ginseng, 107
  and lomatium, 162
  and turkey tails, 53
  and Venus's-flytrap, 235
  and wild indigo, 254–55
impetigo, 171–72
impotence, 48, 49, 54
Indian-pipe, 50
Indian strawberry, 50
infertility, 161
influenza
  and echinacea, 97
  and goldenseal, 114, 119
  and goldthread, 124
  and honeysuckle, 50
  and kudzu, 42
  and lomatium, 161–62
  and pipsissewa, 194
  and sage, 250
  and self-heal, 44
inoculations, reactions to, 254
Inouye, David W., 36
insect bites, 51, 249
insect repellant, 86
insomnia, 49, 185, 283

International Carnivorous Plant Society, 224, 234
Irish moss, 277, 278, 282
irritable bowel syndrome, 42, 43
Israelson, Loren, 4
jack-in-the-pulpit, 25, 32, 34
Japanese knotweed, 41–42
jaundice
  and goldthread, 124
  and Japanese knotweed, 42
  and knot grass, 50
  and pennywort, 54
  and toadflax, 53
  and trillium, 41
jeffersonia, 70
jet lag, 61
joe-pye weed, 139
Jones, Feather, 266, 268
Josselyn, 143
Jules, Erik, 227, 229, 230
juniper, 94, 194
Katz, Sara, 8, 297
kava, 27, 130–38
  on At-Risk list, 11
  harvesting, 135–38
  medicinal uses, 131, 132–34
  side effects, 132, 134
  substitutes for, 136
Keewaydinoquay, 44
Keller, Helmut, 234–35
kelp, 277, 279, 283
Keville, Kathi, 147–48, 297
kidney stones, 217
Kierstead, Julie, 163
King, John, 67, 96, 254
King, Tyler, 146–47
Klein, Robyn, 223, 298
Kloss, Jethro, 1, 186
knot grass, 50
kombu, 279, 283
Krezak-Larson, Kathy, 266
kudzu, 42–43
kundalini, 66
Kuts-Cheraux, A.W., 254
lady's mantle, 229–30
lady's slipper, 27, 40, 139–49
  on At-Risk list, 11
  flower essence, 57, 58

harvesting, 144–49
lifespan, 25, 26, 31–33
medicinal uses, 142–44
substitutes for, 148
land conservation, 18–19, 21, 289, 290–91. *See also* botanical sanctuaries
laryngitis, 50, 62, 74, 216, 217
lavender, 144
Lebot, Vincent, 131
lemon balm, 148
lespedeza, 50
Lewallen, John, 280
Leyel, Mrs. C.F., 184
licorice, 223, 265, 274, 286
Liebmann, Richard, 298
Lightall, J.I., 66, 69
lily, 33, 35
Linnaeus, Carolus, 100, 112, 216
lion's-foot, 50
liriodendron, 70
lizard's-tail, 50
Lloyd, Curtiss Gates, 69, 113
Lloyd, John Uri, 69, 80, 94, 96, 113, 118, 128
lobelia, 29, 150–58
  harvesting, 155–57
  medicinal uses, 70, 144, 150, 152–55, 205, 274
  side effects, 150, 154–55
  substitutes for, 157
  on To-Watch list, 12
lomatium, 27, 32, 159–66
  on At-Risk list, 11
  harvesting, 163–65
  medicinal uses, 161–62, 185
  side effects, 162
  substitutes for, 164
loosestrife, 43
lopseed, 51
lousewort, 32
lovage, 160, 164, 179, 180, 181
Lovett, Ezra, 153
lymph nodes, 254
maidenhair fern, 12, 29
malaria, 48, 53, 169
Maloof, Joan, 36
Mars, Brigitte, 298

marsh mallow, 98, 180, 208
Martin, Hugh, 113
mastitis, 44, 50, 216
Mather, Cotton, 184
Mavor, Sunny, 60
Maximilian, Prince, 205
mayapple, 12, 29, 152
McCargo, Heather, 70, 129
McConnaughey, Evelyn, 280
McGregor, Ronald K., 94, 96
McGuffin, Michael, 117
McKeown, Kathy, 96
Mead, Margaret, x, 9
measles, 223
Medicinal Plant Task Group, 285
Medicine Eagle, Brooke, 74
medulla oblongata, 70
Meehan, Thomas, 182
memory, improving, 49
meningitis, 68
menopause
  and black cohosh, 65
  and ginseng, 107
  and lady's slipper, 143
  and sumac, 45
  and trillium, 227
  and wild yam, 262
menstrual problems
  and black cohosh, 65–68, 262
  and blue cohosh, 80
  and burnet, 47
  and bur reed, 47
  and goldenseal, 114
  and helonias, 128
  and hyssop, 54
  and lobelia, 154, 155
  and nut grass, 51
  and Oregon grape, 170
  and partridgeberry, 185, 186
  and smartweed, 52
  and spicebush, 44
  and spikenard, 212
  and sweet gum, 53
  and sweet melilot, 53
  and trillium, 227
  and wild yam, 262
  and yerba mansa, 267
Meyer, Joseph, 143

milk thistle, 22
milkweed, 198, 199
Mills, Simon Y., 223
Millspaugh, Charles F., 152, 182, 227
mint, 274
miscarriage, preventing, 128, 129,
  185–86, 212
Montgomery, Pam, 298
Moore, Michael, 22, 161–63, 224,
  243, 250, 266–68, 274
Morton, Julia, 184
motherwort, 71, 83, 129, 187, 189, 229
Mountain People, 20
mugwort, 32, 251
mulberry, 51
mullein, 130, 208, 223, 225, 273,
  274, 275
multiple sclerosis, 235
mumps, 44
myrrh, 187, 254
Nature's Way, 116
Nature Conservancy, The, 117
nettle, 22, 179, 273, 275
New England Wildflower Society,
  147, 290
New Jersey tea, 152
Newman, Robert, 125
night-blooming cereus, 27
Nitsch, Twylah, 183
nori, 279, 282
North American At-Risk Flower
  Essence Set, 56–57, 297
nut grass, 51
O'Callaghan, Ellen, 24
oak, 9, 187, 204
olive leaf, 51
onion, 34
Oregon grape, 29, 40, 118, 167–75
  harvesting, 172–75
  medicinal uses, 169–72
  side effects, 169–70
  substitutes for, 172
  on To-Watch list, 12
osha, 27, 32, 160, 176–81
  on At-Risk list, 11
  harvesting, 179–81
  medicinal uses, 178–79
  substitutes for, 179, 180

oxeye daisy, 51
pain relief, 194, 262
palytoxin, 280
parasites, 115, 124
parsley, 32, 36, 160, 177, 219
partridgeberry, 27, 182–90
  harvesting, 188–89
  lifespan, 34
  medicinal uses, 184–88, 262
  substitutes for, 183, 187, 189
  on To-Watch list, 12
passion vine, 130
passionflower, 136, 148
penicillin, 153
penny cress, 51
pennywort, 54
peppermint, 189, 265
perilla, 51
persimmon, 51, 52
Peruvian bark, 187
peyote, 11, 27
Phillips, Michael, 298–99
Phillips, Nancy, 298–99
physiomedicalim, 39
phytolacca, 70
Pilarski, Michael, 163
pine, 275
pinkroot, 12, 29
pipsissewa, 29, 183, 191–96
  harvesting, 195
  medicinal uses, 193–94
  substitutes for, 195
  on To-Watch list, 12
pitcher plants, 232
plantain, 54
plants, medicinal. *See also* herbal
    medicine; individual plants
  biennials, 24
  in China, 4, 39
  clonal, 25
  in England, 5, 39
  gardening, 9, 13–15
  for general wellness, 15
  in Greece, 4–5
  growth stages of, 24–26, 30–36
  identifying, 22
  in India, 4, 39
  organic, 8

perennials, 24–25, 29, 30, 32–34
  wild vs. cultivated, 6, 11
plants, medicinal, scarcity of, ix–x, 2–5,
    6–8, 40, 285. *See also* individual
    plants
  At-Risk List, 9–10, 11, 13, 26–28
  and botanical sanctuaries, x, 10, 15,
    18–23
  and educational programs, 16, 23
  and ethical harvesting, 6–7, 11
  guidelines for consumers, 13–16
  and native plant trail projects, 14, 23
  rescue teams, 287
  To-Watch List, 9–10, 12, 28–30
pleurisy root, 197–202
  harvesting, 201–2
  medicinal uses, 197–98, 199–200
  side effects, 200
  substitutes for, 201
  on To-Watch list, 12
pneumonia
  and bluebells, 47
  and goldenseal, 113
  and honeysuckle, 50
  and lobelia, 154
  and lomatium, 161
  and pleurisy root, 199, 200
  and sea vegetables, 282
poison hemlock, 160, 177
poison oak, 272
pokeroot, 70
pokeweed, 253
posttraumatic stress disorder, 61
prairie dock, 40
pregnancy. *See also* childbirth;
    miscarriage, preventing
  and black cohosh, 65, 66, 68
  and blue cohosh, 80–81
  and partridgeberry, 184, 185, 187,
    188, 262
  and pleurisy root, 200
  and stoneroot, 217
  and wild yam, 262
premenstrual syndrome. *See* men-
    strual problems
prickly ash, 70
prickly pear cactus, 94
Priest, A.W., 265
Priest, L.R., 265

primrose, 34
prostate problems, 52, 54, 193, 283
prunes, 92
psoriasis, 170
psychic abilities, 66, 68
pulsatilla, 71
puncture vine, 52
purslane, 52
pyrola, 192, 195
QBI, 116
quaking aspens, 25
Queen's delight, 29
Queen Anne's lace, 160
radiation, 282
Rafinesque, 113, 227
ragweed, 52
rain forests, 130
raspberry, 179, 186, 187, 189, 229
red clover, 22, 103, 219, 238
redroot, 33
reed, 52
rhubarb, 89
rice flour, 40
ringworm, 51, 73
root beer, 193, 212
Rose-of-Sharon, 52
rosemary, 77, 164, 180, 249
rush, 52
sage (white), 30, 247–51, 275
  harvesting, 250–51
  medicinal uses, 54, 103, 225, 249–50
  substitutes for, 251
  on To-Watch list, 12
sage, garden, 251
sage, lyre-leaved, 51
Sage Mountain, 126
sagebrush, 251
saguaro cactus, 33
sandwort, 52
sargassum, 279, 282
sarsaparilla, 40, 212
sassafras, 205, 212
Saunders, Charles Frances, 184
saw palmetto, 111
scabies, 51
scarlet pimpernel, 52
Schecter, S., 282
schistosomiasis, 154
schizophrenia, 283

Schnell, Donald E., 238
Schofield, Janice, 178, 299
sciatica, 48
scorpion stings, 153
Scudder, John K., 143, 144, 253
scutellaria, 70
sea lettuce, 279, 280
sea palm, 279
sea vegetables, 277. *See also* individual
    plants
  contamination of, 280–81
  diminishing supply, 278–79
  as food, 279, 281–82
  as food additives, 277
  harvesting, 279–80
  medicinal uses, 282–84
seasickness, 61
seizure disorders
  and arnica, 61
  and calamus, 85
  and cow parsnip, 48
  and Indian-pipe, 50
  and lady's slipper, 143, 144
self-heal, 43–44, 270
senecio, 60
senna, 92
sheep sorrel, 283
shepherd's purse, 179, 229
shingles, 283
silene, 33
sinusitis, 42, 102, 217, 273
skin diseases
  and goldenseal, 113, 114
  and kava, 133
  and lobelia, 154
  and sweet gum, 53
  and trillium, 228
  and yerba mansa, 267, 268
  and yerba santa, 274
skullcap, 70, 71, 148, 275
skunk cabbage, 275
slippery elm, 27, 40, 203–9
  on At-Risk list, 11
  harvesting, 207–9
  medicinal uses, 204–7
  and replanting programs, 9
  substitutes for, 208
smallpox, 66, 68
smartweed, 52

Smith, Ed, 8, 93, 94
Smith, Peter, 80
smoking cessation, 85, 154, 274
smudging, 248, 249, 272
snakebite
  and black cohosh, 66
  and bloodroot, 73
  and echinacea, 96
  and hawkweed, 49
  and Japanese knotweed, 42
  and lion's-foot, 50
  and wild indigo, 253
snakeroot (Virginia), 28, 32, 241–46
  on At-Risk list, 11
  harvesting, 244–46
  medicinal uses, 64, 66, 242–44
  side effects, 243
  substitutes for, 245
Snow, Joanne Marie, 299
Sokolski, Katie, 146–47
Solomon's seal, 34
sore muscles
  and black cohosh, 65
  and dogwood, 48
  and lobelia, 150, 154, 155
  and sea vegetables, 283
  and yerba santa, 274, 275
sore throat
  and arnica, 62
  and bloodroot, 73
  and calamus, 85
  and dayflower, 48
  and Indian strawberry, 50
  and lomatium, 161
  and loosestrife, 43
  and mulberry, 51
  and pennywort, 54
  and rush, 52
  and sage, 54
  and slippery elm, 206
  and wild indigo, 253, 254
  and yerba mansa, 268
Soule, Deb, 299
sourwood, 52
Southwest School for Botanical
  Medicine, 224
Specific Medicine Cypripedium, 144
spicebush, 44
spikenard, 29, 210–14

flower essence, 57, 58
lifespan, 34
harvesting, 213–14
medicinal uses, 212
substitutes for, 213
on To-Watch list, 12
spilanthes, 98, 225, 256
spinal problems, 65, 67–68
spotted knapweed, 34
St. Clare, Debra, 60
St. John's wort, 111, 133, 164
stillingia, 12
stoneroot, 30, 215–20
  harvesting, 218–20
  medicinal uses, 215, 216–17
  side effects, 217–18
  substitutes for, 219
  on To-Watch list, 12
Strauss, Paul, 19–20, 83, 299
stream orchid, 12, 30
striped maple, 40
stroke, 61
sulpha drugs, 153
sumac, 44–45
sundew, 28, 139, 221–25, 232
  on At-Risk list, 11
  flower essence, 222, 225
  harvesting, 224–25
  medicinal uses, 222–24
  substitutes for, 225
sunflower, Aspen, 33
surgery, 61
swallowtail butterflies, 241–42, 244, 245–46
sweating, 51, 249
sweet clover, 219
sweet goldenrod, 49
sweet gum, 53
sweet melilot, 53
sweet vetch, 34
sweet wormwood, 53
Sweet, Earle, 225
Sweetgrass School of Herbalism, 223
syphilis, 212
teasel, 31, 32, 34, 53
teething, 143, 144
Thacher, James, 253
Thie, Krista, 299
Thompson, Frances, 4

Thomson, Samuel, 150, 151, 152–53, 205
Thoreau, Henry David, 141
thrush, 45, 54, 124–25
thyme, 98, 157, 180, 212, 225, 274, 275, 286
thyroid problems, 44, 47, 283–84
Tilford, Greg, 125, 160, 288, 289, 299–300
To-Watch List of plants, 9–10, 12, 28–30
toadflax, 53
tonsilitis. *See* sore throat
toothache, 50
tormentil, 270
TRAFFIC, 285–86, 290
Train, Mr. & Mrs. Percy, 161
tree-of-heaven, 53
trichomonas. *See* vaginal infections
trillium, 7, 28, 32, 226–30
  on At-Risk list, 11
  flower essence, 57, 58, 230
  harvesting, 228–30
  lifespan, 33, 35
  medicinal uses, 41, 227–28
  substitutes for,
true unicorn, 11, 28, 35
tuberculosis, 46, 113, 222
tulip tree, 53
turkey corn, 12, 30
turkey rhubarb, 92
turkey tails, 53
turmeric, 112
Tyler, Varro E., 115
typhoid, 253–54
ulcers
  and bloodroot, 73, 74
  and burnet, 47
  and dayflower, 48
  and loosestrife, 43
  and pipsissewa, 193
  and sage, 51
  and slippery elm, 206
  and stoneroot, 217
  and sundew, 223
  and wild indigo, 254
  and yellow oxalis, 51
  and yerba mansa, 268
Ullmann, I., 32

Ulrich, Gail, 56
United Plant Savers, ix, 301
  and botanical sanctuaries, x, 10, 19, 20
  founding of, 8
  Jubilation Committee, 239
  and land conservation, 21
  nursery directory, 287, 291–93
urinary tract infections
  and club moss, 48
  and kava, 133
  and lizard's-tail, 50
  and partridgeberry, 184
  and pipsissewa, 193, 194, 195
  and puncture vine, 52
  and reed, 52
  and rush, 52
  and sourwood, 52
  and spikenard, 212
  and sumac, 45
  and sweet goldenrod, 49
  and trillium, 41
  and yellow oxalis, 51
  and yerba mansa, 268
  and yerba santa, 273
usnea, 172
uterus
  and cattail, 48
  and cockscomb, 48
  and dogwood, 49
  and goldenseal, 114–15
  and helionas, 128–29
  and osha, 178, 179
  and partridgeberry, 184, 185
  and pleurisy root, 200
  and spikenard, 212
  and stoneroot, 217
  and trillium, 227, 228
  and white ash, 54
  and wild indigo, 254
  and wild yam, 262
uva-ursi, 192, 194, 195, 286
vaginal infections
  and cockscomb, 48
  and knot grass, 50
  and lomatium, 161, 162
  and loosestrife, 43

and Oregon grape, 169
and sage, 250
and slippery elm, 205
and trillium, 227
and yellow root, 54
and yerba mansa, 268
valerian, 136, 148, 262
varicose veins, 49, 62, 185, 216
velvet leaf, 53
Venus's-flytrap, 27, 231–40
  on At-Risk list, 11
  harvesting, 236–39
  medicinal uses, 234–35
  side effects, 235–36
  substitutes for, 238
Venus, 233–34
vertigo, 51
violet, 34, 157
Virginia snakeroot. *See* snakeroot
Vogel, Alfred, 93
Vogel, Virgil J., 184
von Bingen, Hildegard, 101
Wagner, H., 254
wakame, 279, 283
wake robin. *See* trillium
Wall, Martin, 300
Warner, Richard, 112
warts, 73, 222
water purification, 85
Weed, Susun S., 300
Weil, Andrew, 75
whiplash, 65
white ash, 54
whitlow grass, 54
whooping cough, 61, 70, 113, 223
Wichtl, Max, 184
wild cherry, 152, 212, 223, 274, 275
wild indigo, 30, 252–58
  harvesting, 255–58
  medicinal uses, 252–55
  side effects, 253, 255
  substitutes for, 256
  on To-Watch list, 12
wild radish, 54
wild yam (American), 28, 259–65
  on At-Risk list, 11
  harvesting, 263–65

medicinal uses, 185–86, 261, 262
  side effects, 263, 265
  substitutes for, 265
Willard, Terry, 22, 70
Williams, Stephen, 184
windflower, 34
Winston, David, 101, 206, 223, 300
wintergreen, 182, 192, 193
witch hazel, 187, 254
Wolsey, Cardinal, 85
wood betony, 136
Wood, Matthew, 200, 272, 300
Woodland Essence, 57, 75, 230, 297
World Wildlife Fund, 285
wormwood, 86
wounds
  and arnica, 61
  and bloodroot, 73
  and eyebright, 102
  and Japanese knotweed, 42
  and pipsissewa, 193
  and self-heal, 44
  and slippery elm, 206, 207
  and snakeroot, 243
  and spikenard, 212
  and stoneroot, 217
  and yerba santa, 275
Wright, Machelle Small, 55
wyethia, 34
xanthoxylum, 70
yarrow, 63, 103, 179, 229
yellow dock, 40, 174, 187
yellow oxalis, 51
yellow root, 54
yerba del lobo, 63
yerba mansa, 30, 118, 266–77
  harvesting, 269–70
  medicinal uses, 267–68
  substitutes for, 270
  on To-Watch list, 12
yerba santa, 30, 272–76
  harvesting, 275–76
  medicinal uses, 272, 273–75
  substitutes for, 275
  on To-Watch list, 12
yucca, 33, 71, 94, 245
Yvinskas, Katherine, 20–21